PRACTICAL DESIGN, CONSTRUCTION AND OPERATION OF FOOD FACILITIES

Food Science and Technology
International Series

A complete list of books in this series appears at the end of this volume.

Practical Design, Construction and Operation of Food Facilities

J. Peter Clark

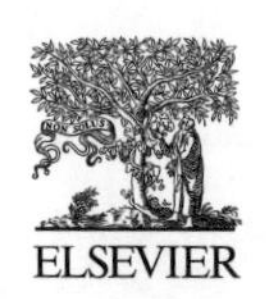

AMSTERDAM • BOSTON • HEIDELBERG • LONDON • NEW YORK • OXFORD
PARIS • SAN DIEGO • SAN FRANCISCO • SINGAPORE • SYDNEY • TOKYO
Academic Press is an imprint of Elsevier

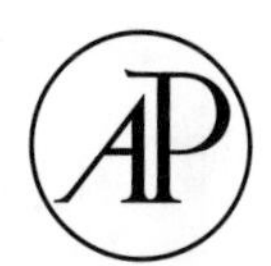

Academic Press is an imprint of Elsevier
30 Corporate Drive, Suite 400, Burlington, MA 01803, USA
32 Jamestown Road, London NW 1 7BY, UK
525 B Street, Suite 1900, San Diego, CA 92101-4495, USA
360 Park Avenue South, New York, NY 10010-1710, USA

First edition 2009

Library of Congress Cataloging in Publication Data
A catalog record for this book is available from the Library of Congress

British Library Cataloguing in Publication Data
A catalogue record for this book is available from the British Library

ISBN: 978-0-12-374204-9

For information on all Academic Press publications
visit our web site at www.elsevierdirect.com

Typeset by Charon Tec Ltd., A Macmillan Company. (www.macmillansolutions.com)
Printed and bound in the United States of America
09 10 11 12 13   10 9 8 7 6 5 4 3 2 1

Contents

1 Introduction

This book was suggested to me by people who knew of my unusual career in research, education, industry and consulting. Most of my professional life has been spent designing, helping to build and consulting on the operation of food plants. I have not seen a text in which these topics are addressed from an industrial or practical point of view as distinguished from an academic or theoretical perspective. Concisely, that is the objective of this work.

There are many sources of information on specific food processes, including some which I have written or to which I have contributed (Valentas et al., 1991; Clark, 2007), so I do not attempt to duplicate that material here. Rather, I try to provide information about designing, constructing and operating food plants that is not typically available elsewhere.

The next chapter tries to set the context for the typical food plant project, whether new or an expansion, by describing a typical corporate structure within the broader food industry. Most companies have similar procedures for initiating and approving a major capital request, so those are described as well.

It is important to understand how corporate management evaluates potential investments and how a new or expanded plant contributes to ultimate shareholder value. Engineers and food scientists may not easily communicate with financial analysts and accountants, but they must learn how to do so. There have been some important but relatively obscure studies by The Rand Corporation on the factors that contribute to poor capital cost estimates, especially for new technologies. These have been valuable to me and so I try to summarize the lessons while also providing checklists to help in estimating capital and operating costs (Merrow et al., 1981).

Practical Design, Construction and Operation of Food Facilities
ISBN: 978-0-12-374204-9

The next section discusses some of the many important, and in some cases unique, features of a food plant. Food safety is a paramount concern and is challenged by the facts that foods are made from agricultural raw materials, which are variable in properties, contaminated by soils, and perishable. Many foods are consumer products while others are ingredients for consumer products. This means that distribution and flexibility are critical concerns affecting siting and design. Finally, while the actual processes are certainly important, and are often the subject of academic research and education, the support facilities are equally essential but are often neglected in thinking about food plants.

Expansions, either physical expansion of a building or expansion of production capacity within existing walls can be a viable alternative to a new facility. Here is introduced, briefly, Goldratt's Theory of Constraints, an effective approach to understanding production lines and to optimizing operations (Goldratt and Cox, 1986). The practical challenges of construction while maintaining safe and sanitary operations are also discussed.

Process development and equipment selection are vast subjects, which can be only treated briefly. However, the intent is to teach an approach and methodology that can be extended to other cases in addition to those described. Food process equipment may be relatively standard, similar to that used in other industries, or proprietary, in the sense that it is highly specialized and intended for a specific purpose. Even standard food processing equipment is subject to some legal and voluntary design requirements. As a result, most are made of stainless steel and are often polished and have smooth welds. Choosing among alternative equipment choices can be challenging, but there are ways it can be done.

Project management and plant operations are the topics of the final two sections. These have more to do with leadership and management than with technical skills, but engineers often find themselves in the roles of managing a design or construction project or of supervising a portion of a plant. Troubleshooting an unsatisfactory operation is usually seen as a technical challenge, but might in fact be a human performance issue.

Appendices I and II discuss some topics that did not fit smoothly in the body of the text, including basic heat transfer and the calculation of residence time in hold tubes. Some flow chart symbols are provided in Appendix III and Appendix IV is a glossary of some of the terms used that may be unfamiliar to a few readers. Finally,

Appendix V is a collection of short discussions of various topics based on the Processing column I have written for *Food Technology* since 2002. These can be used as brief case studies or tutorials.

This book might find use in a senior course in food or biochemical engineering and should also be of interest to new and even more experienced engineers in the food industry. Students of business, project management and executives should also find it helpful.

How to use this book

An instructor using this book as a text in a typical food engineering design course will find the discussion questions and candidate assignments at the ends of chapters provocative and open-ended. They are not intended to be typical numerical equation solving exercises. There are plenty of those in other texts. Rather, they ask the student to make some decisions before even embarking on the assignment. Likewise, the instructor may have to do some homework before specifying assignments that might affect grades. One approach is to take the questions as written. Another is to make some choices, perhaps giving the class 1–4 specific foods, companies or processes, where the question asks the reader to select one, in the interest of reducing variability among responses. In preparation, an instructor might collect flow sheets, trade press articles and business press stories about the food industry to supplement the text and suggested assignments. I recognize that some instructors will not have the industrial experience I have had and so may be uncomfortable expounding on the subject. This should not be a concern. I believe the best learning occurs through action rather than listening, and so strongly suggest that class time be heavily devoted to student presentations and discussion of the open-ended questions. Some supplemental lectures by visitors from industry, such as vendors of equipment or plant managers, could provide additional insight. Approached creatively, teaching a course with this book should be a significant learning experience for all parties.

Readers not taking a formal class can use the questions for self-directed learning. Some readers will be new to the industry, for whom I hope the book is a valuable introduction. Others will have more experience and may differ with some of my opinions. In many areas I discuss, there are few absolutes and there can be many valid opinions. I offer mine on the basis of what I have learned, experienced and observed. I offer them in good faith, I respect those who differ and I welcome correspondence with corrections of errors and suggestions of alternative approaches.

I am grateful for teachers, mentors, clients and co-workers who have accompanied me in my career and whose collective contributions to this book are too numerous to detail but are enthusiastically acknowledged. The wisdom is theirs; the errors are mine. The illustrations were drawn by Chris Fry of Siebert Engineers Inc., Lisle, IL, based on manufacturers' literature, my sketches and other sources. The book is dedicated, with love and gratitude, to my wife since 1968, Nancy, who patiently read every word, commented wisely and perceptively, and generously encouraged me throughout this effort and through all the years of my career.

2

Context for new or expanded facility

Typical corporate structure

Most corporations have a hierarchical structure in which some functions are centralized while others are dispersed. Functions include: marketing, research, finance and accounting, human relations, manufacturing, information technology and engineering. Within these broad functions, there are many specialized areas, such as advertising, sales and brand management. Corporations are constantly rearranging the pieces and reorganizing, suggesting that there has not yet been found the ideal or universal form of organization.

Especially as firms get larger through growth and consolidation, the challenges of communication and control grow exponentially. Public corporations are owned by their investors, shareholders, who are represented by a board of directors. The board's major responsibility is to hire a chief executive officer (CEO) and then to monitor his or her performance; approve compensation for the CEO and other officers; and approve major financial decisions, such as spending, distribution of dividends, borrowing and issuance of stock. The board must also approve attempts to acquire other firms or offers from other firms.

Family-owned firms and smaller companies have most of the same functions, but some may be sparsely staffed. A sole owner plays many of the roles of a board of directors.

Practical Design, Construction and Operation of Food Facilities
ISBN: 978-0-12-374204-9

Major capital expenditures, such as a new facility, would typically be presented to the board, after long scrutiny by lower levels of executives. Once an amount is approved, most boards are quite reluctant to approve additional costs, so it becomes crucial to the career survival of responsible parties that major projects be well-defined, estimated accurately and managed well so as to finish on time and within the approved budget. Helping to achieve those goals is one objective of this book.

Estimates of future capital spending are constantly being made in a typical corporation. From the leadership – the CEO and Board, or the owner – may come guidance that a certain fraction of available resources is to be reinvested in the business to promote growth, reduce costs and enter new markets. From the operating branches of the company may come expressions of need, new product ideas and cost reduction concepts. Collectively, the opportunities to invest are usually greater than the resources available. Choosing among alternatives then becomes a significant strategic exercise.

In contrast to this approach, there are firms with relatively modest capital expenses most of the time that occasionally identify a need for a major investment, such as a new plant, an acquisition or an expansion internationally. For such firms, with sporadic capital spending, there may be less well defined procedures and practices than in those environments where spending is more regular and routine.

In any event, someone, often the Director of Engineering, has responsibility for assembling the capital budget, seeing that it is spent wisely and projecting future needs.

A common mechanism for defining and collecting the approvals of a capital project is the Capital Appropriation Request (CAR), which may have other names and acronyms in some firms. This is a standardized document on which a specific project is briefly described, including a financial analysis of its impact, a schedule is provided and the signatures of approving executives are collected.

Once a CAR is approved, it is usually difficult to get additional money, so it is wise to be conservative in estimating costs. However, too generous an estimate may unfavorably affect the economic impact and jeopardize the project. Later chapters discuss this quandary in more detail.

Food industry overview

Various studies have been published of the food industry from an economic and consumer point of view (McCorkle, 1988; Connor, 1988). While these references are old, they are still accurate in an industry that does not change very quickly. The food industry is the largest by economic impact in the USA, with annual sales of over $500 billion. The industry is very diverse, but major segments include those that process raw commodities into ingredients and foods; those that preserve and modify ingredients into foods and ingredients; and those that produce consumer food products.

Examples of each include:

Raw commodities

- Meat animal slaughter (beef, pork, poultry)
- Sugar milling and refining
- Flour milling
- Oil seed processing
- Corn wet and dry milling
- Dairy processing (milk, cream, butter)

Intermediate

- Baking (bread, cake, cookies, crackers)
- Ice cream
- Confectionery
- Vegetable freezing
- Fruit and vegetable dehydration
- Baby foods (fruit and vegetable purees)
- Dry cake mixes

Consumer products

- Soft drinks
- Beer
- Wine
- Canned soups
- Fruit and vegetable juices, aseptic, canned and hot filled
- Prepared meals (refrigerated, frozen and shelf stable).

These examples are not intended to be comprehensive, but rather are to present a small taste of the diversity and variety of the industry.

Corresponding to the wide range of products are the many processes involved, ranging from the relatively simple size reduction and physical separation of flour milling to the sophisticated biochemical process of fermentation and aging involved in making wine. In between are combinations of culinary and engineering art and science to reproduce on a large, commercial scale the flavor, texture and nutrition of home-prepared dishes and meals.

Food companies can be very large, with sales approaching $25 billion per year, and relatively small, with sales that might not exceed $1 million per year. (See the August issue of *Food Processing* (Putnam Media, Itasca, IL) each year for a list of the top 100 food companies.) In the list for 2007, the top five companies, by food sales in 2006 were:

1. Kraft Foods Inc.	$23 118 Million
2. Tyson Foods Inc.	23 059
3. Pepsico Inc.	22 178
4. Nestle (USA and Canada)	20 688
5. Anheuser-Busch Cos. Inc.	11 888

In contrast, the last five on this list were:

96. J & J Snack Foods	$515 Million
97. American Seafoods Group LLC	510
98. Pierre Foods	488
99. B & G Foods	411
100. Ruiz Foods	400
Ventura Foods	400

It took $400 million in sales to make the top 100. Sales of $1 billion put several firms tied at 74th. The top 48 firms had sales of $2 billion or more.

Consolidation among large companies has made the largest multinational firms very large indeed, with operations all over the world. In the context of designing and operating facilities, one consequence is that such firms need to be cognizant of customs, regulations and cultures very different from those of their home country. As one small example, it is common in many countries to provide one or more hot meals each day to the workforce. Sometimes, dormitories are also provided for a work force that may have moved a long distance to get a job. This means that a food facility may need to have a full kitchen and extensive living quarters on site. These are not commonly found in US food facilities.

Religious and cultural practices often affect what foods arc popular. Muslim and Jewish adherents do not eat pork; Hindus do not eat beef; Muslims avoid alcohol; and Chinese apparently like corn chowder, among other preferences. Such cultural practices affect what food products are likely to sell well in a given market and thus what a given facility is intended to do.

The distribution systems in developing countries may be relatively primitive due to poor roads, lack of refrigeration in homes and stores, and the lack of a commercial infrastructure. These conditions mean that the scale of operation may need to be smaller than it would be in the USA. Products that are shelf stable, as compared with frozen or refrigerated, are better suited for developing countries. Food manufacturers may need to establish their own system of distribution centers and wholesalers, whereas third parties in the USA often handle these functions.

Some facilities may be located to take advantage of local raw materials. Thus, for example, sugar mills are in tropical areas because sugar cane is a tropical crop. Sugar mills produce raw sugar, which is about 97% pure sucrose, and is shipped closer to markets in temperate areas for further refining. Tropical oils, such as palm oil and palm nut oil are harvested and the raw oil produced close to the palm plantations, with refining taking place closer to shipping points on the coasts of Southeast Asia.

Another factor in facility location is the relative density of the raw material and finished product. For instance, potato chip snacks, which have a low bulk density, are commonly made near population centers, while frozen and dehydrated potato products are usually made near potato producing areas.

Wheat flour mills in the USA tend to be located near wheat producing areas and near water ports on rivers, lakes or oceans. Flour users, such as bread bakers are closer to markets. Cookie and cracker bakers may have larger and fewer plants because cookies and crackers are denser than bread and have a longer shelf life.

The customers of food manufacturers are not usually consumers but the stores and food service institutions that serve consumers. About 50% of food consumed in the USA is consumed outside of the home, so the manufacture and distribution of products for food service are increasingly important. These products are different in many ways from those intended for use in the home or factory. Food service products are often refrigerated or frozen, are usually portion controlled, and may be heavily influenced by culinary concepts. This means they are conceived and developed by chefs or people with some culinary training and are meant to be used by kitchen personnel in restaurants, colleges, hospitals and prisons. Consumer food products, in contrast, are often developed by food scientists and food technologists.

Consumer food products tend to be sold in supermarkets, convenience stores and, increasingly, in mass merchandisers. Often these customers have their own distribution systems and centers (DC). Usually, food manufacturers have distribution centers as well, so there can be some redundant handling as a product moves from factory to distribution center to another distribution center and then to the store. Rationalizing the food distribution system is a major cost reduction opportunity, but the ideal solution has not emerged yet.

Some products require direct store delivery (DSD), usually because they are perishable or have such high sales volume that they need frequent deliveries. Bread, milk, soft drinks and salty snacks are examples of foods delivered daily to most stores. DSD is an expensive distribution system because it is labor intensive and because fuel costs have been increasing. DSD driver/salespeople are often paid a commission on sales, which provides a substantial incentive, but adds to costs. Some are company employees while others may be independent contractors who own their equipment. Independent contractors often service vending machines for snacks, soft drinks and confections. DSD once was largely a cash business, with store owners paying on the spot. This is less common now. Managing and controlling a widely dispersed sales and delivery force can be a challenge.

Mass merchandisers have been influencing the food industry because they demand low prices, very good service and, often, special packaging (especially in 'club' stores). They also move very large amounts of product, so accommodating them is a major objective. Food manufacturers often open dedicated sales offices near the headquarters of mass merchandisers so as to service them better.

Reasons for new or expanded facilities

Facilities have finite lifetimes and may need replacement because they are too small, are located in the wrong place, are inefficient, or just have worn out. New facilities may be needed to accommodate a new product or process, provide additional capacity for an existing product or process, take advantage of new technology, serve a new market, or consolidate multiple operations into one location. This last justification often occurs after an acquisition, when cost savings may be captured by reducing overhead and eliminating duplicate operations. New regulations, such as nutritional labeling, allergen labeling and permission to make certain health claims, may lead to changes in processes and packaging.

There are several reasons for larger scale operations tending to have lower unit costs than smaller ones, including labor efficiency, lower supervisory and managerial costs, opportunity for automation and opportunity to purchase larger quantities of raw materials and packaging. Thus, an existing plant may be obsolete simply because it is too small to be cost efficient and incapable of meeting demand. Usually, larger capacity process lines require larger space and, often, there is no extra space in an existing building. Adding space to a building is sometimes an option, but that depends on whether there is land available. In addition, building construction while food production is occurring is challenging. It is not impossible, but it requires care. A separate chapter is provided on this topic later.

Markets change as populations move over time and as demographics change. Likewise, distribution systems, including the location of distribution centers, change, with many distribution centers growing larger with time. DCs can be over 1 million square feet in size with frozen, refrigerated for produce, refrigerated for dairy and dry storage spaces connected by miles of belt conveyor and with scores, if not hundreds, of truck docks.

Perishable products may require specific temperatures and humidity conditions and some products require separation from others because of undesirable interactions. For example, some fresh produce emits ethylene, a chemical that hastens ripening in other fruits and vegetables. Thus, ethylene emitters are separated from those items that are sensitive to ethylene.

Ice cream requires storage at −10°F (−23°C), while other frozen foods can be stored at 0°F (−18°C). Fresh meats are stored at

35°F (2°C), but should be separated from fresh milk which may be held at about the same temperature, but should be in its own space.

Distribution centers are one type of food facility that may need new construction or expansion because of a changing market. Other examples might include growth in the market for a product or product line that cannot be met by existing production lines. Usually, a study is performed to determine where best to put a new line. Influences might be where there is extra space in an existing building, where DCs are located, where raw materials come from and where the product is most needed.

Typical procedures for initiating a project

As mentioned earlier, a capital appropriation request (CAR) or similar document needs to be prepared, sometimes in several iterative versions (preliminary, final) to receive formal approval to commit the money for a project.

A significant part of any capital project is an estimate of its cost. In truth, the cost of a major project is not known until it is complete and all the bills are paid (Merrow et al., 1979, 1981; Merrow, 1989). Nonetheless, it is expected that the cost will be accurately estimated in advance. This is a challenge addressed in the next chapter.

The single most important part of preparing a successful CAR, leading to a successful capital project, is the preparation of a detailed scope document. Even if this document is too large by company policy to be attached to a CAR, it is essential as a foundation for all subsequent design and estimating. A well-prepared scope document is like a news story: it tells who, what, why, where and how. 'Who' is the responsible division or department. Who wants the project, who is paying for it, who is managing it and who will operate it when it is complete.

'What' is a complete description of what is to be made in what quantities and by what process. 'Why' is the project justification – new product, line extension, market expansion, new territory, etc. 'Where' is the chosen location with its justification. 'How' is the project execution plan – who in the company is managing and has decision making responsibility, what outside resources are to be engaged (architect, engineer, construction manager), what is the schedule, what are the known risks.

In preparing the scope document, it is common for many choices to be unresolved. These should be clearly identified with dates for decisions to be made. It is usually unwise to proceed with designs and cost estimates unless the scope document is complete so far as possible. The most common cause of cost overruns in projects is unanticipated changes in scope. The worst of these are those that are not recognized because the scope was not clearly documented and so there was no base against which to measure changes. Preparing a clear scope document does not mean that there will be no changes during a project, but it does mean that the changes will be recognized as such and their impact will not be a surprise.

Many things can change over the course of a project and managers must be flexible. So long as upper management approves – and often they are the source of changes in goals, scale and even location – then a project manager must adapt, but if he does not have an accurate scope document, he or she cannot account for the impact and make a persuasive case for a corresponding change in budget and schedule. Sometimes, scope documents are translated into detailed schedules and budgets, but there is no substitute for a concise, literate narrative that answers the key questions in a form that anyone can understand.

As important as preparing a scope document, estimate, schedule and CAR, is understanding the corporate budgeting cycle. It takes time to approve even small expenditures in a large bureaucracy and it takes a long time to approve large expenditures, in part because the money may need to be raised from outside the company. Thus, every organization has an annual cycle for developing, approving and spending the capital budget. There can be exceptions but, as a general rule, it is a good idea to prepare CARs in a timely fashion, which means doing the preliminary work well in advance. For an engineer, this may mean close communication with business units, research and development, marketing and finance to identify likely future capital needs and then preparing corresponding scope documents, preliminary designs and estimates, even if they rest on a shelf for a while and have to be revised later. Revision is usually easier and faster than preparing the material from scratch, often under severe time pressure.

It is unfortunately common for an engineer to be asked to prepare a CAR, including what is expected to be an accurate cost estimate, on very short notice, because someone has just identified a need for a new facility or expansion. It is unreasonable to expect that such an estimate will be very reliable. If, however, the engineer or the engineering department has prepared a variety of hypothetical scope documents or contingent projects, based on a good understanding of the business and its needs, it is more likely that one of those plans can be adapted to the immediate requirements. At least, if the engineering department is in the practice of preparing scope documents and estimates, they will have the discipline and skills to plan and execute projects well. One goal of this book is to help develop some of those skills.

Discussion questions or assignments

1. Select a major or minor food company (public companies are somewhat easier to research) and diagram its corporate structure. Where does Engineering fit in? Trace the likely path of approval for a major project.
2. Identify a relatively recent food industry project, such as a new plant or expansion, and prepare a scope document for it. Sources include the trade press (*Food Engineering*, *Food Processing*, *Food Technology* magazines), the business press (*Wall Street Journal*, *Business Week*), the Internet and company news releases.
3. Find the most recent listing of food companies by sales (*Food Processing* and *Food Engineering* magazines publish these annually) and analyze the data to answer the following:
   a. Who is the largest in the world?
   b. Who is the largest in the USA?
   c. Who is the most profitable?
   d. What food category is the most profitable?
   e. Who has the highest return on assets?
   f. Who has the largest market value?
   g. Is there a relationship between capital spending and the above factors?
4. The trade magazines sometimes publish lists of capital projects compiled from questionnaires and list the architect, engineer and construction firms associated with some of the projects. Identify as many of these firms as you can and see if, from the lists, you can associate them with specific categories of projects. Do this without contacting the firms, though most have web sites, which list their own perceptions of their

expertise. Compare your observations with their claims. Who would you contact for a meat project? For a beverage project? For a distribution facility?

5. Identify as many of the food facilities as you can in your region, state or city, as appropriate. What do they have in common? Why are they there? Are they large or small? Who do you think are their customers? (Do not ask them.) Based on your research, if you were trying to attract new investment to your area, what type of food industry would you target and why? Prepare a persuasive letter arguing your case.

3 Economic evaluation

Measures of worth

Cash is the lifeblood of a business, so a proposed investment is best evaluated by how it contributes to the flow of cash. Cash is defined in a business context as after tax profits plus depreciation. These terms will be discussed in more detail. The objective is not to duplicate more extensive treatments elsewhere, but rather to enable the engineer to understand and communicate with his colleagues in finance, accounting and management (Valle-Riestra, 1983; Clark, 1997a).

A business such as a food company uses *fixed assets*, such as buildings and equipment, and less tangible assets, such as patents and trade secrets, to produce items for sale. The company pays for its assets with a mixture of *equity* and *debt*, where equity represents money invested or accumulated by the owners and debt represents money borrowed from a bank or other source. In accounting, debt and equity are considered liabilities, offsetting the assets that were purchased, as well as other assets such as money owed to the firm by customers, pre-paid expenses, work in process and retained earnings.

In evaluating a potential investment, companies are interested in how the new asset will contribute to cash flow relative to its cost. There are also investments that must be made, which may not directly contribute to cash flow. These are considered non-discretionary and include projects dictated by customer safety, employee safety and environmental regulations. Even these can be

Practical Design, Construction and Operation of Food Facilities
ISBN: 978-0-12-374204-9

evaluated by the same techniques because, almost always, there are alternatives and the objective is to select that alternative which is most cost effective.

In the normal course of business, a company receives *income* from the sale of products and pays *expenses* associated with making the products and with operating the plant. Expenses may be *direct* or *variable* because they are proportional to the amount of product, or they may be *indirect* or *fixed*, because they are relatively constant, no matter how much product is made.

Examples of variable expenses include raw materials, packaging material, energy and labor. Examples of fixed expenses include management, marketing, taxes, insurance and depreciation.

Profit before taxes is the difference between income and expenses. *Depreciation* is a special category of fixed expense that reduces taxes but is not a true cash flow. Rather, it is an allowance provided in the income tax laws that permits recovery of the cost of fixed assets over their assumed lifetime (Maroulis and Saravacos, 2007).

Depreciation may be calculated in several ways: straight line, meaning an equal amount is taken each year; double declining balance, in which larger amounts are taken early in the project's life, for reasons explained shortly; and various modifications, in which, usually, larger amounts are taken early but not so large as by double declining balance.

The reason that the timing of depreciation is important is the *time value of money*. The time value of money is the concept that a dollar in hand today is worth more than one received a year from now. This is because money in hand can be used to earn more money in the form of interest or profit on an investment. Thus, a dollar invested at interest rate, i, will be worth $(1 + i)$ at the end of one year. At the end of two years, it would be worth $(1 + i)(1 + i)$ or $(1 + i)^2$. It then follows that a dollar received in the future is only worth $1/(1 + i)$ today. More generally, an amount received n years in the future is worth $1/(1 + i)^n$ times the amount, F, today. The symbol, P, is often used for the present value.

Since higher depreciation charges early in a project's life contribute to higher cash flow in the early years, those values are discounted less in computing the *net present value (NPV)* of a project. The NPV is the sum over the life of a project of the discounted cash flows for each year.

An important factor in the calculation is the *discount rate*, i. Considerable debate can ensue over the correct value to apply. The discount rate is meant to represent the potential return of relatively safe alternative investment opportunities, such as government bonds or the cost of borrowed money, which often is fairly close to the bond rate. In practice, the discount rate is adjusted upwards to account for some degree of risk. The discount rate to use in a given company is usually set by the corporate finance department and may vary with time and for different classes of project. It is important to realize that calculating NPV, and other measures of worth, using the time value of money and discount factors is meant for comparison of alternatives and should not be seen as computing an absolute measure of value. In many cases, cash flow contributions, positive or negative, which are identical among all options will be ignored in an analysis so that the focus is on those elements that differ. This means that the result is not a measure of absolute value, but only of relative value. In the case of a non-discretionary investment for which there are only costs and no positive cash flows, the result of an NPV calculation will be negative and the best choice is that with the value closest to zero.

When considering a company's capital budget as a whole and alternatives within it, there are almost always more costs of potential projects than there are funds to invest. Thus, projects are evaluated and ranked with the goal of investing the available funds as wisely as possible. In theory, those projects with a positive NPV using the agreed upon discount rate should be funded. In practice, those projects contributing the most to the company's value should be funded. This would tend to favor larger projects.

Even after applying all the appropriate quantitative measures, there remains an important role for strategic judgment in choosing between new products or markets as compared with extension of existing products. There is comfort in the familiar and risk with the new, but also greater potential from innovation. Publicly held companies are often pressured by stockholders to cut costs and increase profits, sometimes within a relatively short time frame, while an objective understanding of long-term benefit might favor greater investment in projects with greater risk and greater potential.

There are other measures of worth besides NPV which are in common use. One of the simpler ones is *return on investment (ROI)*. ROI is the ratio of profit to capital invested. It is usually computed for the first year and implies that profits are constant with time. It can be misleading, especially for projects with varying conditions and complex investment patterns, but is simple to calculate and easy to understand.

Closely related to ROI is *payback time*, typically the time to recover the investment from profits. It is the inverse of ROI. Neither of these approaches recognizes the time value of money nor the contribution of depreciation to cash flow. Some variations of ROI and payback time use cash flow instead of profits, which is more realistic, but not as conservative. Being overly conservative in evaluating investments can prevent the choice of wise, longer-term projects in favor of shorter-term and perceived to be safer choices. Strategic judgment should prevail.

Internal rate of return (IRR) is defined as the discount rate for which the NPV is zero. It is computed by a trial and error calculation of NPV for various discount rates. If IRR is greater than the value used by the company as a guide, then an investment is acceptable. Projects with high IRR should be funded. However, often relatively small projects can show high IRR while contributing relatively little value to the firm. Also, there are conditions of varying cash flow, such as additional investments over time, for which the calculation of IRR may give ambiguous results. While admittedly rare, the possibility of such a case suggests that IRR be used judiciously. NPV is generally recognized as unambiguous and reliable as a measure of worth for alternative investments.

Estimating capital investment at this stage

To evaluate and compare investments requires an estimate of the cost. However, as pointed out in a series of studies by The Rand Corporation (Merrow et al., 1979, 1981; Myers et al., 1986; Merrow, 1989), even when a project is 95% complete there can be uncertainty about its final cost. How, then, does one make a reasonable estimate early in a project? There are several possibilities:

- Past experience
- Comparable facilities
- Feasibility study
- Detailed design.

A reliable approach is to use past experience, especially with similar facilities. Some companies build essentially the same plant, often using the same designers and contractors, year after year to satisfy steady growth. Even with this much experience, there are differences among the plants because of site differences, lessons learned in the past and changing expectations of flexibility. Site influences include seismic zones (relative risk of earthquakes), environmental regulations, flood plains and availability of utilities. Each of these can affect the cost of what otherwise might be an identical facility. For example, structural requirements are quite different in California than in the Eastern USA, because California experiences frequent earthquakes. Buildings are required to take the anticipated forces of an earthquake into account in California. In practice, this may mean reinforcing concrete block walls, for instance, and fastening equipment to the floor, whereas in other states the equipment might simply be put into place.

Regulatory restrictions on air, odor and water emissions also vary from place to place. Areas subject to smog formation may have more stringent restrictions on emissions of volatile organic carbon (VOC) for example. VOCs are compounds that can interact chemically in the atmosphere to form irritating compounds. Bakeries emit small amounts of ethanol formed during the fermentation of bread and, in many parts of the country, must reduce the amount with fairly costly equipment. Choices include incineration with natural gas, catalytic oxidation over a supported precious metal and cryogenic condensation. Water and odor restrictions also vary, depending on local conditions, waste treatment capability and the proximity of neighbors. Even the sources of benign odors, such as coffee roasting, chocolate and bread baking, may be considered noxious by some neighbors and require controls.

Finally, there is a significant cost to bringing fuel, electric power, water, sewer and rail to an undeveloped site as compared with one where these utilities are present. Of course, there will usually be a difference in the land cost as well between a developed site and raw land. The Rand studies found that one of the biggest contributors to inaccurate cost estimates was not having a specific site in mind.

When cost estimates are performed for a hypothetical site, it is almost always assumed to be flat, requiring little grading and having all utilities nearby. In reality, there are few, if any, such sites to be found. The good ones have been developed; leaving land that almost always has some costly defect, such as poor soils, poor drainage, an environmental hazard that must be removed or sequestered, or an unusual shape. Without a specific site in mind, it is difficult to anticipate what costs might be encountered. It seems to be human nature to estimate optimistically, but this is almost always wrong.

Lacking directly relevant past experience, comparison with other facilities can be useful. Bartholomai (1987) published a useful collection of mostly small plant designs for a variety of food factories and Maroulis and Saravacos (2007) derived some correlations from his data to show relationships of capital costs to projected sales and of total costs to equipment costs. Sometimes, equipment costs are relatively easy to estimate, compared to those of a total project, because the equipment is directly related to the process, while the project has a myriad of other costs and influences. Much of this book is focused on these other influences.

Food plants can cost about $100 per square foot (Clark, 1997a) for the building and support utilities, but these costs can vary dramatically depending on details of the design. Some food plants require refrigeration of the entire space, such as meat plants, and these then have greater insulation requirements. Other plants must be capable of resisting large amounts of water and harsh chemicals, such as dairies. Such plants demand more expensive finishes for floors and walls. Broadly, food facilities can be categorized as dry or wet, refrigerated or not, dusty or not, and handling raw agricultural materials or not. (Raw agricultural materials may include fruits, vegetables, root crops and grains and handling them implies dealing with dirt, insects and other potential contaminants.) Relying on comparable facilities for guidance in cost estimating means understanding the impact of these differences on costs.

If time and budget permit, the most accurate cost estimate relies on a relatively complete and detailed design for a specific site. However, neither cost nor time usually permits this approach and, instead, a feasibility study is performed. A feasibility study is a limited exercise usually performed by a small team in which sites may be evaluated, a preliminary design developed and a cost estimate prepared. It is understood that the design is not final but rather is intended to support a cost estimate sufficient to allow evaluation of the project, hence the feasibility or viability.

One measure of the relative accuracy of cost estimates is the *contingency* that is included. Contingency can be a controversial topic, in the same way that discount rate often is, because both involve judgment. Contingency in a cost estimate is a line item that is meant to account for costs that are not otherwise explicitly identified and for errors in the other items. Contingency is not intended to account for changes in scope, acts of God or other catastrophes. As designs progress, details are resolved and cost estimates become more detailed, contingency as a percentage of total cost can be reduced, but experience dictates that it never disappears. In a feasibility study, contingency might easily be 30% of known costs or even higher. In an estimate derived from a final design, contingency should still be about 10%. Because of a misunderstanding about what contingency is intended to cover, some companies insist that contingency cannot be greater than 10%. This corresponds to the margin of error that many firms allow in project budgets. In preparing a feasibility study estimate, it may be necessary to bury the true contingency to satisfy this type of arbitrary dictate. The point is to understand the limitations of early estimates and to include proper allowances for inevitable errors.

Finally, if a detailed design, or at least a more detailed exercise than a typical study, can be performed, the resulting estimate will be more accurate and can a have a lower contingency. Underlying any estimate must be a clear narrative scope document, as previously mentioned. The feasibility, preliminary and detailed designs make no sense without the scope document. A scope document is meant to be capable of change, as circumstances change, but without the original as a base, the reality and consequences of change are hard to identify.

In summary, a food facility cannot be designed and evaluated without precisely articulating what it is, where it is and what it is to do.

Estimating costs and benefits

Sometimes it is difficult to estimate operating benefits, which is one reason much emphasis is often placed on costs and cost reduction – costs seem easier to quantify. Finance and accounting people are often skeptical about claims of benefits because they may seem like wishful thinking. It is important in estimating benefits to be realistic and to base estimates on historical data whenever possible. For example, a real benefit of a new or expanded facility may be increased sales and thus increased profits. If sales of the firm or of the relevant product line have been steadily growing and capacity of existing manufacturing has been reached or exceeded, then it can be persuasive to project future sales continuing to grow, probably at a somewhat lower rate. The lower rate is suggested because, in reality, most products tend to grow at a reduced rate as they mature.

If the facility is justified by projected sales of a new product with no prior history, it is important to have some test market data, which shows likely per capita consumption, or some other basis for estimating. Justifications based on improved *quality* are difficult to support, though they may in fact exist. Often in the course of design, choices arise that can affect capital or operating costs and which are evaluated by their impact on quality of the product. It may be easier to justify an incremental increase in capital cost by a *life-cycle analysis* than by an assertion of improved quality, simply because it is hard to persuade people that quality increases sales or profits.

Life-cycle analysis refers to the practice of estimating future maintenance and operating costs, discounted to the present, as well as initial cost, in comparing alternatives. A piece of equipment or a building finish with a higher initial cost may be less expensive to maintain, be more energy efficient and be less expensive to operate over its lifetime and thus justify its higher initial cost. Examples include heating, ventilation and air conditioning (HVAC) equipment, boilers, floor and wall finishes and increased roof and wall insulation.

Another benefit from a new or expanded facility might be a reduction in the cost paid to produce a product through a contract manufacturer or co-packer. *Co-manufacturing* is a common practice and there are many companies and facilities dedicated to this service. Using a co-manufacturer permits a company to have fewer fixed assets than it might otherwise have, often allows quick entry to a market and may give a company access to technology and expertise it does not have. Companies that specialize in manufacturing for other companies believe that they have superior management and operation techniques because they are focused on manufacturing, leaving marketing and sales to their clients.

On the other hand, there are some disadvantages as well. The most obvious is that the co-manufacturer expects to make a profit, that is earn some return on the assets that are employed. If a company were to invest in its own assets for manufacturing, it would expect to earn a return on that investment. In fact, it might expect a higher return than does a co-manufacturer. Further, the book value on which a return must be earned may be lower for the existing assets of a co-manufacturer than it would be for a new facility. Many co-manufacturers are privately held and are willing to accept a lower profit margin than are publicly held large corporations.

Nonetheless, many users of co-manufacturers begrudge them their fees and look for ways to avoid or reduce them.

There can be less direct control over quality and practices, since the employees are not those of the customer. Understanding this, co-manufacturers encourage close interaction with customers and often have quality personnel on site from customers. Finally, there is some risk to proprietary information that may be shared between the co-manufacturer and the customer. This last risk is more perceived than real because co-manufacturers who violate confidences will not remain in business very long. On the other hand, co-manufacturers cannot help learning from each assignment and may be tempted to become competitors at some point.

Co-manufacturing makes the most sense when appropriate assets exist and are not fully utilized. It is common that some investment is required, such as for special packaging, but if an entire new line is required then a different justification is needed. If major investment is required, the customer will have to pay a sufficient fee to provide a return to the co-manufacturer. However, it can happen that the co-manufacturer does not demand as high a rate of return as does the customer and, therefore, using the co-manufacturer even with major capital required, makes sense. Also, many co-manufacturers have lower labor costs than their customers and, because of their experience, may be more efficient at operations than their customers are. Finally, using a co-manufacturer may significantly shorten time to market.

For these reasons, many major food companies use co-manufacturers for some, if not all, of their requirements. Likewise, there are many successful co-manufacturing companies, who are typically almost unknown to the public. If part of the justification for a new or expanded facility is cost savings from bringing a product or products in-house, then all the costs should be considered, not just the toll or fee charged by the co-manufacturer.

Another benefit from a new facility may be improved efficiency due to new technology, reduced cost of energy or raw material, or reduced labor cost. At one time, many manufacturers moved from the Northern USA to the South because labor was less expensive in the South. Areas with less active unions are perceived to have less expensive labor. New facilities may have greater automation and thus reduce labor costs. Areas in which electric power is generated with dams may have lower energy costs. Countries outside the USA tend to have less expensive sugar and so some confectionery companies have relocated from the USA. Other costs, such as shipping, may offset some of the expected savings from such a move.

Some of the operating costs are:

- Raw materials
- Energy
- Labor
- Wastes
- Packaging material
- Depreciation.

Raw materials and packaging material constitute, on average, about 70% of the cost of foods (Clark, 1997a). Other costs, including labor, energy and depreciation, are about 10% each. A major influence on raw material costs is yield, that is how much or how little of what is purchased winds up in the finished product. Some yields can be shockingly low. For example, it takes about 10 pounds of milk to make 1 pound of cheese. About 50% of a hog or steer is edible. Other raw materials, such as grains and vegetables, can have similar losses that are essentially intrinsic, that is they occur because of the composition of the material.

There are other sources of yield reductions, in addition to composition of the raw material, some of which can be addressed. Examples include:

- Spillage
- Over-filled containers (giveaway)
- Improper recipes
- Mislabeled containers
- Improper processing
- Contamination
- Out of code (aged) raw material or product.

Good engineering, construction and operation of material handling equipment, such as conveyors, can reduce spillage. Every transfer point is a candidate for leakage and a spill, and therefore a candidate for careful observation and improvement. Material on the floor of a food plant is not only a sign of poor housekeeping, but also of poor maintenance and operation. A useful approach is to have trays or shelves under transfer points, which can catch spills before they reach the floor and possibly permit the material to be added back to the conveyed stream.

Reducing product giveaway is the motivation behind digital scales, which are so accurate and precise that they have been justified by the saving of one potato chip per package. The challenge of product dispensing and filling is that under filling is considered fraud, so all manufacturers over-fill to some extent. Filling is a statistical process in the sense that there is a normal distribution around a target fill weight with most filling equipment, in part because of the natural variability of foods.

Figure 3.1 shows two normal distributions that might result from two fillers, one with a small standard deviation and another with a larger standard deviation. Both are centered on the same mean – 225 grams in this case. Depending on the variability of weights achieved for a given food in a given filler, the target weight is set so that a high fraction of all packages exceeds the minimum allowed, typically the label weight. This means, in practice, three

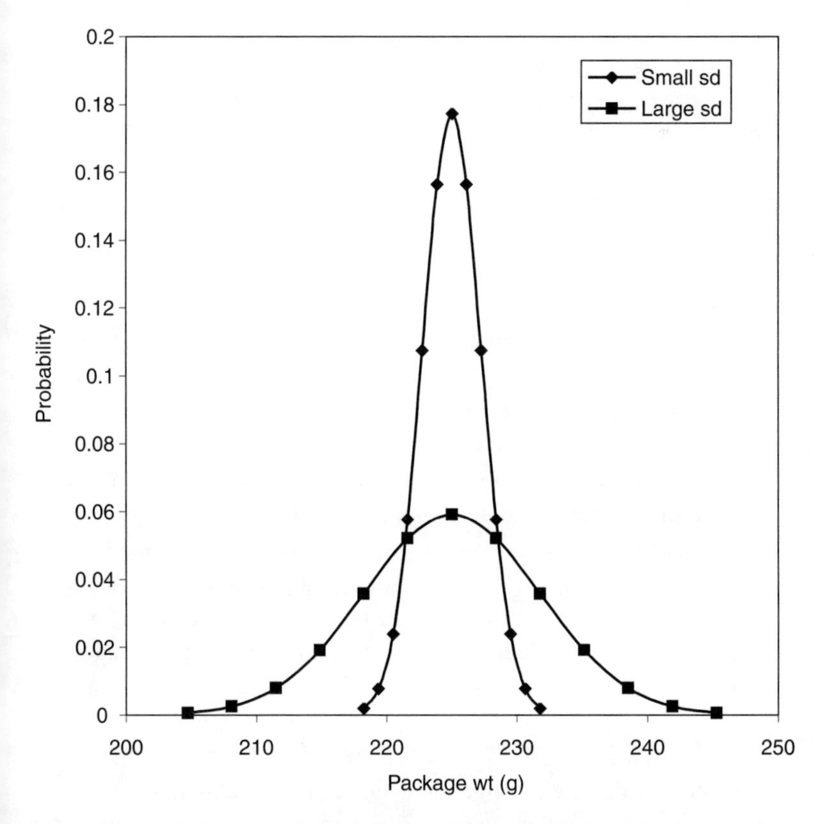

Figure 3.1 Two normal distributions, illustrating effect of different standard deviations

standard deviations greater than the minimum. The smaller the standard deviation, the more narrow the distribution and therefore the smaller the excess fill over the minimum. Digital scales use up to 16 buckets into which product is dispersed and then, very quickly, each bucket is weighed and some combination of four buckets is chosen and their false bottoms released to fill a container so that the contents are close to the target. Referring to Figure 3.1, the filler with more precision (small standard deviation) could be set to deliver about 232 grams on the average while the less precise filler would be set at about 245 grams. Both fillers would overfill on average but the more precise filler would save 15 grams per package compared to the filler with a large standard deviation. In practice, data are taken on a large number of packages, using an in line checkweigher, to establish the distribution and the filler is fine tuned to meet the target with minimal give-away.

Liquid fillers often use precise volumetric pumps or valves to achieve the same goal of small standard deviation and reduced give-away. Pumps and valves are made with close tolerances, but suffer wear with use, so their precision may decline over time. Check weighers are used to monitor package weight and to indicate when maintenance may be required on a filler. Underweight packages are rejected after the check weigher. Underweight packages may be opened and the contents salvaged; they may be sold in a company store to employees, donated to a food bank or discarded, depending on the value of the contents, the amount of packages involved and the availability of outlets. A package may be under filled because of temporary failure of a bucket, valve or pump; because of an empty feed hopper; or because of a variation in product density. Check weight data should be carefully monitored to identify trends that may indicate a process flaw or a need for maintenance.

Recipes may have too much or too little of an ingredient due to human error or mechanical failure of a feeder or scale. Too much use means a yield reduction, at least, and could impact quality. Too little used could impact quality such that a batch is discarded or needs to be redone. A major goal of operation management and automation is to reduce errors in formulation so as to maintain consistent quality and maximize yield.

Food labels are governed by regulations intended to inform consumers and to prevent fraud. Labels may be incorrect because they do not declare an ingredient that is used, deliberately or inadvertently; because the weight is incorrect; because the nutritional information is incorrect; or because the food may contain an undeclared allergen. The contents may be otherwise safe and nutritious, but the product cannot be sold. Mislabeled product may be repackaged, discarded or given away out of commercial channels, such as to a food bank. In any case, it is a source of yield loss or cost increase.

Improper processing may result in over-cooking or under-cooking, poor color, poor shape, poor particle size, poor distribution of a mix, or some other failure attribute. A company establishes quality standards for such attributes and rejects those that exceed the boundaries. Some improper processing can be corrected by reprocessing, but other times the product is discarded. Out-of-specification food is often diverted to animal feed, especially grain-based products such as cereals and pet foods.

Some processes, such as extrusion of snacks, cereals and pet foods, have start-up and shutdown episodes during which out-of-spec material is inevitably produced. Keeping such times as brief and infrequent as possible is a good way to improve yields.

There are many potential sources of contamination of foods. Some are easier to detect than others. Metal and other foreign objects can be detected by X-rays or potentiometric coils like those found at airport security. Metal detectors only detect metal pieces above a certain size while X-rays can also detect glass, wood and plastic, provided the materials are sufficiently different in density from the food. Food may be examined on its way to packaging or after filling. Conventional metal detectors cannot examine metal containers or those laminated with aluminum foil. In fact, metal detectors are used to confirm that small foil pouches of flavor are included in packages of instant noodles.

Packages or streams of food found to contain metal or other foreign objects are diverted for further examination, reprocessing or discarding. Depending on the value of the food, it might be passed over magnets or screens to remove ferrous metal or other foreign particles. It is important, when foreign object contamination is found, to establish the source and cause if possible.

Metal fragments enter food due to wear of equipment parts, by breaking of screens, by careless maintenance and by deliberate or accidental introduction by people. Prevention of such introduction is one reason visitors and workers are asked to remove jewelry and objects in shirt pockets. Typical workers' uniforms do not have shirt pockets nor metal snap closures to help prevent accidental introduction of foreign matter to food.

Other contamination can occur from dripping water, dust, grease or incorrect ingredients. Such contamination may be difficult to detect, so prevention rather than reprocessing is the best protection. As discussed later, the principles of sanitary design are primarily intended to prevent contamination. Places where food is exposed pose the greatest risk, so, often, conveyors may be covered, kitchens and preparation areas may have ceilings, hoods for dust collection are installed at ingredient dumping locations, only food grade lubricants are used, cold pipes are insulated to prevent condensation and seals are routinely inspected for leaks of lubricants.

Finally, ingredients that have exceeded their usable life must be discarded and represent a yield loss. Inventory control with first in/first out practices are important in using ingredients before they become too old. Foods are perishable to varying degree – some absorb water and cake up, some lose water, some oxidize and some discolor. Proper storage conditions are important as well. The ingredient storage area should be dry, temperature controlled if needed, and provide sufficient space for access to stored materials. Purchasing ingredients in the right amounts can prevent loss through aging. The concept is to understand the frequency and amount of use and to purchase accordingly. This may mean paying a slightly higher unit cost for an ingredient than if larger quantities were procured but, by preventing loss through aging, the net cost is reduced.

Energy is a relatively small operating cost for food plants, but controlling it in times of rapidly rising prices is important. Good insulation, efficient refrigeration plants, efficient boilers and intelligent energy integration are all contributors to reducing energy costs. Most food plants burn natural gas because it is clean and relatively plentiful. Some food processes, such as baking, are energy intensive, in the sense that they use a lot of energy, but they may also be energy efficient, because baking ovens are typically well insulated. The highest use of fuel in a bakery is often the boiler, used primarily to make hot water for cleaning. Lighting is an opportunity to use energy efficient fixtures, typically halogen lamps. Mercury vapor lamps are avoided in a food plant because they attract insects.

Food plants vary widely in their dependence on labor. Meat processing is very labor intensive, while some other plants operate with very few people. A later chapter discusses plant operations and people management in more detail. It is sufficient here to say that people are extremely important in a food plant and that, even though they may be a small cost, they can make or break an operation. In particular, food processing still relies heavily on the skill and craft of its workers because the product is ultimately judged by its taste and other sensory properties. Modern practice is to hold line operators responsible for the quality of their production by training them in quality standards and then requiring them to evaluate products on a regular schedule.

Wastes include water and solid wastes as well as air emissions. Food plants can use large volumes of water, especially for cleaning. Wastewater discharges are treatable but can be relatively strong and may have a wide range of pH and fats, oil and grease (FOG). FOG is worrisome because it can solidify in sewer lines. It is good design practice to have separate sanitary and process waste lines, which are connected to a sewer through an air break, typically in a catch basin. The air break is to prevent backflow of sewage into the process area, and is achieved by having the waste lines from the plant enter the catch basin near the top, while the sewer connection is near the bottom. A catch basin is a cylindrical vessel built beneath grade level and accessible through a man way. Volume of the vessel is based on achieving a minimum residence time for the heaviest flow rate, typically seen during cleaning. Residence time with the vessel half full depends on the amount and properties of waste, but should be several minutes. Heavy solids drop to the bottom, below the sewer connection. FOG floats to the top. FOG and heavy solids are periodically removed by an outside service and disposed of as solid waste. If the removal of FOG is not sufficient to meet discharge requirements, then it may be necessary to install an air entrainment separator or dissolved air flotation unit, in which small air bubbles help float FOG to the surface, where it can be skimmed and trucked away.

Most food plants discharge their liquid wastes to a municipal treatment plant for a fee. It is important to confirm that the municipal plant has adequate capacity and that the fees are fair. Even when the treatment plant is adequate, it is wise to practice water conservation in the plant. Typically, the plant must buy water and also pay for waste treatment. If water is a significant part of the product, it is wise to measure and document exact usage because, often, water consumption and waste discharge are assumed to be closely related. For example, a soft drink or fruit juice plant may purchase much more water than it discharges as waste, because so much of what it buys is used in the product.

Clean in place (CIP) systems, in which water and cleaning solutions are recovered and reused, not only reduce labor but also save water and reduce discharges (see Seiberling, 1997). Other water conservation measures include having 'dead man' nozzles on hoses so that they only run when attended and selecting equipment with low water use. Using a cooling tower to recycle and reuse cooling water is another good practice. A cooling tower is a device that reduces the temperature of a water stream by evaporating a portion through contact with air. The air may be circulated by fans or it may be moved by natural forces – wind and natural convection as the air temperature changes. A cooling tower is constructed of corrosion resistant materials and sometimes uses chemicals to reduce scale and corrosion. Fresh water is added to compensate for that lost by evaporation.

Solid food wastes are often taken by farmers to use for animal feed. If so, they should be stored carefully and protected from contamination. Wet solids may spoil quickly and so should be removed often. It is rarely economic to dry such wastes, but sometimes this is done. Examples include spent grains from brewing; start-up and shutdown residues from cereal, snack and pet food extruders; and citrus peel from juice plants.

In isolated areas, food plants may need to treat their own wastes and provide their own potable water. A common approach, where land is available, is to spray the wastewater on land planted in grass or other crops. Soil permeation properties, wind and temperature all affect whether land application is appropriate. Land application is not practical in freezing weather, but is suitable for seasonal canneries, which typically are mostly idle in the winter. It is also important to understand the source of incoming water and to be sure it does not become contaminated by the land application. Incoming water is often raised from wells whose aquifer could become contaminated.

Water for use in foods must be potable, meaning it complies with minimum standards for safe drinking. This may not be adequate for a particular process. For example, drinking water is often chlorinated, but for use in beverages, it may be treated with activated carbon to remove the chlorine taste.

Finally, depreciation has been previously discussed. It is listed here as a cost to remind that the capital investment matters. Depreciation is one component of fixed cost or overhead, as distinct from variable costs, such as labor, energy and raw material. Typically, unit fixed costs are reduced as capacity utilization increases, which is one reason more food plants consider seven-day operation and multiple shifts. The same facility can produce more, so long as there is a market, and the fixed cost component of each unit produced goes down, because there is little need for more management, and depreciation remains constant, as do other components of fixed cost, such as taxes and insurance.

In evaluating a project, all the anticipated benefits and costs must be estimated. This only is reliable for a specific site, because utility, labor, energy and raw material costs all vary with location. It is important in estimating benefits to be creative without exaggerating and losing credibility.

Discussion questions or assignments

1. Obtain the general parameters for a relatively new food plant from such sources as trade publications, *The Wall Street Journal* and the Internet. Calculate all the measures of worth that you can, stating any assumptions you find you must make.
2. Compare three projects on such parameters as cost per square foot, cost per unit of production, and cost per dollar of sales. Discuss the differences and similarities as related to product category, scale and any other characteristics you can identify.
3. Research the unit costs of utilities in your area (community or county). Compare to national averages. Is yours an attractive area for a food plant? Why or why not?

4

Design of a new facility

The design and construction of a new facility is a relatively rare event in the career of most food professionals. A major expansion is much like a new plant except that the site and some supporting facilities may already be in place. This chapter discusses some of the issues that arise in a typical new plant project. A food professional may be a member of a team responsible for selecting and supervising various consultants involved or he or she may be such a consultant, drawing on education and experience. For the most part, there has been little published in this area (Clark, 1993a,b,c, 2005a,b; Maroulis and Saravacos, 2003; Lopez-Gomez and Barbosa-Canovas, 2005).

Site selection

For a new facility, one of the first issues is where it is to be located. This is the art and science of site selection. Site selection starts broadly, identifying a country or region and then focuses more narrowly until a specific piece of property is identified. One can think of choosing a time zone, then a state, then a Zip code and, finally, an address. What are some of the influences and how does one make choices?

One of the more significant influences is location of a firm's existing and potential markets. Some companies are initially regional and aspire to a more national presence. Others already have a national presence in the USA and seek international markets. Supporting existing markets is a distribution system with distribution centers (DC), customers and delivery systems (trucks,

Practical Design, Construction and Operation of Food Facilities
ISBN: 978-0-12-374204-9

rail, sales and delivery people). Moving into a new market requires integration with the existing distribution system and may require additional facilities, such as warehouses and depots. Adequacy of transportation systems can be a major factor, because raw materials and packaging materials must be obtained and finished products distributed by ship, rail or truck. As will be discussed later, some plants are near ports while others need not be.

If a firm is starting new, building a facility may not be the wisest strategy until its product line is proven. Typically, a new venture arranges for production by a third party or uses an existing facility while getting its products established. Sometimes this arrangement may be maintained for many years. Usually, when considering a new facility, it is because a product line is well established and alternative sources of production are inadequate or may be considered too expensive. This usually means that the distribution system is well established and can be extended to a new region as needed.

In the USA, the Midwest is a popular location for food manufacturing because that region is a source of many raw materials and it has an extensive transportation system of rivers, rail and highways. Other popular locations include the Northeast, because of proximity to large population centers and California because it is a large market in its own right, grows many raw materials and is expensive to supply from other regions of the USA because it is a long way from the Midwest and is separated from the rest of the country by mountains.

Raw materials, relative product density and product shelf life are additional influences on location. Raw materials may be agricultural products, live animals, partially processed materials (such as coffee beans, meat or raw sugar), or ingredients such as syrups or flavors. Water is often an ingredient in foods, so a plentiful source of potable water is always a consideration.

If raw materials are perishable, bulky or seasonal, it often makes sense to locate processing plants close to the source. Thus, tomato processing plants are often very close to the farms where tomatoes are grown. The products, tomato sauce, tomato paste, ketchup and canned tomatoes, being shelf stable and concentrated compared to the fresh fruit, can be stored and shipped. Meat processing used to be concentrated near rail yards in Chicago and Kansas City so animals could be received and meat shipped in refrigerated rail cars. In recent years, meat processing has moved closer to where cattle and hogs are fed, in the mountain west for cattle and in the corn belt for hogs. Wineries are almost always placed near vineyards. Frozen and dehydrated potato plants are usually located near potato growing areas, most in the northwest, while potato chip plants are located near markets because their products have a low bulk density and relatively short shelf life.

Bread is typically baked close to markets for much the same reasons – low density and short shelf life. These characteristics affect the cost of shipping and over how far a distance it makes sense to ship. Processed foods with longer shelf lives and higher bulk density can be manufactured almost anywhere because it is reasonable to ship the products long distances. Site selection for such products is dictated by the overall distribution system and strategic considerations.

Once a broad region is selected, then specific states and communities can be considered. There are a number of factors that can apply:

- Taxes
- Labor supply
- Energy supply and cost
- Water supply and cost
- Solid and liquid waste disposal capacity and cost
- Incentives
- Transportation (roads, rail, ports).

Taxes vary widely across the USA and across the globe. In addition to federal income taxes, there are state and local taxes on income, personal property and real estate. Some states charge a tax on inventory of finished goods as of a certain date, which may make those states less attractive than their neighbors who may not have such a policy. Companies often reduce inventory near such dates to reduce their tax burden. Real estate and employment taxes are often used by local governments to support schools and other services. Because they are imposed by local governments they may be negotiable to an extent. Abatements or freezes on assessments are often offered as inducements for plants to locate in certain communities.

Labor supply and cost matters more to labor intensive industries such as meat packing than it does to a more automated factory.

However, all food plants require some labor and the required skill level is increasing, as plants are more automated and equipment is more sophisticated. Immigrants are often the source of large labor pools and so there are pockets of south-east Asians and Hispanics in the Midwest working in meat plants and other food processors. Labor costs in the South were traditionally lower than those in the Northeast, leading to a migration of such industries as textiles from New England to the South. Food manufacturing is typically less sensitive to labor costs than to other costs, such as raw materials, so relocation just to reduce labor cost is less frequent in the food industry. However, in selecting a specific state or community, the availability of sufficient labor is a concern.

Since management of a plant may need to relocate from other sites or be hired specifically for the plant, the desirability of the location as a place to live is also a serious factor. Thus, the quality of schools, amenities such as recreation and culture and relative levels of education will be considered.

Most food plants are not energy intensive, but some can consume large amounts of fuel or electricity, especially if they are refrigerated, have ovens or have large amounts of frozen storage. Energy costs have been increasing and are quite variable across the USA, especially for electricity, depending on whether an area has access to hydroelectric power (the least expensive) or must rely on natural gas, coal or nuclear. Large users of power can usually negotiate favorable rates, but may be required to accept interruptions in supply, which may or may not be tolerable to a food plant. There are energy saving and reduction technologies, which help reduce a plant's energy footprint, but controlling the cost of energy is always a consideration.

Food plants can use large amounts of water for cooling, cleaning and as an ingredient. Water in a food plant must be potable, meaning suitable for drinking safely, but even when it is, it may be more or less suitable for use in foods. Beverage plants, for instance, treat incoming water to remove turbidity (suspended matter) and chlorine. Locally available water may have excessive hardness or unsuitable flavors, even if it is suitable for drinking. If water is relatively expensive, it may make sense to have a closed cooling water system to avoid discharging water that is merely heated up. In a closed system, warm cooling water is exposed to air in a cooling tower, where some evaporates and reduces the temperature of the bulk of the water. A small amount of fresh water is added to make up for losses by evaporation. Chemicals may be added to reduce scale formation and to minimize corrosion of the tower and piping.

Solid and liquid waste disposal can be an issue. Food plants can produce large amounts of both liquid and solid waste. While it is biodegradable because of its food origins, it may also be vulnerable to rapid decomposition, producing odors and attracting insects, birds and rodents. The recommended approach to liquid waste is to discharge to a municipal treatment plant for a fee. Where there is no adequate plant, the food plant may need to treat its own wastes. This can require a substantial investment and an ongoing operating expense. Food plants in rural areas, such as fruit and vegetable canneries, have often used land disposal to treat liquid wastes by spraying on fields planted in grass or other forage crops. This has become less common as housing has encroached on these once-isolated plants.

Land application depends on permeable soil, predictable winds and mostly mild climates. Because many canneries did not operate beyond the harvest, the impact of winter weather was not important.

Modern food plants required to treat their own liquid wastes may use conventional activated sludge processes or industrial waste treatment processes, such as anaerobic digestion. Activated sludge uses high concentrations of aerobic bacteria to consume the organic matter in a waste stream. Excess microbial mass is separated by gravity and disposed of by spreading on land or by anaerobic digestion. Sludge is bulky and may have high concentrations of heavy metals and other toxic substances that are not consumed by bacterial growth, making its safe disposal a challenge. Anaerobic digestion uses a different family of bacteria, in the absence of air, to convert organic matter in a waste stream or in sludge to carbon dioxide and methane. This gas may be recovered for its energy value or burned for disposal. Anaerobic digestion is slower than the aerobic process of activated sludge but produces the useful by-product gas and relatively little undigested sludge.

Often, a plant's sewage charges are based on incoming water consumption. If the plant puts a large amount of water in its product, it is wise to meter sewage separately, so as not to be charged for waste disposal that it does not use. Soft drinks, beer and reconstituted juice plants are such cases.

Solid wastes may be taken away by farmers to use as animal feed or they may be dried to stabilize them before removal.

The only other alternative is landfill, which may be expensive and limited in capacity. Packaging material wastes, such as empty bags and trim from packaging that is made on site, may be recycled but are often burned or land filled. A good food plant design aims at reduction of liquid and solid wastes, but there always are some, and the costs and capability of disposal of them can affect site selection.

Transportation systems can influence the size and location of a plant, especially in some developing areas, where roads are so poor that distribution areas are restricted and so plants must be smaller than they would be if located in the USA, with its Interstate highways.

Finally, states and communities may offer incentives beyond tax concessions to induce a plant to locate in their area. The motivation is increase in jobs and, eventually, in the tax base. Incentives may include:

- Free or low cost land
- Free or subsidized training for workers
- Frozen tax assessments
- Reduced tax rate for specified period
- Cooperation in securing zoning and permit variances, if needed
- Assistance in relocating personnel
- Infrastructure improvements, such as paving a road
- Concessions from utilities on rates or upgrading supply
- Others specific to the case.

Negotiating incentives is an art practiced by specialized consultants. Many areas have development groups for regions, states and towns, which publicize the advantages and benefits of their area. They can be sources of incentive opportunities but, ultimately, it is the political leadership that determines how aggressive an area may be in attracting new investment. If all else is equal among several candidate areas, a firm considering a new location might do well by letting it be known that several candidate areas are being evaluated. This promotes competition and may improve the eventual incentive offers. Incentives should not tip the scales when other factors are not equally attractive because usually the incentives are temporary, while other factors may be permanent in their effect.

In considering a specific piece of property, once a region, state and community have been chosen, the factors are practical and mundane:

- Cost
- Size
- Soils
- Neighbors
- Utilities
- Location.

Within a given area, cost of raw land is not likely to vary widely, but the more desirable the location and the more developed it is, the more expensive it will be. Going a few miles out of town can reduce the cost, all else being equal, quite a bit. Size is obviously critical – the land should be about four times the footprint of the plant to allow for truck circulation, parking, set back from roads and some expansion. If major expansion is contemplated, then the amount of land should be increased for a given original plant size. It is generally better to buy sufficient land in the first place than to depend upon getting more later if it is needed. The price will certainly increase over time and that vacant parcel may not be available when the need arises later. If land disposal of liquid waste is planned, then even more area is required. Some large companies acquire land in various areas well in advance of a specific need to provide choices when a new facility is planned.

Building cost is influenced by the structural strength of the soil and the terrain. Level land with good soil is in short supply in the USA because many of the desirable plots have already been built upon. This means that one can safely assume some form of soil issue with almost any candidate property. Some will require grading; some will require removal of past contamination (brownfields); and some will require removal of soil and replacement with engineered fill because the soil is weak or wet. Most food plants are built with slabs on grade, so the load bearing strength of the soil is critical. If it is inadequate, there may be a need for driving piles to support the building or the poor soil may be removed and replaced with fill that is appropriate. Brownfields are sites that have experienced some environmental contamination, such as leaking chemicals, buried storage tanks for gasoline, or past use as landfills. Depending on the exact conditions, the contamination may be removed or enclosed to prevent further spread. It is wise to inspect a property during or after a rain to observe drainage and detect potential flooding issues.

Food plants are not usually bad neighbors, but some do emit odors, noise or dust, so it is best if residential areas are distant from the plant site. It is also important not to have bad neighbors, who might be a source of contamination or other hazards, such as a chemical plant or landfill. Where a food plant might become a nuisance, costs must be budgeted to reduce the impact, perhaps by landscaping, baffling for noise reduction or other controls, such as incineration of stack discharges.

The degree of development can affect cost of the property and of the plant. It is most convenient if major utilities are at the property line, such as high voltage power, water, natural gas and sewer. If these must be brought any significant distance, the respective utilities will charge their costs unless they can be persuaded to abate those costs as an inducement. Likewise, it is best if a road provides access to the property, but this may not be the case where a large plot is subdivided, in which case potential roadways are usually planned but not necessarily paved. Usually the seller or developer will provide access roads, but if this has not yet been done, there may be a delay in the start of construction.

Real estate professionals emphasize location in determining value of land and it certainly has an impact. A good location gives convenient access to transportation routes, maybe has a rail spur if needed, is relatively easy for workers to reach and, as mentioned previously, has the services and characteristics desired. Public transportation is not common in rural areas, so an employer may need to assist workers in getting to work by subsidizing buses or even, in other countries, by providing dormitories and cafeterias.

Size

The size of a new facility, and hence its cost, is probably the single most critical decision to be made. If a firm has several existing plants and is expanding essentially the same business into a new area, then it probably has a good idea of the capacity and capability of a plant of a given size. Many companies build almost standard facilities to accommodate growth and expansion. The more difficult challenge is when a product is new and there is uncertainty about needed capacity. In this case, it might be wise to build a minimum sized facility with provision for expansion in the future. This brings up some other issues that must be resolved.

Capability

As discussed earlier, a new plant is considered to accomplish a given mission in a given area. Executing that mission then involves a number of other decisions, including:

- Number of lines
- Warehouse or not
- Distribution center or not
- Expansion in the future
- Flexibility.

The number of lines and flexibility are closely related but separate issues. Often a plant makes several products or families of products, perhaps various package sizes or different manufacturing processes, as in candy where a plant might have starch molding, tableting and panning. Sometimes processes share common facilities or equipment, such as a kitchen or mix room. Other processes may have common packaging lines, as in bagging, canning or pouching. One challenge is to decide how independent any line or group of connected equipment should be. Will it be self-sufficient and able to operate without reliance on another line or will it share some equipment or services? A case can be made for either approach.

The more equipment is shared, the lower the investment and the higher the utilization of capital resources. On the other hand, sharing resources may mean that some lines cannot operate while others are and this can limit the capacity of the plant. Ultimately, food process design usually results in careful compromises that are deemed to make sense for a given company in a given business. There is no one answer that fits all cases. A common solution is to have shared support facilities such as ingredient preparation and dedicated processing and packaging lines that are optimized for certain products and package sizes. In any event, the overall process design is chosen (Maroulis and Saravacos, 2003; Clark, 2005b; Lopez-Gomez and Barbosa-Canovas, 2005).

Other characteristics of the facility are then decided. Most food plants have separate warehouses for raw materials, finished goods and packaging material. Raw materials and finished goods are separated to reduce the risk of contamination, since many raw materials are agricultural products that may be dirty. Depending on the overall plant layout, raw materials and finished goods may be handled in separate parts of the plant. Storage conditions can also vary, as in ice cream, where raw milk and cream are refrigerated, while ice cream is frozen.

Packaging materials should be treated as if they were ingredients because they come in contact with food and can be contaminated. Different materials have different requirements. Glass containers may be cold upon arrival in winter and need to be carefully warmed up to prevent condensation of water and thermal shock when they are filled with hot food. Paper for labels, cartons and pouches needs to be stored in controlled humidity to acclimate to the plant environment and then perform properly in packaging equipment. Metal cans need to be protected from moisture to prevent corrosion. Plastic foil also needs to be stored in a temperature and humidity controlled environment and all packaging materials need to be protected from dirt and other contaminants. In addition, because packaging materials are used towards the end of a typical line, it may be convenient to store them nearer to the point of use than at either end of a plant. Sometimes packaging materials have a dedicated receiving door. Soft drink plants often move cans directly from a truck to the line, in part because the cans are relatively bulky and are used in large quantities.

A modern plant tries to minimize the amount of area devoted to storage by carefully controlling inventory, using 'just-in-time' purchasing and delivery practices and producing closer to order than to inventory. Finished goods storage can be minimized by promptly removing finished goods as soon as a truck can be filled. The products may go to customers, to a company distribution center (DC) or to a customer or third-party DC. One way to ensure that inventory is kept low is not to build much storage in the first place, but this may be resisted by plant operations people who would rather produce efficiently and not be concerned about whether they had made too much. Making to order may mean that less than a full shift of production is sufficient, which is a departure from traditional practice of scheduling full shifts, whether the product is needed or not. So, an early decision is how much, if any, finished goods storage to provide.

For a multiproduct company, a distribution center both receives and ships the full line of products. DCs are usually located to serve regional markets and may or may not be adjacent to a plant that produces some or all of the products. If a new site is also to be a DC, then it does not need a finished goods warehouse, but it will need additional truck docks to receive outside shipments and will now have a more complex order picking function. Especially when entering a completely new market, as in another country, it may be advantageous to construct a DC with a factory so that the market can be served initially from one location, with one management team. There is, of course, additional cost in building a larger facility, but warehouse space is generally less expensive to build than is factory space.

Capability of future expansion is almost always required, but how much must be decided. It is not uncommon to double the size of a plant over time. There needs to be sufficient land for such expansion and the design should anticipate where and how it will be done. Certain features of a plant are difficult and expensive to move, so these should be located on a face of the plant not designated for expansion. Such features include docks, labs and offices. Provision for their expansion should also be made. Likewise, support facilities need not be fully sized for the ultimate capacity, but provision should be made for their expansion when necessary, typically by leaving extra space in various places, such as machine rooms, maintenance shops and electrical switch rooms. Expansions are discussed further in the next chapter.

Flexibility is a profound topic and will be considered more than once. Here, in discussing initial design scope decisions, the impact is to consider whether the plant needs to make many short runs of various products in different size packages or longer, more standardized runs. Many choices flow from this decision. For example, a line with much of its equipment on casters that can be rolled into place or out as needed is very flexible, but may be less efficient than a large capacity, fixed line. A flexible line needs extra space to store equipment that is not in use. Flexible lines may be down more often for changeover and cleaning and so are less productive. However, a flexible strategy can reduce inventory and may be more profitable than a more dedicated line. Again, there is no single answer for all circumstances, but there does seem to be a trend toward more flexibility.

Overall layout

Overall layout, the way equipment is located with respect to other pieces, is dictated by efficient flow of materials and people. The usual options, for one level, are:

- Straight through
- U-shaped
- L-shaped.

Straight through layout has generally straight and parallel production lines in which raw materials enter one end and finished products emerge at the other end. One advantage is relatively easy expansion by adding similar lines so long as there is sufficient space. Another advantage is that there are aisles between and alongside of the lines for people and fork trucks.

In order to minimize distances that materials or finished goods are transported, it is common that raw materials be received and stored at one end and finished goods be stored and shipped from the other end. This puts trucks on two sides of the building and requires two sets of receiving and shipping clerks and two areas for truck drivers to wait. As previously mentioned, it is not necessarily a disadvantage to have storage of raw materials and finished products separated, but there can be extra expense in building sufficient truck docks with their equipment (lights, levelers, locks, doors) in two locations. When all the doors are in one area, they can serve double duty for shipping and receiving. Having them all in one area also means an additional face of the building is free for potential expansion.

Arranging lines in parallel can be difficult if they are of unequal lengths. If they all start together, then some will end before others. This can result in wasted space and extra transport distances. Some processes can have parallel lines for part of the process, as in baking ovens, but must fan out when they come to packaging, which occupies a much greater floor area than do the ovens. In some bakeries, packaging is put on two or more floors so as to minimize the footprint of the building.

An alternative process layout is 'U'-shaped, where lines reverse their path so that they begin and end on the same side of the building. This allows for shipping, receiving and storage to be in one general area, allows truck docks to be used more efficiently and may save clerical and material handling labor. On the other hand, it is physically difficult to arrange similar lines this way and moving people along a line or between lines is more difficult.

A variation is 'L'-shaped, in which lines have one turn of 90 degrees. This can result in a more square shaped, rather than long and narrow, building. It has similar advantages and disadvantages to the straight through option, but can accommodate lines of different lengths.

Another issue is that of levels in a building. The least expensive way to build is to have one level or floor, but there are circumstances in which multiple levels can be advantageous. Certain types of food processes are traditionally multilevel, including flour milling, ready to eat breakfast cereal and pet foods. These have in common that they use solid raw materials and produce solid products. Solids are easy to handle by gravity flow, so often these processes convey raw materials to a top floor by elevator or pneumatic conveying, then transfer between subsequent operations by dropping through chutes. Even meat packing used to operate in multilevel buildings, relics of which still exist in Chicago's Union Stockyards. Animals walked up ramps to the kill floor at the top and primal cuts and by-products were conveyed by gravity until they emerged on the ground floor.

A multilevel building has a compact footprint, but bears extra costs for its structure, for the floors and for transporting of people and material among floors (elevators). They also can make communication among the workforce difficult in modern, automated plants where there may be relatively few people on each floor. Elevators, in particular, are seen as expensive and often unreliable, requiring maintenance and becoming a threat to interrupt production by breaking down. The common solution is to install multiple elevators, adding to cost.

A popular compromise in food plant building design is a high bay structure with equipment placed on a relatively open structural frame that is separate from the structure of the building. The frame has walkways and work places where people need to be, but is sufficiently open that the platforms do not qualify as floors, which can affect building code requirements for fire protection and also can influence tax assessments. There is often debate between making work platforms of open grid or solid plate. Solid plate is generally preferred because it prevents dirt from shoes or spills falling and contaminating food on lower levels. Where the food is confined and protected, open grid can be used for its lighter weight. However, it is hard to clean.

Partial mezzanines are another approach to achieving some of the benefits of multilevel and gravity flow without the disadvantages of a full floor. With a mezzanine, some equipment or storage bins are elevated, access is by stairs and equipment can be located below. A common example is dry mixing, where the mixers are located above loading or packing stations. In considering any partial floor or mezzanine, it is important to understand local building and fire codes, because these can affect exit door requirements, fire protection, insurance and tax assessments. Companies want work platforms to be considered part of the equipment and not part of the building whenever possible because buildings are often assessed in part on their floor area. Equipment is also subject to more rapid depreciation than is a building for tax purposes. The space under a work platform needs its own lighting and fire protection. As a general rule, enclosed work spaces need two separate exits for people in case one is blocked in event of an emergency.

In summary, the process, the scale of equipment and the flows of people and materials will dictate the three-dimensional arrangement or layout. This in turn will strongly affect the overall shape of the building. Other influences on the shape include the other functions that are present in addition to the process, the specific site, local requirements and other architectural considerations. Lately, a desire to be 'green' and sustainable may also influence building design.

Green design and LEED (low energy and environmental design) are efforts to reduce the energy and carbon footprints of a facility by being efficient in lighting, heating and air conditioning (HVAC), using recycled materials and using other design elements as appropriate. Some features that contribute to sustainable design include:

- Lighting in warehouses that is controlled by motion sensors, so it is only turned on when people are present
- Low solvent epoxy coatings
- Heat recovery from oven and boiler stacks
- Water reuse and recycle
- Low inventory ammonia refrigeration systems
- The use of sustainable materials in office finishes.

It is difficult for a food plant to satisfy many of the goals because relative to commercial or institutional buildings, industrial buildings in general and food plants in particular are relatively energy intensive and have constraints on their design that limit the LEED features. Primary among these limitations is sanitary design.

Sanitary design

Sanitary design refers to those building design features that may be unique to a food plant and are intended to reduce the risk of contamination by biological, physical and chemical hazards (Jowitt, 1980; Troller, 1983; Imholte, 1984; Clark, 1993b, 2007). Some of the same principles are found in pharmaceutical plants. Hazard analysis critical control points (HACCP) refers to a rigorous approach to identifying, anticipating, making provisions to correct and documenting potential hazards to people from food. It also provides a framework for food plant design. Food plants convert agricultural raw materials and other ingredients into edible and safe foods and beverages while protecting foods from spoilage and from posing a hazard to humans. Hazards may be microbiological, such as *Clostridium botulinum*, *Escherichia coli O157:H7*, *Salmonella* or *Listeria monocytogenes*, organisms that can cause disease; or they may be physical, such as glass, wood or metal; or they may be chemical, such as pesticide residues, cleaning chemicals or unapproved additives. Critical control points are identified in the process which, if properly achieved, will control hazards. Procedures are devised and documented to respond to deviations from control points. These are primarily the concern of operations. The task of sanitary design is to minimize risks of contamination and to make easier the challenges of cleaning and maintaining the plant and equipment.

Since microorganisms require water and food to live, one approach to reducing their presence is to deny them these essentials. This leads to the principle that, if a plant is normally dry, keep it dry, because it is difficult to remove water once it is present. Plants that are normally wet anyway, because they process liquids, must be designed so that water does not accumulate and so that they can be easily cleaned. In practice, this means designing so that floors drain quickly and using materials and finishes that are resistant to cleaning chemicals, water and heat.

Most food equipment is made of stainless steel because it is resistant to corrosion and can be polished so that food and dirt cannot easily cling to it. In addition, welds must be smooth, corners rounded and the equipment designed so that it can be taken apart and inspected. These requirements follow from the second essential of microbial life – food. In the course of food processing, many foods form films on surfaces with which they are in contact. These films can harbor microbes. If the surface is rough, the film is difficult to remove and it may be hard to detect whether the surface is clean by inspection. Some types of equipment can be cleaned in place (CIP) by passing strong hot cleaning solutions through at high velocities, but inspection is still required to ensure that the cleaning process is successful. Often food equipment is designed so it can be disassembled without requiring tools or, at the most, one or two simple tools, such as a wrench.

Some equipment can only be cleaned by hand washing – clean out of place (COP) – in special sinks. The conversion from COP to CIP was one of the great advances in food plant design and permitted the growth in size of dairies, in particular, by reducing the labor needed for sanitation (Seiberling, 1997).

For the same reasons stainless steel is used in equipment, it is often chosen for building mezzanines and work platforms in food plants. At first, this seems extravagant but, in the long run, it is a good decision. Stainless steel does not require painting, as would carbon steel structural members. Unprotected mild steel or carbon steel will corrode in the wet atmosphere of most food plants and the rust could become a food contaminant. Paint can chip and become a contaminant. Painted surfaces require recurring maintenance. Galvanized (zinc coated) carbon steel is an acceptable structural material, but poses its own challenges. Structural members can be galvanized in a shop but, when they are assembled by welding, the coating is removed at the welds, creating a location for corrosion unless the coating is replaced in the field. It is generally best to use stainless steel for structures in a food processing area. Some plants have gone so far as to use stainless steel panels for floors, walls and ceilings. This may be a bit extreme for most cases, but is justified when conditions in the space are so severe and the food so vulnerable that the durability of stainless steel is required.

Doors, drains, pipe hangers and even electrical conduit should be made of stainless steel in a wet environment. A common convenient structural unit, a perforated metal channel with the ends bent in, should not be used in a food plant because it is hard to clean. Contractors like it because it is familiar and easy to use to make pipe and conduit hangers. Instead of it, supports should be solid bars or angle members, with the angles pointed down so that the piece does not trap dirt. Pipe and conduit that runs along walls should be set about one inch away from the wall using special clamps or stand-offs so that the space behind can be reached for cleaning.

In a dry plant, where dust is a concern, metal does not need to be stainless steel, but flat surfaces should be minimized. It is common to encase vertical columns in concrete bases with sloping tops, to make curbs at walls with sloping tops and to cove or curve the intersection of floors and walls so that that area is easier to clean. Dust is a concern in a dry plant because it can harbor insects, attract rodents and birds and be a potential explosion hazard. Many food dusts from flour, sugar and starch are explosive in certain concentrations, which can occur in confined spaces, such as ductwork and equipment. A slight spark or static electricity can set off an explosion and the initial shock can create a second dust cloud, which may do even more damage.

Dust in a food plant is commonly controlled with a central dust collection system, which is a vacuum pneumatic system with connections to hoods over bag dump stations, mixers and other locations where dust can be generated. There are one or more receivers with replaceable filters on the exhaust, which should discharge outside the plant. The filters must regularly be inspected and replaced. The discharge must be inspected and must comply with air emission regulations. Dust collected in the receiver is discharged to a bag or drum for disposal. The amount collected should be observed and the air flow in the system carefully balanced to achieve the desired compromise between elimination of dust in the air and yield loss. The dust collection system can exceed the explosive concentration limit in its ducts and receivers and so all electrical equipment must be spark-proof and the entire system correctly grounded, so static electricity does not build up and create a spark. The dust collection system must be inspected and cleaned periodically because dust can build up in ducts to the point that the system is no longer effective.

Insects, rodents (rats and mice) and birds are concerns because they can spread microorganisms, insect parts are considered foreign matter in food and their droppings are also contaminants. Evidence of rodent infestation is enough to cause a food plant to be shut by public health authorities. Designing for protection against rodents is a challenge because they are attracted by the abundant food present in the food plant, they can go through very small holes and they can gnaw through wood and some other materials. Food plants should have a rodent control program using traps placed by a professional and regularly serviced. There should be a clear path around the inside and outside perimeter of a food plant to allow placement of traps and to prevent rodents from being diverted into the plant by obstructions. Rodents are nearly blind and find their way by feeling surfaces with their whiskers, so if they encounter an obstacle along a wall they turn into the plant, where they can cause contamination. It is a continuing challenge to keep the perimeter paths clear, as it is tempting to use that space for casual storage. Normally, the inside perimeter path is painted distinctively to remind people that it is not to be blocked.

Insects are controlled in part by devices that attract them with ultraviolet light and then kill them with electricity. Air curtains at doors to the outside are used to keep potential contaminants, including insects, from the outside from entering the plant when the doors are opened. An air curtain is created by a strong fan forcing air through a downward facing slot nozzle at the top of the doorframe. The fan turns on automatically when the door is opened. An air curtain can also help keep high humidity air from entering a freezer and thus reduce frost formation in the freezer. (Freezers should not have doors opening directly to the outside, but rather should have vestibules or small rooms between their entrances and the outside. These vestibules can be used as coolers.) If a space in a food plant becomes infested with insects, it may need to be fumigated by a licensed professional, using approved chemicals. Typically, even approved chemicals are toxic to people and great care must be taken to ensure that no residues enter the food. An alternative to the use of chemical pesticides is the use of heat to kill insects and their eggs. This is achieved by heating the space – which might be the entire plant – to 140°F (60°C) and holding for 24 hours. Such prolonged heating might damage computers and electronic controls unless they are protected with cooled enclosures or are shut down. Achieving such temperatures is usually beyond the capability of normal heating systems, so if heat sterilization is contemplated, the system must be designed accordingly.

Wood, paper, plastics and glass are potential sources of foreign matter contamination and so should be minimized in food processing areas where food is exposed. Thus it is good practice to transfer materials from common wood pallets to captive plastic pallets for use within the plant. Better still is to have a separate space where bags and drums of ingredients are emptied into totes or other reusable and sanitary containers, keeping paper and plastic bags away from the food. This also separates a source of dirt – the outside of containers holding ingredients.

Glass should not be allowed in a food plant, which can mean minimizing windows or putting windows high on a wall (clerestories) so they are less likely to be inadvertently broken. When foods are packed in glass containers, care must be taken in material handling to prevent breakage. This means synchronizing conveyors and fillers so containers do not jam or contact each other. Samples are collected in plastic containers rather than in glass and mercury in glass thermometers are replaced with electronic instruments.

Lighting in a food plant may be fluorescent, high intensity halogen or incandescent bulbs. Mercury vapor lights should not be used because they attract insects. Glass bulbs must be shielded so that if they break, glass is not scattered. Different lighting levels are needed in each area, ranging from 15–20 foot-candles where the objective is safety, as in warehouses, to 40–50 foot-candles where inspection occurs. Lighting spectrum should simulate sunlight so food appears most natural. For LEED or sustainable design, lighting can be controlled by movement sensors, in places such as warehouses, where people are not always present, so it is only on and consuming energy when people are present.

Floors, walls and ceilings should be smooth and impervious so they can be easily cleaned and will not retain dirt and dust. A good material for walls and ceilings is fiberglass-reinforced polymer panels. Insulated metal panels with enamel coatings are commonly used for partitions and sometimes for outside walls, but they are vulnerable to puncture by fork trucks. Concrete masonry units (CMU) coated with high quality epoxy paint are commonly used for structural partitions. It is important to use higher grade CMU with smaller pores and then to seal those before applying the epoxy. CMU should be laid so that seams between them are continuous in the vertical direction – an uncommon masonry pattern – but this permits water to drain easily and not get trapped in the intersections between units laid in the normal, overlapping pattern.

Floors may be made of brick, tile, terrazzo or coated concrete. Brick was traditional for food plants and is still used in dairies and other operations where truck traffic is heavy and floors are often wet. The grout used to lay the brick must resist acid and basic cleaning solutions as well as extremes of temperature. Tile is less common and is suited to lighter traffic areas. Terrazzo, a monolithic concrete with aggregate filler, is durable and resistant, but relatively expensive. A common choice offering a good balance between cost and durability is a filled epoxy coating over concrete. The filling of aggregate in the coating (small stones or sand) is to adjust the thermal expansion of the coating to match that of concrete so the coating resists exposure to live steam, hot water or cold refrigerant. Otherwise, the coating can easily be stripped from the floor when exposed to extreme temperatures because of differences in the rate of thermal expansion between concrete and the coating. Paint or sealant is the least expensive floor treatment, other than leaving the concrete bare, and is rarely adequate for a food plant except in warehouse areas.

Wet areas need floors that slope to drains and enough drains to remove water quickly. Drains may be hub or trench and should be stainless steel until they join the main sewer. Hub drains are familiar circular openings covered with a grating or sometimes a plate with a perimeter slot. One drain per 200 square feet ($18.6\,m^2$) of floor area is common. Trench drains are shallow cuts in the floor covered with a removable grate, sloping to a connection to under floor drain pipe. Sanitary drains (from rest rooms) should be separate from process drains until they are outside the plant, where they may be combined in a grease trap that also serves as an air break, so that waste cannot flow back into the plant. Floating fats and oils and sinking solids are periodically removed and disposed of in landfills.

Trench drains can have high capacity for flow, but because of the extensive open grating, they need extra provisions for cleaning, because they can harbor microorganisms and spread these in aerosols. Aerosols – suspensions of small drops of water in the air – are created when hoses are used to clean floors and equipment. It is poor practice to use hoses while food is exposed because of the risk of contamination. One approach to cleaning trench drains is to connect the CIP system to the drain so it is cleaned as if it were another piece of equipment.

Ceilings are a frequently debated feature of food plants. Sometimes they are required to enclose a space completely to control temperature, humidity, odor or dust. In buildings where the roof is supported by trusses, a ceiling over processing areas protects against dirt and dust from the hard-to-clean metal supports and from leaks. An ideal roof for a food plant uses pre-cast double tees, which need not be painted and have few surfaces on which to catch dirt and dust. A new plant can be specified to have pre-cast construction, if it is available in the area, but many existing buildings have less expensive metal trusses, or more rarely, wooden trusses. Trusses are nearly impossible to clean and so a ceiling of fiberglass-reinforced panels may be needed. The cost of pre-cast concrete construction varies with area of the country due to differences in supply, competition and demand.

The disadvantage of a ceiling is that the space above it is often forgotten and can become dirty. The remedy is routinely to inspect and clean the top of the ceiling by removing some panels for access. Lighting and fire protection is usually required above and below the ceiling, depending on local codes. Some ceilings are made of panels that are strong enough to support people walking on them. This permits easy access for servicing piping and ductwork running above the ceiling.

Spaces that may pose hazards such as dust explosions or excessive noise (compressor rooms, boiler rooms, hammer mills) often have special construction requirements, including blast proof doors, blow out panels to the outside and reinforced CMU walls. These requirements may be dictated by local codes.

Since raw materials are a major source of potential contamination, it is important to separate raw materials and their containers from exposed finished product. There is also increasing concern about allergens and preventing allergenic materials from contaminating foods in which they do not belong. Separation is achieved by partitions, by balancing and controlling pressure and airflow and by controlling access by people. The most common food allergens of concern are:

- Peanuts
- Wheat
- Milk
- Eggs

- Tree nuts
- Fish
- Shellfish
- Soy.

Ninety percent of food allergies are associated with these categories. People are protected by labels that declare whether a food contains known allergens or whether it was made in a plant that also processes allergens. It is a serious matter to produce a food containing allergens without properly declaring their presence on a label.

Airflow should be counter to the flow of product, so it contacts clean product first. People may be issued distinctively colored uniforms so that it is easy to see if they are where they belong. Hand washing and footbaths are often used before entering an area where food is exposed. Often overlooked is the fact that maintenance mechanics enter and leave all parts of a plant and so may transmit contaminants. They must be trained to keep themselves, their tools and their vehicles clean. It is common to use color-coding for brushes, shovels and other tools so those used for raw materials or inedible waste are not used to contact finished products or edible rework.

Finally, one of the most important principles of good sanitary plant design is to allow enough space for safe movement and easy inspection. It is always difficult to justify space in the design phase because equipment dimensions are rarely well known and so initial layouts seem poorly filled, but as time goes by and details are filled in, space always gets tight. At the same time, costs almost always rise and the easy way to cut costs seems to be to reduce size. This is usually a mistake.

At the risk of some redundancy, it is worth presenting many of these same principles in another form. The American Meat Institute (AMI) formed a Facility Design Task Force, composed of representatives from meat packers and engineering firms, with the mission, 'Establish sanitary design principles for the design, construction, and renovation of food processing facilities to reduce food safety hazards'. They identified eleven principles listed and defined in Table 4.1 (American Meat Institute, 2004).

Meat plants are typically cooled to below 50°F (10°C), which is why the principles address HVAC, fog formation during sanitation (from the hot cleaning solutions interacting with cold air) and the

Table 4.1 Facility Design Task Force Mission

Facility Design Task Force Mission: Establish sanitary design principles for the design, construction, and renovation of food processing facilities to reduce food safety hazards.

Final FDTF Principles & Expanded Definitions 5/4/04

Principle 1: Distinct hygienic zones established in the facility
Maintain strict physical separations that reduce the likelihood of transfer of hazards from one area of the plant, or from one process, to another area of the plant, or process, respectively. Facilitate necessary storage and management of equipment, waste and temporary clothing to reduce the likelihood of transfer of hazards.

Principle 2: Personnel & material flows controlled to reduce hazards
Establish traffic and process flows that control movement of production workers, managers, visitors, QA staff, sanitation and maintenance personnel, products, ingredients, rework and packaging materials to reduce food safety risks.

Principle 3: Water accumulation controlled inside facility
Design and construct a building system (floors, walls, ceilings and supporting infrastructure) that prevents the development and accumulation of water. Ensure that all water positively drains from the process area and that these areas will dry during the allotted time frames.

Principle 4: Room temperature & humidity controlled
Control room temperature and humidity to facilitate control of microbial growth. Keeping process areas cold and dry will reduce the likelihood of growth of potential food-borne pathogens. Ensure that the HVAC/refrigeration systems serving process areas will maintain specified room temperatures and control room air dew point to prevent condensation. Ensure that control systems include a cleanup purge cycle (heated air make-up and exhaust) to manage fog during sanitation and to dry out the room after sanitation.

Principle 5: Room air flow & room air quality controlled
Design, install and maintain HVAC/refrigeration systems serving process areas to ensure airflow will be from more clean to less clean areas, adequately filter air to control contaminants, provide outdoor make-up air to maintain specified airflow, minimize condensation on exposed surfaces and capture high concentrations of heat, moisture and particulates at their source.

Principle 6: Site elements facilitate sanitary conditions
Provide site elements such as exterior grounds, lighting, grading and water management systems to facilitate sanitary conditions for the site. Control access to and from the site.

Principle 7: Building envelope facilitates sanitary conditions
Design and construct all openings in the building envelope (doors, louvers, fans and utility penetrations) so that insects and rodents have no harborage around the building perimeter, easy route into the facility or harborage inside the building. Design and construct envelope components to enable easy cleaning and inspection.

Principle 8: Interior spatial design promotes sanitation
Provide interior spatial design that enables cleaning, sanitation and maintenance of building components and processing equipment.

(*Continued*)

Table 4.1 (*Continued*)

Principle 9: Building components & construction facilitate sanitary conditions
Design building components to prevent harborage points, ensuring sealed joints and the absence of voids. Facilitate sanitation by using durable materials and isolating utilities with interstitial spaces and stand offs.

Principle 10: Utility systems Designed to prevent contamination
Design and install utility systems to prevent the introduction of food safety hazards by providing surfaces that are cleanable to a microbiological level, using appropriate construction materials, providing access for cleaning, inspection and maintenance, preventing water collection points and preventing niches and harborage points.

Principle 11: Sanitation integrated into facility design
Provide proper sanitation systems to eliminate the chemical, physical and microbiological hazards existing in a food plant environment.

need for good drainage. Dry processing facilities do not have such concerns, but otherwise, the principles apply to most food plants and provide a concise summary of the topic.

Security

In any manufacturing facility, there is concern for employee safety, prevention of theft and prevention of sabotage. Food manufacturing raises the additional concerns of food safety, prevention of deliberate contamination as well as inadvertent contamination and the safety of visitors. Thus, there are good design and operational practices that address these concerns. Sadly, this is an evolving area, so existing plants may need to revisit their conditions and practices. New plants need to anticipate possible changes in the future.

Training and education of employees is the first priority. This is a never-ending task as there can be high turnover in food manufacturing. Employees should know who belongs where, should wear their picture identification and challenge anyone who does not and should personally observe safety and access rules. Employees should understand that a risk to their company is a personal risk to them, of not having a job, at least. Past instances of deliberate contamination have often been attributed to disgruntled employees. Thus, good employee relations can be considered a first line of defense. This need not mean abandonment of discipline nor of sound business practices in compensation, but it does mean that investment in employees can be preventive of serious problems.

Security in design includes such features as a perimeter fence, gates at vehicle entrances, card-controlled access to interior spaces, limited access for truck drivers and control over visitors. One consequence of limiting access for truck drivers is the need for a rest room and lounge where they can wait while a truck is loaded or unloaded. A perimeter fence prevents casual trespassing, which carries the risk of liability for injury to a visitor – even one without permission to visit. Fences can be easily penetrated and so are not the sole precaution taken against unauthorized entry. Access to the plant should be limited and guarded.

Visitors need to show identification and are usually escorted by an employee. Contractors and consultants need identification, are instructed in plant policies and may be limited in where they can go unescorted. Visitors and employees remove jewelry (except for plain wedding bands), remove anything from pockets above the waist (to prevent objects from falling into food) and wear hair and beard nets. Visitors and employees usually wear company-issued smocks, which may be color-coded. Smocks do not have buttons, which can fall off, but rather use snaps or ties. Shoes should be closed and, in some plants, may have steel safety toes. Some plants require bump hats or hard hats because they may have low equipment or other potential hazards.

Food manufacturing, especially meat packing, can be relatively hazardous because some tasks are repetitive, sharp tools are often used and there are many pieces of moving equipment, such as conveyors. Workers' tasks should be analyzed for repetitive motion risks and people cross-trained so they can be rotated away from making the same motion for too long. Visitors should be cautioned against touching or contacting equipment or food, except where specifically permitted. Tobacco, other food and glass containers are not usually permitted in a food plant. A break room/cafeteria is usually provided, commonly equipped with vending machines, but sometimes with catered food. Smoking is only permitted outside of the plant. In other countries, several free, hot meals may be provided each day to all employees. While seen perhaps as an amenity, there is also a safety and security aspect to providing a place for eating and relaxation. In any event, provision for such a space must be provided.

In developing a food process and specific plant layout, it is important to identify each place where food is exposed and vulnerable to deliberate or accidental contamination. Measures that can be taken include securing hatches and entrances to tanks, covering conveyors, directing video cameras at such locations (and then monitoring the image!) and having responsible employees at such locations. People are the best observers of quality in foods, so inspection by visual observation as well as by instrumentation and laboratory analysis is needed at many points in a process. Such inspectors and observers are also guardians as well.

As with the HACCP plan, where the needed response to a deviation in the process is determined ahead of time, it is important to anticipate and prepare for breaches of security or safety. For example, employees need to know what to do and where to go in the event of a fire or severe weather. Where tornadoes occur, a place in the plant needs to be designed for and designated as a shelter. There needs to be a rallying point in the event of an evacuation, as may be required if ammonia leaks from a refrigeration system. There needs to be coordination with local authorities for response to fire or other emergency. Some plants employ nurses for care of minor injuries, in which case a room needs to be provided for supplies and treatment.

Fire officials need to know if there are any hazardous chemicals on the premises, such as tanks of oil or areas where dust accumulates. Supervisors need to be trained to account for people in an evacuation and to shut down equipment safely in an emergency. Often plants have a public address system for paging, which can also be used for announcements and instructions, but food plants can be too noisy for these to be heard well. Many plants also have a radio system for contacting individuals. Closed circuit video monitoring is useful to observe operations, reduce pilferage and prevent tampering. Obviously, it is only useful if the screens are watched.

Support facilities

Support facilities refer to the areas of a plant used for purposes other than direct manufacturing. These include space and equipment for utilities, space for employees to change and eat and offices and labs.

Common utilities include:

- Steam
- Electric power
- Compressed air

- Water
- Fuel
- Sewer
- Refrigeration
- Hydraulic fluid
- CIP chemical
- Nitrogen or carbon dioxide.

Steam is usually raised in a boiler. Good practice is to have at least two boilers, each capable of providing about 75% of the required total load, so that the plant can operate, perhaps at reduced capacity, if one boiler is down for maintenance or suffers a failure. Boilers for food plants normally produce steam at 100–150 psi, which is reduced as needed at the point of use. It is rare to need much higher-pressure steam in food processing. Steam is normally distributed in carbon steel pipe with threaded connections. Good practice installs steam traps at low points in the lines to remove condensate. Discharge of steam traps should be direct to drains or to condensate return systems. Condensate is recovered both to save heat and to save specially treated water. Boiler feed water may be softened to reduce scale formation, which costs money. Steam and condensate in carbon steel pipe picks up rust and corrosion products, so if discharged to the floor, it will quickly stain the floor.

Culinary steam is specially generated for direct contact with food. It is common to inject chemicals into boiler feed water to prevent corrosion and scale formation in the boiler and piping, but these chemicals are not intended for food use. Culinary steam is raised in a heat exchanger using high-pressure steam to heat purified water. The culinary steam is filtered and piped in stainless steel to where it is used. To minimize the cost of stainless steel piping, culinary steam is normally generated near where it is used.

Boilers are often fired with natural gas, but may use coal, fuel oil or waste material. Fuels other than natural gas may require special boilers. Boilers that use wastes, such as paper, wood or crop residues, need special controls to compensate for the variable heating values of such fuels. With the rising costs of fossil fuels and the increasing emphasis on sustainability, it may become more common for food plants to use unconventional fuels in steam boilers. A high-pressure, stationary boiler usually requires a licensed operator in attendance. This can be a specially trained member of the maintenance staff who may have other duties. Steam below 15 psi does not require a licensed operator and is often adequate for many food processes.

Other heat sources for processing include closed loop hot water and hot oil systems. These use steam or fuel to heat a circulating medium, such as water under pressure (so it can exceed 212°F, 100°C) and heat-stable oils, which can exceed 500°F (260°C). Circulating fluids may be preferred over steam because they do not pose the potential hazards of steam and, in the case of oil, can reach higher temperatures than are practical with steam. They also can provide good temperature control in processing equipment. While boilers are usually located in a relatively central place, circulating systems are usually located close to the use point to minimize distribution costs and are considered part of the process.

Boilers should be located on an outside wall with access to outside air for combustion and with room to pull tubes if necessary. Often, a large louvered panel is used both for air intake and potential access. An air emissions permit is usually required for the boiler stack. Most natural gas does not require treatment of its combustion products before discharge, but coal or waste fuels may, depending on their sulfur content and the efficiency of the boiler.

There are situations in which a food plant can get steam from an outside source, such as a co-generation plant or a neighbor with excess steam. This can save on capital, but makes the plant dependent for an important resource on another party. It might be wise in such a case to install a stand-by boiler or to establish in advance a source from which to obtain a replacement boiler. There are firms that promise to deliver a boiler on a trailer in less than 24 hours.

Electricity is usually supplied to the site by a high voltage line from the local utility. The plant needs to install a step down transformer and then an electrical distribution system with several voltage levels – 440, 220 and 120 are common. The higher the voltage, the less expensive the wiring and the more efficient the conversion of electricity to useful work in motors on equipment or to light. Equipment and areas of the plant are usually wired separately so individual pieces can be isolated. Switchgear and motor starters generate heat and so should be in rooms that are ventilated. Much of the switchgear is only rarely accessed and so can be located relatively remotely.

Lockout procedures must be established and people trained in their use for safe maintenance and operation of the equipment. Only those authorized should touch electrical controls. Each person is issued a lock and key and is responsible for personally shutting off power to a device on which he or she intends to work. All moving equipment should have emergency stop controls (E stop) in easy to reach locations.

Control and communications wiring is normally relatively low voltage and should be isolated from power wiring. Wire in a food plant is normally contained in metal conduit, which protects it from accidental damage, water, dust, insects and rodents. Conduit should not be over-filled. Local codes usually dictate good practice. Conduits should not be installed too close together for ease of cleaning. Conduit should be one inch (2.5 cm) away from walls, for the same reason, and hangers should be of the same sanitary design as is used for utility and process piping, that is no perforated channel, no all-thread rod. In some plants, putting wire in cable trays is acceptable, but these are difficult to clean. The benefit is lower cost and easy access.

With the importance of computers to modern manufacturing plants, it is important that a power source be reliable. One approach is to have power supplied from two independent sub-stations so that at least one will always be available. This is not always possible to arrange. Another approach is to have a stand-by electrical generator fueled by natural gas or diesel fuel. Often, the generator is supplemented by a large battery uninterruptible power supply (UPS) that detects a drop in incoming voltage, supplies power temporarily and switches to an alternate source.

Few food plants are self-sufficient in electricity, but this may become more common in the future, especially for situations where the plant also can use the waste heat from a generator. This is called co-generation. The generator may be driven by a gas turbine or large diesel engine. In some areas, local utilities are required to buy surplus power generated by private parties. Unless otherwise required by law, the utilities may not pay a very high price, because most utilities want to discourage co-generation, since it means a loss of business for them. The threat of investing in co-generation is often effective in negotiating favorable electricity rates for a new or expanded plant.

Compressed air is almost always required in a food plant because it is used in many controls and instruments. Air compressors are noisy and so should be isolated, often in the same room as boilers and refrigeration equipment. Compressors also generate heat and saturate compressed air with moisture, so compressed air should be cooled and dried. Air to be used in instruments should be oil-free, meaning an oil-free compressor is used or there is a filter on the compressed air to remove lubricating oil mist. Intake for air should be directly from the outside to avoid compressing conditioned air (if it were taken from inside the plant) and to reduce noise. Compressed air systems normally have a storage tank to buffer surges in use. Typical pressures are about 100 psi with reduction at use points. Compressed air is usually distributed in carbon steel pipe with threaded fittings, but may use copper or plastic tubing after reduction.

Water is important in food processing as an ingredient, for cooling and for cleaning. Water must be potable, meaning suitable and approved for drinking, but even potable water may require additional treatment to remove chlorine and suspended matter. As previously mentioned, boiler feed water is often treated by ion exchange to remove hardness (calcium and magnesium salts that can form scale). Water for cooling may be reused either for cooling again, by returning to a cooling tower, or for other purposes, such as cleaning. Water in a closed cooling circuit may have chemicals added to reduce scale and corrosion, in which case care must be taken that such water does not contaminate food.

Water may be supplied by a public or private utility or from a well or surface water source, such as a lake or river. If the firm supplies its own water, then it is responsible for testing and treatment to ensure that it is potable and suitable for processing. Water quality often varies with seasons and weather, though water from an underground source varies less than that from other sources.

Most of the water that enters a plant eventually is discharged to a sewer and then to the environment. The exception is water that is used in the product. If this is substantial, it is prudent to meter incoming and discharge water separately and to negotiate fees based on actual use. Otherwise, it is common to base sewer charges on incoming water rates on the assumption that these are approximately equal. Water may be distributed in carbon steel pipe, plastic pipe or copper tubing. In process areas, ingredient water should be distributed in stainless steel tubing.

Fuels were discussed earlier in regard to the boiler. Fuels may also be used in ovens, dryers and some other equipment. The normal choice is natural gas because it burns cleanly. Where natural gas, which is mostly methane, is not available, liquefied petroleum gas (LPG), which is mostly propane or butane, may be used. Natural gas is supplied by underground pipe from a utility company. LPG is delivered by truck to above ground pressurized storage tanks. Fuels are normally distributed in carbon steel pipe to use points, at which the pressure is reduced as needed. There is a difference in heating value between natural gas and LPG, so burners need to be specified for the specific fuel. For direct contact with food, as in ovens or dryers, it is uncommon to use other fuels, but wood and coal have been used and for special purposes, such as smoking meats, wood (as saw dust) is preferred.

Sewer service was discussed previously in considering sites. The preferred approach is to discharge to a municipally owned and operated treatment plant. Both sanitary (from rest rooms) and process wastewater can normally be handled by such plants, because food process wastes are biodegradable, though they may be strong, meaning higher in biological oxygen demand (BOD) and suspended solids than conventional sanitary wastes.

Inside the plant, sanitary and process wastes should be kept separated in their own cast iron pipes. Under floor drains are combined outside the plant in a grease trap/air break. This is a chamber in which the separate drains enter at a high level and the connection to the treatment plant is made at a lower level. The chamber permits fats, oils and grease (FOG) to float to the top, from which they are periodically skimmed by specially equipped trucks and disposed of as solid waste. Heavy solids may sink to the bottom, from which they are removed as needed. The separation of inlet and outlet in the chamber construction prevents wastewater from flowing back into the plant and possibly contaminating food and equipment.

In some plants there is a need for a central hydraulic power system. This is a network of carbon steel pipe in which a special oil is circulated under high pressure and then returned after use to a supply tank, from which it is pressurized and used again. The high-pressure oil is used to drive special motors and other equipment by reducing its pressure through small turbines. It is important that the system be kept very clean, as tolerances in the motors are tight. Hydraulic power has been used where there is a lot of water, creating the risk of shorts if electric motors were used, and for driving conveyors where speeds are continuously modulated, simply by varying the flow of hydraulic fluid to each motor.

Where one or more central clean-in-place (CIP) systems are used, there may be central storage and distribution of cleaning chemicals, which is another support system. Common cleaning chemicals are sodium hydroxide, also called caustic soda, hydrochloric or nitric acid and a sanitizer, which might be an iodoform, quaternary ammonia compound or another substance. Caustic and acid are received as concentrated liquids, which are hazardous and corrosive. They are stored in plastic or stainless steel vessels surrounded by concrete dikes, in case of leaks or spills. Chemical storage should be separate from other areas and access restricted to those properly trained and with a need for access. Concentrated chemicals are delivered to use points in plastic or stainless steel pipe. They may be diluted in line or after arrival. The use points are small tanks with pumps and associated piping for a section of the process. Properly diluted acid and caustic are circulated through the piping and equipment, normally returning to the tanks for reuse after filtering and replenishment of used chemicals.

Nitrogen or carbon dioxide may be used for cryogenic freezing or for blanketing storage vessels, as inert gas. Either gas is normally delivered as a pressurized liquid by truck and stored in highly insulated steel or stainless steel vessels. Often the storage vessels are supplied by the gas vendor. The liquids are very cold, so distribution lines must be insulated to reduce condensation and ice formation. If only used for blanketing, typically of oil in storage to reduce oxidation, it might be cost efficient to install a nitrogen generator, which recovers nitrogen from atmospheric air by using special membranes. In cryogenic freezing, the liquefied gases allow rapid freezing at very low temperatures.

Welfare facilities

Welfare facilities refer to those spaces devoted to supporting the people and equipment in a food plant. Among these are:

- Lockers and rest rooms
- Machine rooms
- Maintenance shop and parts storage
- Equipment storage
- Break and eating space
- Meeting, conference and training rooms.

In addition, most plants have other spaces for offices and laboratories, including:

- Executive and management offices
- Team rooms

- Sales, accounting and personnel offices
- Shipping and receiving offices
- Quality laboratories
- Research and development laboratories
- Nurse's station
- Company store.

The area devoted to these functions is determined by the number of people served or occupying, by corporate standards and by functional requirements. For example, each employee should have a full length locker if they are required to change clothes before going to work, as many food plant employees are. The locker rooms need also to have showers, space for clean and used uniforms, hand washing stations and toilet stalls.

It is common to provide one or two cots in the women's locker room.

Machine rooms house refrigeration compressors, boilers, air compressors, pneumatic conveying blowers, electrical switchgear and, perhaps, telephone and computer equipment. Often such equipment is noisy and can give off heat. These spaces are ventilated, but usually not air conditioned, except for more delicate equipment such as telephone and computers. It is helpful to have overhead doors to the outside for ease of installing and removing the often large and heavy equipment.

A boiler room needs a source of combustion air, which should be from the outside, often through louver panels, which can be removed for access. Likewise, it is best to supply air compressors and pneumatic blowers with outside air, rather than plant air, which is often conditioned – heated or cooled. Air compressors should have aftercoolers and oil filters because a common use is for instruments and air activated controls. Pneumatic blowers also should have aftercoolers unless the heat of compression is considered useful. Space over machine rooms is often used for storage, because height requirements are usually less than elsewhere in the plant.

A maintenance shop should be equipped with appropriate machine tools, welding equipment, small parts storage and tool storage. Control of parts and tools can be challenging, so access to the shop is usually restricted to those authorized. It is also a dangerous place for those not properly trained. Larger equipment storage may be offsite unless the equipment is frequently used. Modern food lines often have easily replaced units that are rolled in/rolled out as needed. These need to be put somewhere safe and convenient.

There was a time when it was common for food plants to provide hot meals on every shift and in many international sites it is still common. In the USA, the trend is towards vending machines serving snacks, soft drinks, hot drinks and some prepared foods. The machines are commonly serviced by an outside vendor, who then needs daily access. Smoking is no longer permitted in most food plants, so employees who wish to smoke must go outside to a designated area. If this is provided, it should be sheltered so it can be used in inclement weather.

Spaces for management and other support personnel can range from strictly functional for a medium scale plant to quite opulent for a corporate headquarters adjacent to a plant. It is still common in US firms for the space allowed for an office, and the quality of furnishings, to be commensurate with rank – larger and fancier for those with more responsibility. However, there is a counter-trend in which offices are more egalitarian or even eliminated altogether in favor of open arrangements or bullpens, some without even having partitions. The choice is a matter of corporate culture and usually has been established well before a new or expanded plant is considered. However, the exercise of considering the design of such space could be the impetus for re-evaluating the usual assumptions.

With or without executive and management private offices, there is always a need for conference rooms and spaces in which visitors, vendors and employees can meet privately. These are usually equipped with speakerphones, white boards, computer network connections, tables and chairs. A good practice is to have several such rooms of varying size, ranging from one in which most employees can be accommodated to one suitable for a meeting among two or three people. Increasingly, companies are organizing their workforce in teams with a relatively flat structure, as distinct from the traditional hierarchy with several levels of supervision. Essential to the team approach is providing a space in which each team can meet, work together and communicate. These spaces are not available as conference rooms because the team needs to be able to leave work in progress on white boards, store papers and references and otherwise leave and return as needed.

Mid-level, as distinct from management or executive, personnel work in sales, accounting, human resources and some other functions that need work space, normally cubicles defined by partitions. They have phones, computers and some storage. A common mistake is to make these spaces too small, with inadequate allowance for inevitable expansion. There are rules of thumb about how much space is sufficient for these functions. Suppliers of modular office furniture often provide the service of designing such spaces in the hope of selling furniture.

Shipping and receiving needs one or two small offices, depending on whether shipping and receiving are together or separated. There is also a need for a small lounge where visiting truck drivers can wait while their vehicles are loaded or unloaded. The lounge should have a small toilet room so the drivers need not go into the main plant.

Quality assurance needs a small laboratory where typical tests can be performed. The exact space and furnishings depend on the specifics of the plant – volume and variety of products, tests that are required and number of technicians. Many quality tests are performed on the line by operators using simple equipment such as scales, but other tests, such as fat content, moisture and salt need more conventional laboratory space and equipment. In addition to lab benches, cabinets for storage and instruments, the lab space needs work space for the technicians to hold a phone, computer and files. Further, there needs to be space to retain samples for at least the life of the products plus some safety allowance. Typically, samples are retained from every lot.

Separate from the quality lab should be any research and develop ment (R&D) space that is required. Often all R&D is performed at corporate headquarters or another facility, but some plants, especially those that are the sole plant of a firm, may have R&D on site. It is important that R&D not interfere with the normal operation of the plant, so it is helpful to have a pilot plant as well as a development lab. A pilot plant is a small space with small-scale equipment that is flexible and can simulate the full-scale production processes. Pilot plants can be expensive investments but they pay for themselves by permitting development work to proceed without using production scale equipment, over-time labor and excessive amounts of raw material.

Finally, many plants have a company store for employees and sometimes for the public. Practices vary by company, ranging from fairly elaborate stores that stock a company's full line, to small counters where employees can pick up designated quantities of locally produced products. Sometimes, the store is used to dispose of off-spec but safe product, perhaps mislabeled or close to the end of its code date. In some industries, it is a long-standing tradition that workers are entitled to a given amount of product each month.

This brief description of the spaces and functions in a new plant is not meant to be all-inclusive, but rather to inspire thinking about these issues early in a project, where they can be accommodated efficiently and allowances made in the budget. Too often, they are not considered and then are either ignored or designed poorly. Properly considered and designed, they contribute positively to morale, safety and quality.

Discussion questions or assignments

1. Pick a food company from the top 100 (see the August issue of *Food Processing*, Putman Media, Itasca, IL). Where do they have facilities now? Where in the USA might they go next? Where internationally? Why?
2. Pick a state or region. What incentives do they offer plants that might locate there?
3. What does raw land in your area cost per square foot? What does developed industrial land suitable for a food plant cost? What do existing industrial buildings of about 100 000 square feet (9290 m^2) cost?
4. Find the costs of utilities in your area or another that might be assigned or of interest. Do costs change with volume of use? Are there shortages or surpluses?
5. Where does water come from in your area or another of interest? What is the water analysis? Would it need treatment for use in a typical food plant? In a beverage plant?
6. What fuels are available in your area or another area of interest?
7. Pick a company of interest. Describe the corporate culture. How might it influence the design of offices in a new food plant?
8. Pick a food product. What are the required quality tests? How are they performed? What equipment is needed? Can any tests be done at the line? Can they be done automatically and in line?

5

Expansions and conversions

Compared with building a new food plant, expanding an existing facility or converting an existing building may offer some significant advantages. There are also challenges that must be recognized and overcome. Some of the possible benefits of expansion include:

- Support facilities may exist
- Labor supply may exist and be experienced
- Might be the right location
- Raw materials may be available
- Distribution system may be in place.

Advantages of expansion

Each advantage will be discussed briefly. First, in an existing facility, the support functions described in the previous chapter may already exist. Often, when a plant is built, expansion is anticipated and so additional land is purchased, electric and fuel services are oversized for the immediate needs and space is allowed in locker rooms and offices. This adds to the initial costs and may represent a wasted investment if the expansion never occurs. But, when the need for expansion does occur, it is helpful to have some assets already in place. In reality, most food plants are expanded to some extent eventually, so it usually makes sense to anticipate this in the original design.

An existing and functioning plant has a labor pool and thus a supply of experienced people. With an expansion, there is a need

Practical Design, Construction and Operation of Food Facilities
ISBN: 978-0-12-374204-9

for new supervisors as well as line employees and support personnel, such as in maintenance. It is easier to add these than to start from scratch. An expansion offers opportunities for people already employed to gain more responsibility and for them to recruit their families and neighbors to new positions. Expansions that add jobs are almost always welcomed in communities and present an opportunity to negotiate additional incentives and concessions, such as continuing tax abatements or freezing assessments.

Selecting the right location for a food plant is a complex exercise, but by expanding an existing facility, presumably most of the factors that influenced the original choice still apply and it is not necessary to repeat the effort. This is an assumption that should be carefully examined: would we locate here if we were not already here? Circumstances do change – demographics, the economy, climate and transportation systems, among others. However, it is rare that major influences change dramatically over a short time and so what was once a good location decision probably still is.

Likewise, sources of raw materials do not usually change greatly and so an expansion can depend upon the same supplies that the existing plant uses. Sometimes, an expansion involves a completely new product line or process rather than more of the same. In that case, new sources of new raw materials may be required and should be considered in deciding whether to expand at a particular site. Large companies have many facilities distributed across a country or region and so have many choices about where to make a new investment. For them, selecting among existing facilities is much like choosing a location in the first place. The same influences apply concerning markets, distribution and costs but, with existing facilities, some costs may be reduced, because of the previously mentioned factors – existing space, labor and infrastructure, among others.

Finally, an existing facility already has a distribution system in place, which an expansion probably can use, unless the new product is somehow different from those already being made. There have been manufacturing facilities in which products with different shelf lives and distribution systems were made, but it is more common for a given facility to manufacture products that are relatively similar to each other. That is, a bakery would not ordinarily be the first choice to make dairy products or frozen foods as new products, though there can be exceptions to such a generalization. Thus, an existing plant may need to add some storage and truck docks to handle increased volume, but its location with respect to the market would be an advantage since it has established relationships and was chosen in the first place at least in part because of distribution considerations.

Challenges of expansion

Needless to say, there are challenges to expanding a food plant. Some of these include:

- Space
- Construction during operation
- Utilities
- Labor
- Waste treatment.

If sufficient space was not provided in the original construction, then it must be added for an expansion. A well-designed plant, as previously mentioned, should anticipate expansion and allow for it by providing one or more walls with few obstructions or obstacles to expansion. Typical obstacles are truck docks, offices and machine rooms. These are expensive to demolish and replace. Sometimes, the concept is to expand internally into storage space and then add additional storage area if needed, because storage space is typically less expensive to construct than is production space. In either case, there is a wall that eventually will need to be penetrated or removed. It is common to leave the wall in place as long as possible to permit construction to occur on one side while production continues in the original plant.

Construction during ongoing operations is a major challenge. Construction is dirty work – it generates dust, requires a large crew of outside workers who are not usually trained in sanitary food operations and puts a demand on utilities and roadways. Careful planning is a key to success. Construction firms need specially to train their labor and supervisors in the unique requirements of food manufacturing. Entrances for construction workers and equipment should be separate from those used by production workers and vehicles, and the workers should stay out of the operating food plant unless absolutely necessary, such as when making utility connections.

Construction firms are always concerned about their workers' safety, but to that concern they must add concern for food safety.

So far as possible, construction activity should be physically separated from food operations. Efforts must be made to minimize dust, odors and other potential contaminants. Often this involves erecting temporary barriers of plywood and plastic film. Even at a cost premium, it is common to minimize the time required for construction so as to reduce the extent of interruption. This is accomplished by using additional shifts of workers and careful planning and scheduling of activities.

Another challenge to expansion is the adequacy of utilities and other support facilities. As previously mentioned, it is good practice to over-size some support functions in the original design, but cost pressures or simply overlooking this aspect may mean that utilities must be improved to accommodate an expansion. This may be more or less routine or it can be a major undertaking. Adding additional electric capacity is usually fairly easy (if the capacity exists at the utility company), but adding more natural gas or water capacity may involve installing underground piping over a long distance, in some cases. Anticipating these issues in the original design and construction can prevent significant costs later.

While an existing labor pool can be an advantage for an expansion, in other cases the labor supply may be tight and become stressed by the addition of positions. Labor costs may go up, additional training may be necessary and provisions for transportation from distant towns may be required. The addition or loss of other employers in the area can influence the labor situation for a food plant in ways that may change after a plant is built. That is, the labor supply may have been adequate when the plant was built, but other circumstances may have affected the supply. Labor is rarely a dominant factor for most food plants, but it is always important. An area that had few unions and relatively low wages might have attracted the food plant in the first place. The same characteristics might then attract additional employers in the same or other industries so that by the time an expansion is considered, labor supply may be tight and costs may have increased. Such a situation might help to justify increased automation in the expansion design. If the labor supply is too tight or too expensive, the proposed expansion might not be financially feasible at that location.

Finally, waste treatment capacity may pose some restrictions on expansion and then require additional investment by the food plant. Solid and liquid waste treatment and disposal are subject to regularly increasing restrictions and costs. Municipal wastewater treatment plants that were adequate when the food plant was first constructed may have become over-loaded and require expansion to accommodate the food plant expansion. The food plant may be expected to help pay for such an expansion. In the same fashion, solid waste landfills are running out of room and towns are shipping solid waste increasing distances. All these factors motivate careful measures to reduce solid and liquid wastes in food manufacturing and investment in pretreatment to reduce loads and costs. Pretreatment of liquid wastes may include screening to remove suspended solids; dissolved air flotation to remove fats, oils and grease; and biological oxidation to remove some dissolved solids.

Overcoming the challenges

Assuming the benefits of an expansion are persuasive, the key to overcoming the challenges is careful planning. Problems that are anticipated are relatively easy to solve and budget; the surprises are what cause delays and cost overruns. Some of the techniques for overcoming the challenges of expansion include:

- Training of plant and construction workers
- Physical barriers
- Scheduling
- Additional investment in utilities.

In addition to the construction safety and food safety training that contractors should provide to their employees, the food plant needs to train its people to handle the special circumstances of an expansion project. They should know that construction people are not normally allowed in the plant and challenge any they observe out of place. Separate rest rooms and eating spaces may be provided to the construction workers to facilitate the separation of people. Plant employees should know about the dangers of construction equipment and how to protect themselves. Construction site management normally requires workers and visitors to wear hard hats and other protective gear. When necessary, plant people may be designated to assist construction by helping with utility and process connections, providing access to utility service entrances and by adapting their processing schedules. As is true in many other circumstances, good communications among all parties can reduce the stress of an expansion project.

Physical barriers between areas under construction and the operating plant can reduce food contamination risk, improve safety and improve security. When the expansion of capacity involves a physical addition of space, the existing wall is the physical barrier until it must be penetrated or removed. Eventually, doors and piping must penetrate the wall or it may be entirely removed. Penetrations are typically cut as late in the schedule as possible and then blocked temporarily with plywood or plastic film until construction is complete. If expansion is into interior space, such as that once used for storage, there may or may not be an existing wall. If there is, then existing doors are kept closed during construction. If there is no wall, as may occur when adding a line in a process area, then usually a temporary barrier is erected using plywood or plastic film. Plastic film is inexpensive and easy to install but is subject to tearing. Even with physical barriers, additional attention to housekeeping and cleaning in the operating plant is necessary because construction dust is inevitable and insidious in its ability to disseminate itself.

Scheduling is an overlooked tool in managing an expansion project. Many food products and processes are seasonal in their operation, because of availability of raw materials or variation in demand. Some examples are canned and frozen fruits and vegetables, which typically are processed during relatively short harvest seasons, and some confections, which have just a few sharp peaks in demand around holidays. In such cases, it is logical to plan expansion construction for off-season or times of reduced demand. Some canneries are almost entirely rebuilt during their off-season because they are worked so hard during the season.

Sometimes products can be produced in advance and stored to permit a lengthy shutdown during construction. In other cases, production may be concentrated in one or two shifts, instead of three, allowing construction to occur when production is not operating. Where possible, production might be shifted to other facilities or to co-manufacturers to permit shutdown during construction. In general, anything that can be done to reduce manufacturing during the time of heaviest construction will reduce the risk of contamination and of interference with both manufacturing and construction.

As previously mentioned, investment in utilities in advance of the need will usually facilitate expansion. There are various ways to accomplish this economically, including leaving adequate space for additional service, laying lines that are not used at first and over-sizing supply lines and equipment, such as transformers. For example, under floor sewer and drain lines might be laid in a storage area, but not connected until that space becomes a process area. It is less expensive to lay the lines during construction than to cut the floor later to add the lines. In the case of electricity, it is usually sufficient to allow space for additional service, which can be added later, when needed. The general principle is to plan ahead, anticipate the possibility of expansion and make prudent investments and allowances of space as appropriate.

Getting more out of an existing line

Expansion of a plant's capacity may be required because of growth in demand of existing products or to accommodate new products. New products may be made on existing lines or might require a new process. If the need arises from growth of existing products or of new products that can be made on existing lines, the question arises of how to get more capacity from an existing line. To do so might alleviate the need for an expansion or at least defer it for a time.

Every process line has a bottleneck or step that restricts its capacity. It is not always obvious what that step is. Goldratt and his colleagues have developed the Theory of Constraints to address the issue of improving a line's capacity and performance (Goldratt and Cox, 1986; Goldratt, 1990, 1994). Often, a food process line is designed around a major piece of equipment, such as an oven in a bakery, an extruder in a snack plant or a filler in a canning or bottling line. Equipment before or after the major piece usually has excess capacity, which is not normally used. For example, the mixing tanks ahead of a filler may function as holding tanks most of the time, because the actual time to formulate and mix a batch is less than the time it takes to empty the tank through the filler. One approach to increase capacity might be to get a faster filler.

However, understanding the capacity of a line involves more than listing the rates or operation of each step. One must also look at the time required between runs of different products. This is called changeover time or down time, because during it, no product is made. Some down time is inevitable in food plants because most lines require cleaning of some sort between different products or time to adjust to different package sizes. It is almost always true that down time in food plants is greater than it could be under ideal circumstances. Management and, increasingly, teams of workers strive to approach those ideal circumstances by studying operations and reducing inefficiencies.

Some traditional manufacturing practices reduce the efficiency of food plants and may lead to the apparent need for expansion prematurely. For instance, it is common to schedule runs of a given product in increments of complete shifts or of multiple hours, regardless of how much product is actually needed. Excess production is stored in inventory, at a cost and at some risk of loss, because the product may age, depending on the product. Ideally, inventory should be minimized and production driven by sales but, for various reasons, this is rarely the case in foods. One challenge is that a line driven by orders might have frequent changeovers and more down time while reducing inventory. Traditional measures of manufacturing efficiency penalize down time.

The Theory of Constraints says, among many other things, that profit should be the ultimate measure of operations rather than most of the usual measures. Thus, it often is more profitable to make only as much of a given product as is required, even if that means idling a line before the end of a shift. The reason this may be true is that it costs money to maintain inventory. Many foods are perishable and deteriorate in storage. Even long-lived products may experience losses because of changes in requirements, changes in packaging that makes an older product obsolete and a reduction in quality during storage. The net effect can be that a plant's profitability may actually increase by reducing production, reducing inventory and scheduling production to fill orders rather than to fill inventory.

It might appear that seasonal products, such as fruits and vegetables require large inventories because of limited availability of raw material except during harvest. However, many commodities can be stored in bulk and packaged to order and others can be obtained from the opposite hemisphere during off-season. Thus, it is usually possible to reduce inventory and optimize production operations. This may mitigate the need for an expansion.

Optimal scheduling of production can also improve operations. For many mixes of products made on the same line, there can be constructed a compatibility schedule which shows what products can be run in sequence without risk of harmful cross-contamination. This requires consideration of allergens, flavors and colors. It is common to sequence darker products after lighter colored ones and products containing allergens after those that do not. Such scheduling permits fewer and shorter clean-ups between runs. In sequential batch processes, where each operation must be completed before the next, analysis can determine which is the limiting process and suggest ways of improving efficiency. One approach is to identify and improve each bottleneck. As one is removed as the limitation, another becomes the restriction. Sometimes the investment to remove restrictions and increase the net capacity of a line is much less than the cost of a new line.

In many operations, work in progress (WIP) builds up insidiously. This is often an indication of a bottleneck, as WIP builds behind the restriction when other elements with higher capacity operate faster than the restriction step can. The correct approach is to reduce the rate of operation of the earlier steps to maintain a better balance of rates. This is counterintuitive. One consequence of reduced WIP is a reduction in space requirements, which could then defer an apparent need for expansion. It is a poor use of funds to add space simply to store WIP rather than find ways to reduce WIP.

Another consumer of space in many food plants is rework or off-spec material that is designated for reprocessing. There are many reasons for rework, including start-up and shutdown of equipment, mislabeling, under filling of containers and misformulation (too much or too little of an ingredient). Provided the food is not contaminated and is fit to eat, it may be possible to salvage it. Food in containers requires that the containers be opened, the food removed, a correction made if necessary, then the food refilled into new containers. Only foods with a valuable ingredient, such as sugar or chocolate are usually salvaged. Off-spec candy, for instance, is dissolved in hot water, filtered with powdered activated carbon to remove colors and flavors and reused as a syrup in new candy. Off-spec chocolate candies are melted, milled and added back to chocolate in some cases.

Rework is rarely a constructive addition to food. It may do no harm, but great care must be taken to ensure that it does not impact quality. It used to be common to use collected ice cream rework in chocolate ice cream, in the belief that the strong flavor and dark color would mask the other flavors and permit recovery of the butter fat and sugar. Likewise, it was common to add rework jelly candy to licorice-flavored jellybeans under the same rationale. Current thinking recognizes that these practices made poor chocolate ice cream and inferior black jellybeans. A more common practice is only to add rework material to its own kind, that is vanilla back to vanilla ice cream, red jellies back to red jellies and so forth.

Any rework takes up space in addition to posing some risk to quality. When efforts are made to segregate rework so as to only add like to like, the situation gets worse – it takes even more space because there are more separate containers. It is usually rewarding to analyze the sources of rework in a food plant and to make serious efforts to reduce or eliminate it. Not only is the space taken up for storage of rework reclaimed, the quality of food is improved and cost is reduced because material is not being processed twice. Reduction of rework in containers also eliminates the expense of lost containers and the labor involved in handling the rework.

If efforts to reduce rework do not eliminate it, serious thought should be given to disposal rather than salvage. Disposal could be by donation to a food bank, such as Second Harvest, so long as the food is safe and nutritious. This not only reduces the space demand and the cost of salvage, but also could result in a tax benefit. The net effect of rework reduction and a new policy towards salvage could be a deferral in the need for expansion.

Automation of a line that is dependent on labor might increase net capacity at less expense than an expansion. Automation may range from mechanization of tasks performed by manual labor to sophisticated computer integrated manufacturing (CIM), in which connection of machine level controls to higher level computers can reduce manual entry of data, improve accuracy of information and help to optimize operations by providing more timely and useful information (Clark and Balsman, 1989). Such information is essential if manufacturing is to respond to orders rather than produce to inventory levels. New production lines are routinely computer controlled and highly automated, but older lines need to be retrofitted, which can be a challenge. Selective investments in such improvements may reduce the apparent need for an expansion.

It has happened that slowing a line increases production and defers the need for expansion. That may seem surprising, but it makes sense. Over time, lines are slowly improved, even as the equipment wears and ages. A point is reached where the line speed stresses the capability of one or more pieces of equipment. A common example is packaging using polymer film to form pouches. As speed increases, the film can stretch, jam, fall out of register (alignment of the graphics) and cause machine stops and defective pouches. Reducing speed until reliability is restored will usually result in an increase in net production.

Another common situation results from incremental reductions in manual labor on a line where people are sorting materials by visual inspection and hand labor, such as in meat, poultry or seafood processing. Usually there are high value and lower value products being separated, such as red meat from white meat in tuna processing. Red meat goes to pet food, while white meat has higher value as human food. Labor reductions appear to increase productivity, but may actually reduce profit because the separation efficiency declines when people are working faster. Restoring people, which would seem to increase cost, actually increases profit because yield of high value products increases.

Finally, selective replacement of older equipment with newer, more automated and more efficient units may significantly improve capacity. This may be the consequence of a bottleneck analysis that identifies the opportunity and benefits.

Converting an existing building for food use

Converting an existing building to use as a food processing facility is fairly common and often tempting because it would seem to be less expensive than building a new facility from scratch. Sadly, it is not always less expensive and it usually involves some compromises in design and construction. However, done properly, with experienced leadership, creative reuse of an existing building can be a satisfactory solution to a need for additional capacity.

What are our choices?

Having satisfied ourselves that we need the additional capacity and having chosen a location, what are our choices for additional capacity? If time and cost are not constraints, a new building, designed and built specifically for the need is often the ideal solution. But time and cost usually *are* constraints. If a need for capacity is demonstrated, then the sooner it is available, the more valuable it is as a contributor to cash flow.

The initial costs of a purpose-built facility and of a converted building may be similar, but a purpose-built facility may have a reduced salvage or re-sale value, because it may have unique characteristics that are not needed nor valued for other potential uses. Industrial real estate tends to deal in generic buildings that are most often used for storage and distribution activities. These buildings are simple boxes with flat floors and high enough roofs to permit stacking of pallet loads 3 or 4 high. Modern industrial buildings often have 30 feet (9 m) clear height while older buildings may have about 25 feet (7.6 m). These are taller than most food processes require, so a purpose-designed food plant might have a lower clear height in some areas, in an effort to economize building cost. This is a false economy when considering future re-sale value. A knowledgeable architect will not allow a food client to be so short sighted in designing a new plant.

It is rare that a plant previously used for food processing becomes available, but it does happen. Such a building may have floor drains, though not usually exactly where they ought to be. There might be some refrigerated or frozen storage, which most food plants need. Walls and ceilings might be of sanitary design – or might once have been. Walls and doors are unlikely to be where they are wanted and an older plant, especially if it has been unoccupied for a while, may be in poor shape. Real estate agents, not understanding the uniqueness of food processes, will present an existing food plant as the answer for any food client. This is not often true.

Much more common on most real estate markets are new or used generic warehouses or distribution centers. These can be quite large – 500 000 square foot (46 450 m^2) buildings and even larger are frequently found. If a food plant needs that much space, the company might be well advised to design and build (or have built for it) a greenfield plant. More likely, the food company needs a portion of such a building. This means either finding a smaller candidate building, sharing the large building with one or more other occupants or taking the entire space and finding another use for the excess area. Controlling the entire building permits the food company more influence over the nature of other tenants, though most leases will allow some right of review so that competitors or potentially noxious neighbors are not introduced.

Finding a 'right sized' new or used building is ideal, but there still are challenges. Most food plants want to have the potential to expand, but most industrial buildings are designed to occupy as much of a given piece of land as is permitted. The typical generic building also usually has about one truck dock for every 5000–6000 square feet (464–557 m^2). Parking for cars is also usually limited because buildings designed as warehouses are assumed to have relatively few employees and few visitors. Food manufacturing can be relatively labor intensive, with several hundred employees not unusual. In shopping for a new or used existing building to usc as a food plant, it is important to know how many truck docks are needed, how much car and truck parking is needed and how much expansion is anticipated. Most likely, a larger building than is initially required will be chosen, to accommodate future expansion. The extra space can be used as storage or left undeveloped until needed.

Other characteristics

Most buildings designed as warehouses or for light manufacturing have relatively light roof structures, to save costs. These are typically made from metal trusses or, in California, laminated wooden beams. Such roofs are not designed with any extra load carrying allowance, whereas food plants often have piping and refrigeration units that are routinely hung from the roof or mounted outside on the roof. One of the more or less inevitable costs of converting an existing building to a food plant is strengthening the roof structure or providing separate structural steel for piping and equipment.

Another predictable cost is cutting the floor and installing process drains, because existing buildings rarely have floor drains and, if they do in some areas, they will not be where they are needed for the new use. A frequent issue is whether to also slope the floors in areas of heavy water use. Good Manufacturing Practices (GMP) require no standing water in food contact areas, so this often means sloping floors toward hub or trench drains. Replacing a large amount of existing floor can be expensive and hard to justify, but may be the correct long-term decision. If it is not done, then measures should be taken to reduce water use and to provide squeegees to workers for removal of spills, prevention of falls and to reduce the potential biological hazard of standing water.

Sometimes a newly constructed building is left with no finished floor so that the first occupants can define and have provided what they want.

Finally, lighting, fire protection and utilities, such as electricity, water, sewage and fuel, must be evaluated and often need to be upgraded. It is common that walls need new paint or panel covering and, whether new or old, the floor will need a food grade coating. Taken all together, the upgrades and improvements required in converting an existing building to food use are not very different from those encountered in building a new plant. One big difference is that most of the work occurs inside the structure, is not dependent on the weather and can start anytime, while site work and steel erection for a new building must wait for construction season (where that applies).

Discussion questions or assignments

1. Identify, compare and discuss the critical issues in a new food facility project and an expansion of an existing food facility, assuming the same product and capacity.
2. Prepare an agenda for a briefing meeting of a construction crew starting a food expansion project.
3. Prepare an agenda for a meeting with the plant staff about to start an expansion project.
4. Select a food product. Describe its seasonality. When would be the best time to expand a plant that produces it? How would the plant satisfy its customers during construction?
5. Select a food process. What is likely to be the bottleneck? How could that restriction be removed? What is the next bottleneck?
6. Select a food process. Where is rework likely to be produced? How could it be reduced? How do you think it is handled now? What would be a better way?

6 Process and equipment selection

The food industry is immensely varied in the processes and products that can be encountered. People develop deep and specific expertise in various segments of the industry, typically, by working for many years in that segment. Some of this expertise is captured in industry-specific texts, a small sample of which is provided in the following list, referring to the list of references:

- Bartholomai (1987) (various foods)
- Boulton et al. (1998) (wine)
- Lewis and Young (2002) (brewing)
- Lopez (1975) (canning)
- Matz (1988) (baking)
- McGee (1984) (multiple foods)
- Tetra Pak (1998) (orange juice)
- Valentas et al. (1991) (several foods)
- Van Arsdel et al. (1973) (food dehydration).

There are many others. The point is that for any given food or segment, there are sources of specific information, which are not duplicated here. Rather, this chapter tries to present a general approach to process development, process design and equipment selection that should apply to any specific case (Maroulis and Saravacos, 2003; Clark, 2005a,b; Lopez-Gomez and Barbosa-Canovas, 2005).

Practical Design, Construction and Operation of Food Facilities
ISBN: 978-0-12-374204-9

Process development and design

Process development refers to the exercise of creating a means to manufacture a given food in a given quantity. It involves the selection and sequencing of process steps from a repertoire of unit operations. Unit operations, the working tools of chemical engineers, include such steps as mixing, heating, cooling, pumping, size reduction and chemical or biological reactions. To develop a food process, one envisions all the steps necessary to convert raw materials into finished products and communicates this sequence in the form of a flow diagram. Some flow diagrams for familiar foods are shown in Figures 6.4–6.6. These are briefly described to show the relationship between the symbols on the flow diagram and the operations they depict.

Aseptic processing/pasteurization

Aseptic processing refers to heat treatment of a fluid sufficiently to sterilize it, holding for a specified length of time and then cooling before filling into a separately sterilized container in a sterile environment. It is a special case of fluid thermal processing (David et al., 1996). The flow diagram is in a form called a block flow diagram, where simple blocks represent unit operations and arrows represent a transfer without indicating how the transfer occurs (Figure 6.1). In the case of aseptic processing, the transfers are by pumps through pipes or tubing. Aseptic processing is an alternative to retorting of foods in hermetically sealed containers, such as cans or jars. It is routinely applied to dairy products, juices, soups,

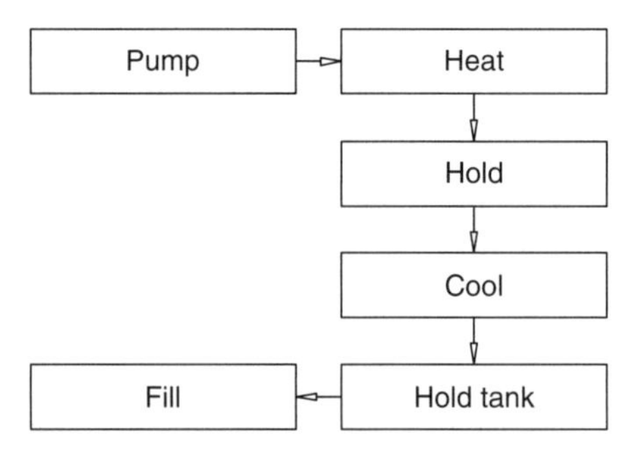

Figure 6.1 Block flow diagram for aseptic process

baby foods, sauces and other pumpable foods. It is also applied in fermentation industries to media before inoculation. The heat exchangers for heating and cooling may be plates, shell and tube or concentric tubes. Another approach is to use direct steam injection. In that case, cooling is by flashing into a vacuum chamber so that excess water from the added steam is removed by evaporation.

In some aseptic systems, and other thermal treatment systems with similar flow diagrams such as pasteurization, some of the heating and cooling is performed in a special heat exchanger called a regenerator, where the cool incoming stream is heated by the hot product stream. This is a way of saving energy and does not require much extra investment because the same amount of heat is transferred as if all the heating and cooling were performed by external streams, such as steam, hot water or cold water. Because temperature driving forces may be reduced in regeneration as compared with using external streams, the required heat transfer area may change. It is not possible to achieve 100% regeneration because heat exchangers need a finite temperature difference driving force, but some systems achieve over 90% energy recovery. (The basic principles of heat transfer are reviewed in Appendix I. More extensive descriptions are found in McCabe and Smith, 1976 and Geankoplis, 1993, among others.)

Examining even a simple flow sheet such as the block flow diagram for aseptic processing can reveal some of the potential issues. First, a desired feed rate must be chosen. Next, the target temperature and hold time must be specified. It is common for such systems to operate at from 15 to 100 gallons per minute (GPM) (about 57–378 L/min). Why would that be? Well, as we will see later, many filling systems operate at 100–600 units per minute. For a 12 ounce (about 350 ml) container, this is a range of 9–56 GPM. Containers may range from 2 to 128 ounces (about 59–3785 ml). For any given system, the processing and packaging capacities need to be selected so that the combination achieves some chosen goal and so that processing, which tends to be harder to modulate or vary in rate, produces more slowly than packaging, which usually can start and stop as needed. This is an important concept, which will be discussed again. For now, the point is that basic parameters of a process system need to be identified. Once that is done, other properties can be calculated. In this case, the flow rates of heating and cooling media can be calculated from heat balances. To do so requires knowing or specifying the inlet temperatures of available streams and choosing outlet temperatures. In heat exchanger design, there is a trade off between the cost of the heat exchanger, which is a function of the heat transfer area and of the type of construction, and the cost of the heating and cooling media. The lower the flow of the heating or cooling medium, the more its temperature will change – rise in the case of cooling or fall in the case of heating. If the heating medium is steam, the temperature does not change, but to achieve a larger temperature difference, and thus a smaller heat exchanger, it is necessary to use higher-pressure steam, which requires more expensive construction of the heat exchanger and, possibly, of the steam generation system.

A common approach for liquid heat transfer systems, such as hot water, cold water, glycol or hot oil, is to choose a flow rate of the medium about three times that of the process feed stream. This gives a moderate temperature change for the media and maintains a reasonable temperature driving force in the heat exchanger. An additional consequence of stream flow rates is the impact on heat transfer coefficients, which increase with flow rate. Heat transfer coefficients are also dependent somewhat on viscosity and other fluid properties, but these do not vary much for most foods.

Additional design decisions include whether or not to use regeneration, what types of heat exchangers to use, how to control the system and how to achieve proper hold time. Why would one not use regeneration? Because the incoming cool feed is not sterile while the hot exit product is sterile (or pasteurized), it is important to ensure that the product stream is at a higher pressure than the feed stream. However, since there is a pressure drop through the system, this means there needs to be a booster pump on the hot product stream. The concern about pressure gradient is to be sure that if there is a leak through a heat exchange surface, the clean product flows to the dirty product and not the other way. Thus, a concern for food safety influences a process design detail. Regeneration requires more complex piping, may increase heat exchange area and requires an additional pump.

If regeneration is used, the amount intended is selected and this then determines the allocation of heating and cooling duties among the sections. It is common with plate heat exchangers to have all three sections on the same frame with special separators defining each section. One of the advantages of plate heat exchangers is the ability easily to change the configuration. Plate heat exchangers can have high pressure drop, but are easy to disassemble for cleaning and inspection. They require periodic replacement of gaskets, which seal the spaces between plates. Proprietary designs are offered which are said to improve heat transfer coefficients (Figure 6.2). Other types of heat exchangers may be less expensive but also less flexible. The shell and tube heat exchanger that is common in other industries is less common in food processing because it can be difficult to clean and inspect and is not very flexible. Once it is built, its heat transfer surface is fixed, whereas plates and modular concentric tubes can adjust their heat transfer surface as needed. A triple tube heat exchanger has a tube inside a tube inside another tube. Process fluid flows in the annulus between the innermost tube and the middle tube while heating or cooling medium flows inside the innermost tube and in the outside annulus (Figure 6.3). The advantage is that the process fluid flows in a relatively thin cross-section, which improves heat transfer. It is common for the triple tubes to come in standard lengths which can be connected in series or in parallel and can be taken apart for inspection. A series arrangement can create high pressure drop, which is alleviated with a parallel arrangement, but care to ensure even fluid distribution must be taken in the case of a parallel arrangement.

The ability to inspect food equipment is a requirement because of the need for frequent cleaning and verification that cleaning has been effective. Most food processing equipment is designed to be

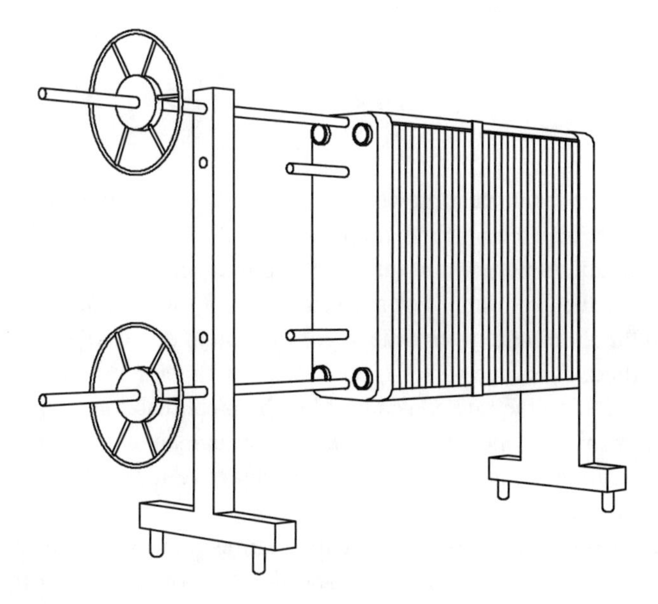

Figure 6.2 Plate heat exchanger

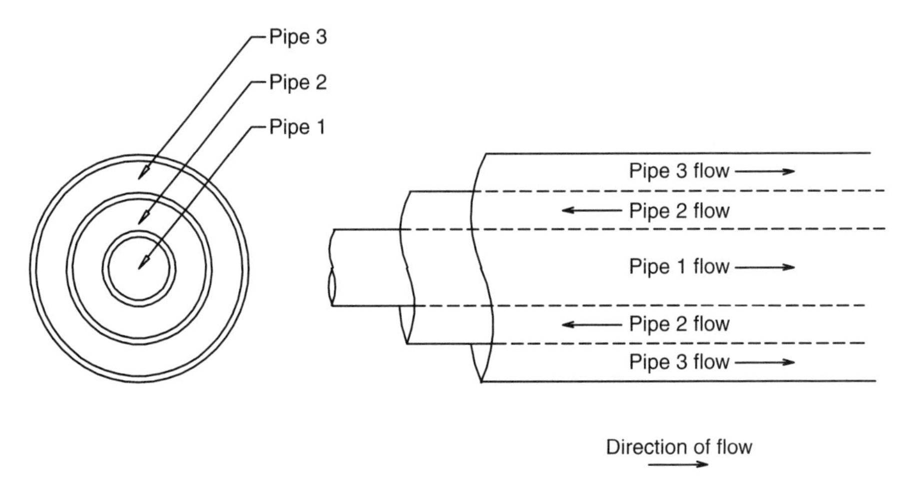

Figure 6.3 Triple tube heat exchanger

Table 6.1 US Federal Pasteurized Milk Order (PMO) temperature versus time

Temperature (°C)	Time (s)
63	1800.00
72	15.00
89	1.00
90	0.50
94	0.10
96	0.05
100	0.01

taken apart for inspection when necessary. Straight tubes are easier to inspect than a coil, for example.

Another subtle point about aseptic processing arises when considering the hold tube. For a given temperature, it is necessary to hold the fluid for a given time to ensure that all spores of pathogens are killed. This time varies exponentially with temperature because it is related to the rate constant of biochemical reactions. The exact relationship depends on the target microorganism and the food and is determined experimentally. A representative table of values for milk is given in Table 6.1.

Most processors use higher temperatures and longer times, but milk is sensitive to overheating and the creation of cooked flavor. The conditions given are sufficient to reduce pathogens in milk to a very low level, but they do not make milk sterile. Spoilage microorganisms can survive, although in reduced numbers. That is why milk needs to be refrigerated and why, even with refrigeration, it will eventually spoil. The point is that for a given food, a hold time is chosen based on the target temperature. The required length of hold tube is calculated by dividing the volume of the tube by the flow rate, in consistent units. There is, however, another complication. If the flow regime is laminar, as it often is for viscous foods, then the hold time required is not the average but rather that for the fastest moving portion of the fluid, which is at the center of the tube. In Newtonian laminar flow, the fastest moving portion travels at twice the average velocity, so the calculated tube length must be doubled compared to that calculated for the average velocity. (See Appendix II for further discussion of hold times.)

In turbulent flow, the average velocity and the fastest velocity are nearly the same. For non-Newtonian fluids, such as power law fluids – and many foods are well described by the power law – the flow profile in laminar flow is flatter than that for Newtonian fluids, but the highest velocity is still substantially more than the average. Now, what happens if the flow rate differs in practice from that assumed for design? This is not uncommon. Flow rates can change because products change; because another part of the process imposes limitations; because demands change; or for other reasons. If the flow rate is lower than the design rate, then the actual hold time will be greater than required and the process will be safe, but the product may be over-cooked. If the flow rate is increased over the design rate, then the hold time will be reduced and the process may be inadequate for safety. This means that, in a well-designed system, there must be a means of adjusting the hold tube length, if the flow rate is allowed to change. One way is to have several hold tubes and a means of connecting the appropriate one for a given flow. Another approach, usually used in milk pasteurization, is to seal the controls on the feed pump so flow rate cannot be changed.

Finally, the process must be controlled, which means providing instruments that measure the critical variables, such as temperature, and connecting them to valves that control the flow of heating and cooling media. In pasteurization and aseptic processing, the outlet temperature of the hold tube is the most important variable. This is used to control the flow of heating medium and also to activate a bypass valve, which diverts product back to the feed tank if its temperature should fall below the target value. The outlet temperature of product from the final cooler is used to control the flow of cooling medium. The pressure of heated product from the booster pump is measured to ensure that it is higher than the pressure of the raw feed in the regeneration section. Typically, the feed pump is a positive displacement pump with variable speed drive. The feed rate is measured and used to set the pump speed. It is common to record the critical values of outlet temperature and feed rate. Interlocks are used to ensure that the correct hold tube is connected for a given flow rate. Interlocks use proximity switches and logic to check that connections are proper.

Orange juice

The orange juice flow diagram (Figure 6.4) is more graphic and shows a little more detail than does a block flow diagram. Orange juice is one of the more valuable and popular juices and employs a variety of processes that are also seen in the manufacture of other products (Tetra Pak, 1998). Oranges and other citrus fruits are seasonal, tropical crops with relatively long seasons. In the USA, oranges are grown in Florida and California; grapefruit is grown in Florida and Texas; and lemons are grown in Florida and California. Internationally, oranges are grown in Brazil, Italy and Israel. Ninety-five percent of Florida oranges are used to make juice and most of this is concentrated.

Important quality aspects of orange juice are sugar content, acid level and the ratio of the two parameters. Color and pulp level are other quality attributes. Color is standardized by mixing fruit from early and late in the six-month season. Pulp is controlled by removing it during processing and adding back as desired.

As seen in Figure 6.4, fruit is hand picked from trees, loaded into trucks and delivered in bulk to the processing plant. Fruit is unloaded by dumping, often into water, which cushions the fall and helps to wash off surface dirt. (Tomatoes and potatoes are handled in a similar way in their respective processing plants.) Oranges are graded by inspection for defects, a sample of each truck is taken to measure juice yield and the fruit is stored in bins until needed. Bins of various quality may be blended to produce a consistent juice.

Extraction of juice from the fruit uses one of two types of machines – a rotary reamer or a finger crusher. The goal is to maximize juice recovery without getting an excessive amount of peel oil

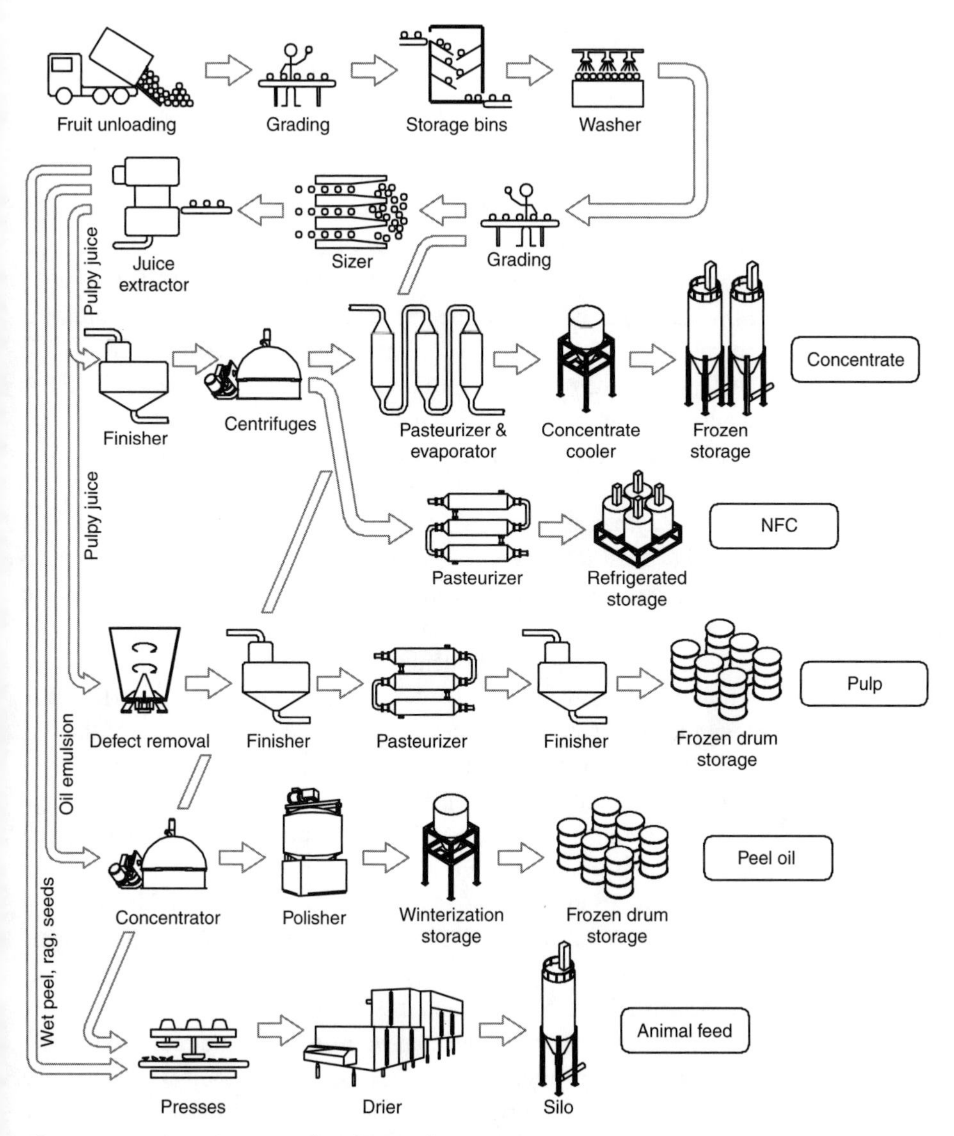

Figure 6.4 Schematic process flow diagram for orange juice

in the juice. The peel oil is a valuable product in its own right, but too much in the juice contributes a bitter flavor. For either type of extractor, the fruit must be sorted by size. At the extractor, the peel is washed with water to collect the oil, which is recovered using centrifuges to break the water–oil emulsion.

The rotary extractor works by cutting the fruit in half, putting each half in a properly sized cavity and then pressing the cut side against rotating burrs, which crush the juice sacs and release the juice. The empty peels are discharged on a conveyor. The finger extractor inserts a perforated tube through the skin and then crushes the fruit around it with intersecting fingers. The juice is forced out the tube and the peel is discharged on a conveyor. The machines are proprietary and are usually leased, not sold. A third approach is used in Europe in which the whole fruit is abraded to release the peel oil and then the fruit is crushed to release the juice. Often the objective is to maximize peel oil recovery; by USA standards, the juice may have lower quality.

Most juice is concentrated by evaporation in multi-effect evaporators after pasteurization. Pasteurization is primarily intended to inactivate enzymes that can hydrolyze pectin, a natural gum that helps keep juice particles in suspension. The heating of evaporation, even though temperature is reduced by vacuum, also inactivates spoilage microorganisms, such as yeasts and molds. Pathogenic bacteria do not thrive in the relatively acidic environment of most fruit juices. Though not shown on the flow diagram, some concentrate has pasteurized single strength juice added back to restore some of the flavor lost during evaporation. In addition, flavor systems using peel oil and essence, recovered from the vapor generated by the first stage of evaporation, may also be added to some products. Orange juice concentrate is stored frozen in drums or in bulk tanks. Most is used industrially at about 80% solids in the manufacture of juice based drinks and reconstituted with water at dairies for delivery as refrigerated single strength juice. Concentrate for retail sale is lower in solids because of the added single strength juice.

A finisher is a wiped surface perforated cylindrical screen that retains pieces of juice sacs and seeds. These, along with peels are pressed and may be dried for animal feed or sold wet, if a close-by market exists. Finishers are used in other food industries to prepare purees and to remove solids from juices and slurries.

Press liquid from the wastes and water from the oil recovery may be evaporated to citrus molasses and added to the animal feed stream. As is often true in the food industry, an effort is made to find some value in every part of the raw material. Only about half the weight of fruit is juice; the rest is peel, oil and other potential waste.

Juice that has not been concentrated (NFC – for not from concentrate) is a premium product because it has more flavor than reconstituted juice from concentrate. However, it is more expensive to ship because of the extra weight and volume. Nonetheless, it is produced in large volumes and is stored frozen or refrigerated. Refrigerated aseptic storage uses large polymer bags or epoxy coated steel tanks. The bags are sterilized by irradiation and the tanks are sterilized by filling with a solution of sterilizing chemical. Filling is necessary because simply spraying on the surface does not treat the air in the tank, while filling and then displacing the sterilent with filtered nitrogen does. (Invention of this technique was cited in awarding Philip E. Nelson of Purdue University the World Food Prize in 2007.) Ships with multiple aseptic tanks of about 1 million gallons convey NFC from Brazil to Europe routinely.

Other juices, such as apple, grape and tomato are also popular and are processed in similar ways, though with special adaptations as appropriate. For example, heat treatments will vary depending on the food's biochemistry and microflora.

Dairy

Figure 6.5 shows a generalized dairy process in which milk is received, fractionated, some parts are recombined and others are processed into products such as butter, cream, ice cream, yogurt and cheese. Milk is a complex and versatile raw material. In the USA, most dairy products use the milk of cows, but other animals can also be a source, including goats, sheep, horses and water buffalo. Cow milk has about 3.5% butter fat, about 3.5% protein, about 5% lactose and less than 1% salts. The balance is water. Milk is an unstable emulsion and, if allowed to sit undisturbed, a high fat layer of cream will form. Milk must be considered a potentially harmful substance because it can be contaminated with pathogens that can cause human illness. The naturally occurring bacteria in milk will also cause it to spoil if allowed to grow. The objective of dairy processing is to preserve the high nutrient content of milk, reduce the potential health hazards, preserve it from spoiling, preserve desirable flavor and maximize economic value.

Historically, much of milk's value was realized in butter, the concentrated fat. For this reason, milk is often purchased on butterfat content and cows are bred and selected for producing high fat milk. However, butter is less important as a dietary fat because

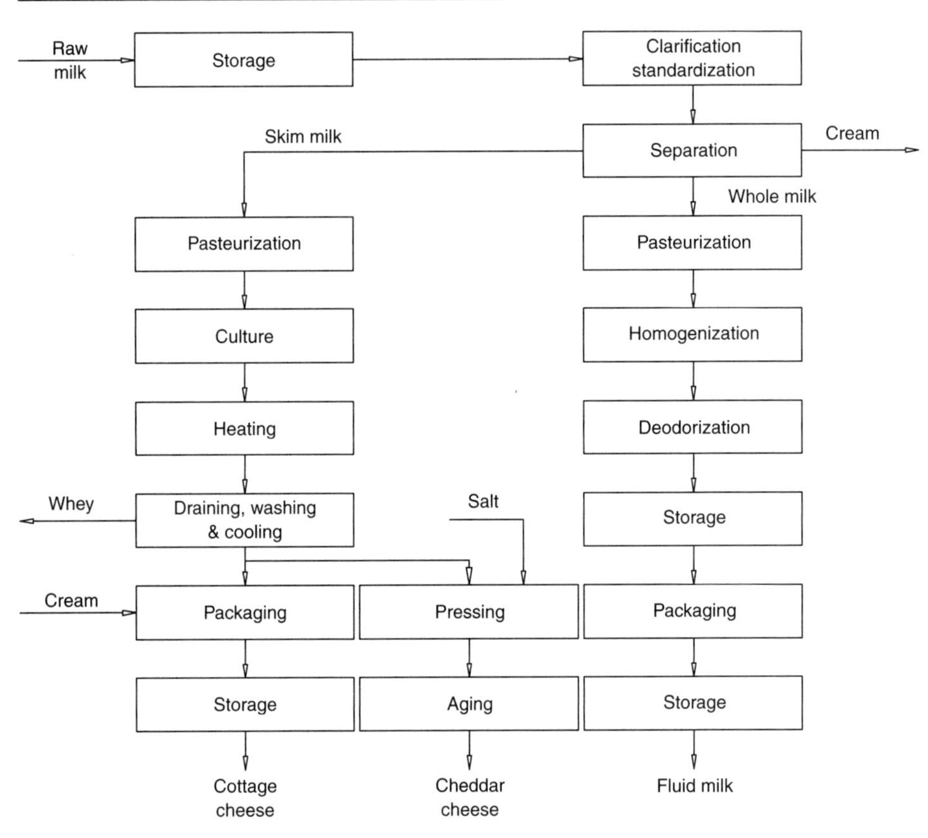

Figure 6.5 Block flow diagram for dairy processing

it is saturated and often avoided by people concerned about the potential impact on heart health of saturated fats. Fluid milks with reduced fat content have become popular and butter is often in excess supply.

Raw milk is received in bulk tank trucks that typically pick up supplies from several dairy farms on a regular route. The farmers milk cows twice a day and store raw milk in refrigerated tanks on the farm. Milk must be refrigerated to keep it from spoiling. Raw milk is tested for unauthorized antibiotics and transferred to storage tanks. The truck is cleaned and released. A dairy usually has several storage tanks because they must be emptied and cleaned every 72 hours to prevent build up of harmful bacteria, even at refrigerated temperatures.

Raw milk is separated into skim or non-fat fluid milk and cream using centrifugal separators. Some cream is added back to skim to make fluid milk of various fat contents, ranging from 0 (skim) to about 3.5%, called whole milk. Unused cream is processed separately. The critical process for all dairy products is pasteurization, named for Louis Pasteur, who first identified bacteria as a cause of disease and spoilage. It is a relatively mild heat treatment to kill all pathogens and most spoilage microorganisms. Because heat can cause undesirable flavor and color development in milk, pasteurization is only as severe as it needs to be. Pasteurized products need refrigeration, because all spoilage microorganisms are not removed. Even with refrigeration, pasteurized products have a finite shelf life. The conditions specified for pasteurization were discussed in the section on aseptic processing and pasteurization. The time required to inactivate a given fraction of microorganisms at a given temperature decreases as temperature increases.

Milk can be sterilized by heat treatment at higher temperatures and for longer times than those used for pasteurization. That process is called ultra high temperature (UHT) processing. Sterile milk is shelf stable, that is it does not require refrigeration until after the package is opened. Sterile milk may taste cooked to some people because of the higher heat treatment.

Cheese is made from milk or cream by causing protein to precipitate into curds, leaving behind most of the water and dissolved sugars and salts in a liquid called whey. The curds can be used nearly as they are, giving cottage cheese and other fresh cheeses, or they can be further compressed and aged to give the enormous variety of cheese products. Cheeses differ in the amount of salt added, the amount of fat in the starting material, the nature of added microorganisms, such as molds to give blue cheese, the amount of aging and the conditions of aging. Cheese making can be artisanal, with much hand labor, or highly automated.

Ice cream is a complex system of fat, ice, concentrated sugar solution and air to create a popular dessert and treat. Fat content can range from less than 10% (for low calorie products that cannot be called ice cream) to about 18% for super premium indulgent products. Ice cream mix is pasteurized after blending, but the equipment used must be specially designed because the mix is more viscous than milk or even cream. Flavors and inclusions, such as nuts and fruit are added at the exit of continuous freezers, which are swept surface heat exchangers cooled usually by ammonia. One consequence is that inclusions can be a source of contamination if ice cream is abused by thawing and refreezing because while the mix is heat treated, the inclusions usually are not.

Yogurt is a specially fermented product made from skim or whole milk. The starting material is sterilized after pasteurization to remove all potentially competitive microorganisms. Yogurt may be fermented in bulk tanks or in individual containers. In either case, the inoculated mixture is held at ideal growth temperatures for the desired bacteria. Some yogurts have added gelatin, inclusions such as fruit, flavors and artificial sweeteners, while others have few or no additives.

The whey from cheese making has been a significant waste, but because it contains some soluble protein and lactose, it often is concentrated through membranes, fractionated and dried to yield valuable food ingredients. The water after most of the solubles are removed can be safely discharged.

Dairy processing is another illustration of separation of food components and maximization of value through targeted processing.

Cereal

Ready to eat (RTE) breakfast cereals were developed as early health foods and have become profitable and popular convenience foods today (Valentas et al., 1991; Fast and Caldwell, 2000). There are many varieties of cereal, made from various raw materials, sweetened and unsweetened, with inclusions and mixtures, with added nutrients and not, and with various target audiences (kids, adults, women). The flow diagram shows that all processes involve mixing, cooking, forming, drying and, sometimes, coating and additions. Originally, these operations were performed separately, sometimes in batches and sometimes in a mix of batch and continuous operations. One of the more significant developments was the application of extrusion, which combined the operations of mixing, cooking and forming into one piece of equipment (Figure 6.6).

Extruded cereals often are made from flours rather than from whole grains and the cooking process is much faster than traditional batch cookers allow. One consequence is that extruded cereals have different flavors than batch-cooked cereals. Often, extruded cereals are sweetener coated, which helps improve their flavor.

Other flow sheet examples can be found in Bartholomiai (1987) and Maroulis and Saravacos (2007). Preparing a flow sheet, even

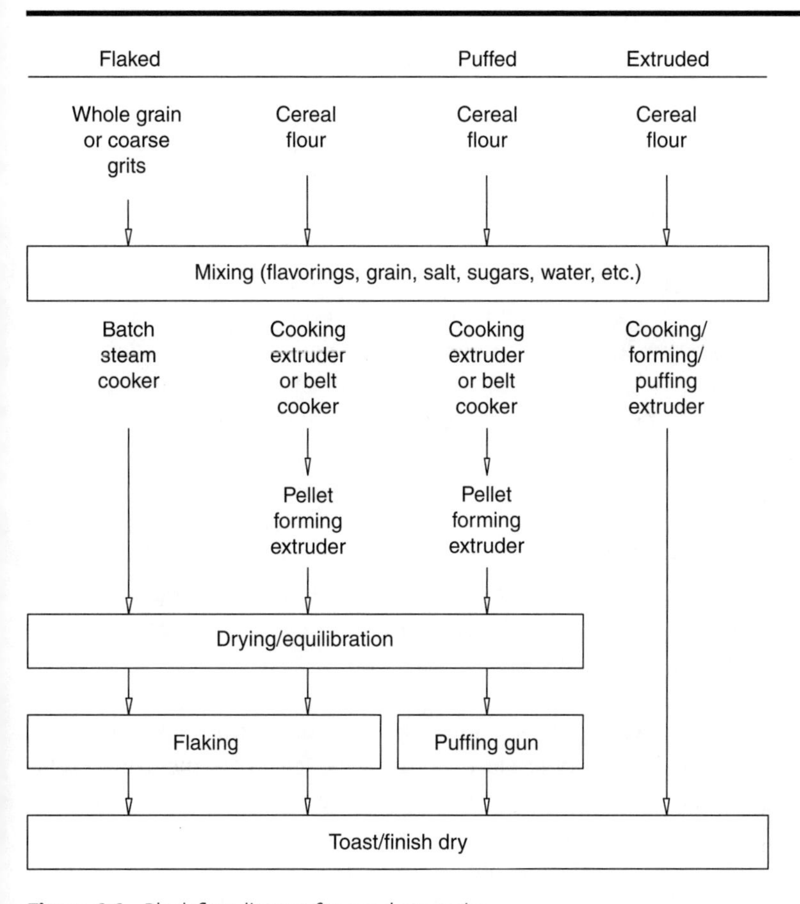

Figure 6.6 Block flow diagram for cereal processing

a simple block flow diagram, is the first step in developing and designing a food process. It is important that a flow diagram be complete. All the unit operations should be shown, as well as all the streams, especially the waste streams.

Categories of food processes

Some broad categories of food processes are illustrated by these examples:

- Thermal treatment
- Forming and cooking
- Separation
- Mixing and formulating.

Thermal treatment

Thermal treatment is often used to help preserve foods by reducing or eliminating all pathogens (disease causing microorganisms) and spoilage microbes. Food-borne disease is a serious problem in the USA and elsewhere. Historically, one of the great concerns was botulism, caused by the toxin produced when *Clostridium botulinum*, a very common microbe, grows under anaerobic conditions in low-acid foods. *C. botulinum* is a spore-forming bacterium, which means that it can protect itself against relatively high temperatures. The process of canning involves heating foods in hermetically sealed containers under pressure so that the food eventually reaches 121°C (250°F), where it is held for a time that depends on the specific food, and then cooled (Holdsworth and Simpson, 2008). These conditions are sufficient to kill *C. botulinum* spores and most other organisms as well. Properly canned foods are shelf stable for years, though their organoleptic (sensory) quality usually deteriorates with time due to slow biochemical reactions.

Containers used for canning include metal cans, glass jars, plastic trays and flexible plastic and foil pouches. Hermetically sealed means that the material and the closure will not allow gas to penetrate. Metal cans are sealed by a double seam formed by bending the edge of the lid and body of the can together. Glass jars are sealed by threaded caps, which have a deformable sealant or gasket. Trays are sealed by heating the edge of a flexible film lid to adhere to the edge of the tray. Pouches are sealed by heating a thermoplastic layer so that it adheres to itself. Canned foods usually have a vacuum or reduced pressure inside, formed by the condensation of water vapor during cooling. The vacuum causes the lid of a can or jar to deform and the presence of this deformation is an indication of proper sealing.

The conditions required to achieve commercial sterility, in which spores of *C. botulinum* are killed, impact the sensory quality of most foods adversely. Texture can be mushy, color can darken, off-flavors can be produced and desirable flavors may be lost. For these reasons, thermal processes are determined by experiment and calculation to be no more severe than necessary (Ramaswamy and Singh, 1997; Singh and Heldman, 2001 and many others).

Forming and cooking

Almost all solid foods are reshaped or formed during their processing. Some broad categories include:

- Size reduction (slicing, cutting, dicing, grinding, milling, shredding)
- Sheeting (rolling a dough into thin sheets)
- Rounding (shaping dough into loaves)
- Flaking (crushing softened whole grains or grits between rolls)
- Molding (forcing dough or melts into shaped cavities)
- Stamping (cutting shapes from a sheet)
- Extrusion (forcing a dough or soft mass through shaped orifices or between rolls)
- Casing cooking (placing a meat mixture in a flexible tube of natural or synthetic material and cooking to form a solid, such as lunch meat)
- Meat fabrication (cutting large pieces of meat into smaller and more useful pieces)
- Starch molding (depositing a concentrated sugar and gum solution into cavities formed in a bed of starch to form a wide range of confections).

These and other similar unit operations have some correspondence with the same operations applied in other industries but, in foods, they may have some special characteristics. Dicing and slicing are examples, derived in a sense from a chef's knife skills, but applied on a large scale by specialized machinery. While consistency of shape and high yield is one objective of automated dicing, it also is usually desired that the end product not seem too 'machine made' even though that is exactly what it is. This poses a challenge to the equipment designer who also needs to manufacture a relatively standardized unit that can be applied to a wide variety of raw materials, themselves variable in shape and hardness. The solution in the case of typical dicing equipment is to have easily changed cutting rotors and adjustments that permit a user to control the three dimensions of a cut piece as desired. Knives are also wear parts that must be regularly replaced, and so designs must permit this to be done quickly and safely.

Knowledge of the available unit operations and the equipment options with which to perform them is a critical skill of the food plant designer or food process developer. All of the forming operations listed can be performed by specialized food processing equipment except for meat fabrication, which is still mostly a manual operation, done by people with knives.

Separation

Separations in food processing are usually based on physical properties rather than chemical properties. Examples are separation by size, density, shape and solubility. Some common unit operations in this category are:

- Screening (sorting dry powder mixtures through various sized screens, which are made of metal, plastic or cloth)
- Finishing (separating solids from liquids using cylindrical screens, which are usually swept by a rotating paddle)
- Elutriation (blowing air through a mixed powder to fluidize and separate by shape and density)
- Filtration (separating solids from liquids by applying pressure against a porous medium such as heavy cloth, metal screen or paper)
- Membrane separations (reverse osmosis, ultrafiltration, microfiltration – distinguished from each other by the molecular weight cut-off range achieved). Membrane separations are distinguished from other filtrations because membranes are usually made of polymers with very fine pores, while conventional filtration uses clothes or fine metal screens
- Evaporation (converting a volatile solvent to vapor by addition of heat. In foods, the solvent is usually water)
- Drying (water or other liquid is vaporized and removed by heating, sometimes under vacuum)
- Freeze drying (water is frozen and then sublimed – converted from solid to vapor – by maintaining a very low water vapor pressure and gently heating)
- Freeze concentration (water is frozen into ice crystals from a liquid solution, such as juice, coffee, tea or wastewater, and then separated by filtering, centrifugation or settling)
- Extraction (usually transferring a solute from one liquid phase to another, but also applied to the recovery of juice

from fruits and vegetables by pressing, which is a more properly considered expression)

- Leaching (dissolving a solute from an insoluble matrix, such as sugar from sugar beets or coffee solubles from ground and roasted beans)
- Expression (removing a juice or other solution from a solid matrix by applying pressure)
- Distillation (separating volatile compounds from each other by applying heat and, usually, multiple stages of mass transfer between liquid and vapor phases)
- Crystallization (removing a high melting or lower solubility compound from a mixture either by cooling or by concentrating the mixture until the solubility limit of the target compound is exceeded)
- Centrifugation (using rotation at high speeds to apply higher gravitational forces and achieve separation by differences in density and shape)
- Settling (using the normal force of gravity to separate solids from liquids).

Separation equipment used for foods may differ from that used in other industries by the requirements of sanitary design and adaptation to the specific properties of the foods involved. Sometimes unit operations are combined, as in sugar refining, where evaporation is used to create a super saturated solution from which pure crystals of sucrose are grown with gentle agitation. Periodically, the slurry of molasses and sugar is dropped to a centrifuge, where the crystals are separated and washed with water. The molasses may be returned to the evaporator or sent to a second or third evaporator/crystallizer for recovery of another crop of crystals. Sugar is one of the purest high volume chemicals made because of the effectiveness of crystallization as a separation process.

Freeze concentration is really a crystallization process and so produces a very pure water. However, because the highly concentrated solution that remains when the water is crystallized is viscous and clings to the ice particles, valuable soluble solids may be lost to the ice stream or the water product may be contaminated by the impurities. For these reasons, freeze concentration has elaborate washing steps which add complexity to the equipment and reduce efficiency.

Many separation processes benefit from using multiple stages or repetitions of the operation. Often, this is done in a counter-current fashion, where two streams move in opposite directions through the stages. Extraction, leaching and distillation are examples of this practice. The principle is that almost any separation cannot be 100% effective; that is the removal of a solute from one liquid stream to another or of a solute from a solid to a liquid is typically expressed as a fraction of theoretical completion. The fraction is determined by the ratio of the flow of the two streams and by solubilities in the respective phases. There is always a trade off between degree of completion and practicality. For example, using an infinitely large volume of water to extract ground coffee might lead to almost 100% removal of coffee solubles, but it would result in a very dilute solution that would not taste like coffee and would cost a lot to concentrate.

Using more practical ratios of the phases and contacting partially depleted solids with 'fresher' solvent permits high recovery at more useful concentrations. The cost (there is always a cost) is in extra equipment and in more complex flow patterns. In many practical cases of solid leaching and liquid/liquid extraction, three stages often are optimal.

Interestingly, the same principle of stagewise operation can apply to operations where the concept may be less intuitive. For example, in size reduction by milling or grinding (mentioned previously as an example of forming), a distribution of particle sizes is usually produced. This is a statistical or stochastic process in which particle sizes are distributed about a mean size with a characteristic standard deviation. The objective of such an operation is usually to achieve a distribution about a given size with neither too many fines (very small particles) nor too many large ones. Large particles can be reground or remilled, but fines may be lost. If size reduction is conducted in one step, yield may be very low because of the production of excessive fines. A better way is to use several stages, often three, in which the fractional size reduction for each step is relatively small. For many particles, screening is used to separate overs, target-sized and fines. In the early stages, 'fines' may be close to the target and can be removed as product. Overs are recycled. A mid-size cut goes to a second and third stage of size reduction and the same screening separation is repeated. The flow pattern can become complex when there is a potential market for several size ranges. Flour milling uses successive size reduction and separation to produce white flour, whole wheat flour, bran and several other by-products.

The lesson is that in considering unit operations to comprise a food process, it is important to realize that many operations benefit from individual optimization, especially the use of multiple stages.

The benefits of counter-current operation can be illustrated by washing, a common procedure in many food processes. Washing is a relatively simple solid/solid separation facilitated by a liquid such as water, sometimes with added chemicals, such as detergents or caustic. One solid is surface soil and the other is the food raw material. (Cleaning of equipment surfaces is a related subject.) An example is the processing of clams.

Clams are dredged from the floor of oceans and bays and delivered in bulk to processing plants located near docks. The clams are covered with mud and, if they are alive, are tightly closed. The first processing step is to wash off the mud. Externally clean clams are then shucked, or caused to open, by heating with steam or open flames in a conveyor oven. Recently, it has been observed that high-pressure treatment causes clams to open and also reduces the amount of resident microbes. Opened clams are then ground so that the meat and shells can be separated by density. The mix is suspended in a clean brine and the meat floats while the shell fragments sink. The meat is then washed, to remove the brine, and cut into pieces. It is washed again and then frozen for subsequent use in soups and other foods.

As described, there are three steps of washing, each of which might use fresh water, which is then discarded. Even though the contaminants came from the ocean or bay in the first place, there are regulations against discharging contaminated water to waterways. The only washing step that really needs to use fresh water is the last; washing off the brine and the mud could just as easily use the water that has already been used. At the cost of some piping changes, the volume of water and the volume of waste discharged can be reduced by a factor of about three, simply by introducing fresh water at the end of the process and reusing it in earlier washing steps.

Counter-current flow not only reduces the volume of a resource such as water, but it also increases the concentration of the solute or soil. This can reduce the cost of recovery or concentration or, in the case of waste treatment, reduce the cost of treatment because the volume is reduced and the concentration is increased, which generally improves the efficiency of treatment.

The same sort of economy can be realized by reusing cooling water elsewhere in a process. Cooling water may be warmed up but is rarely contaminated and so it can be used where fresh water might otherwise be found.

Separation processes rely on some physical or chemical difference between the phases involved. There is a very large range of operations that exploit the specific differences applicable to any given food process. It is difficult to be expert or even knowledgeable in all the possibilities, but it is important to at least be aware of some of the options and to understand the ways in which many of them can be optimally applied. In particular, it is usually worth asking whether a given operation benefits from multiple stages and whether it can apply counter-current flow.

Mixing and formulating

Mixing and formulating are usually the first steps in a food process. This is the step or steps where a recipe is assembled. Because of the enormous range of possible food products, almost every conceivable combination of phases can occur:

- Solids with solids
- Solids dissolved in liquids
- Liquids dissolved in liquids
- Immiscible liquids (emulsions)
- Solids suspended in liquids (slurries)
- Gases in liquids
- Liquids in solids (doughs).

There really are two important aspects of mixing – providing the correct amounts of an ingredient and then incorporating the ingredients together. The first part is where the formulation or recipe is controlled. Techniques may range from scooping a powder by hand from a drum or bin to completely automatic dispensing of liquids and solids from storage tanks and bins. Liquids and solids may be dispensed by weight or by volume. Dispensing by volume is usually less expensive and sufficiently accurate, but it relies on materials having a consistent bulk density. Liquids usually are consistent in density and so volumetric meters are frequently applied to liquid ingredients such as water, oils and syrups.

Other meters use the Coriolis effect, in which a fluid moving through a curved tube exerts a force on the tube that correlates with the mass flow rate. Such meters can be very accurate but are sometimes sensitive to entrained gas in the fluid (Figure 6.7).

Formulation of many foods is done in batches using tanks or vessels that may range from 200 gallons up to several thousand gallons. Choosing the right size of batch to make is one of the early decisions in a design. Considerations include how long it takes to assemble and mix a batch, how fast the rest of the process operates, how much risk a company wants to take and the size of available equipment. Some food processes make the same product for long stretches of time while others make many different varieties. The correct batch size will be different for these cases. Long runs favor relatively large batches or even continuous formulating and mixing, while the need for frequent changeovers may favor small to medium sized batches. In any case, there needs to be a place in which a formula is assembled.

The collection vessel or batch tank can be installed on load cells, which are an electronic means of weighing the tank and its contents. If the tank is used as a scale, only one ingredient at a time can be weighed, which can lengthen the time for assembling a mix. If ingredients are separately measured, they can be loaded simultaneously. Even in this case, load cells are useful as a final check that the correct total batch has been made. They can also be used to calibrate the separate ingredient delivery and measurement systems.

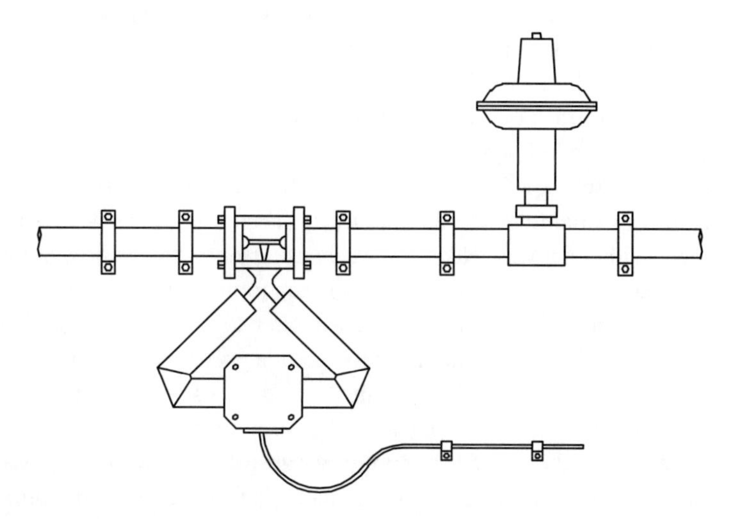

Figure 6.7 Coriolis flow meter

Measurement and delivery of solids is more challenging because of the many ways in which flowing solids can behave. Solid powders can be cohesive, meaning they tend to stick together which leads them to clog openings in bins and bridge over feeders, interrupting flow. Very fine solids can flood as they get aerated and become difficult to control. Some solids are abrasive and cause excessive wear on feeders. Mixtures of solid particles can segregate when they flow due to differences in particle size and density.

Sometimes solid ingredients are added in integer numbers of bags or drums to avoid the challenges of handling them in bins and conveyors. In such cases, the formula may need to be adapted for convenience. Occasionally, the supplier of ingredients in containers is asked to fill a certain weight so the containers can be used as units in formulating.

Many solids are conveyed pneumatically, meaning they are blown through closed pipes or tubing with compressed air from blowers. Pneumatic conveying may use pressure or vacuum. Pressure conveying means the air is supplied at pick-up points while vacuum conveying means the pressure at the receiving point is reduced by a blower. Pressure conveying is convenient when delivering a bulk solid ingredient to several use points. Flour and sugar are routinely delivered this way to multiple mixers in a bakery. A pneumatic conveying system has many significant components. First is the solids storage bin. This must be designed so that the solids flow within it smoothly without a build up on the walls and without flow interruption at the discharge. The bin must be vented so air displaced when filling with solids can be released and so that air can re-enter when solids are withdrawn. The vent must have a filter to prevent dust from being released to the environment and to prevent dirt from re-entering (Figure 6.8, typical pneumatic system).

At the discharge, the solids need a feeder which can dispense the powder smoothly into the air stream. Feeders are star wheels or screws with relatively close tolerance clearances between rotating parts and the fixed chamber to prevent air from entering the bin. In vacuum systems, air enters through a filter to prevent contamination, but the filter should not have too great a pressure drop. Pressure blowers add heat to the air and increase moisture saturation, so it is good practice to have coolers and dryers after the compressors. The reason is that heat and humidity can affect many food powders, causing sugar to cake, for instance. Blowers and compressors are noisy and so are usually isolated in machine rooms. It is good

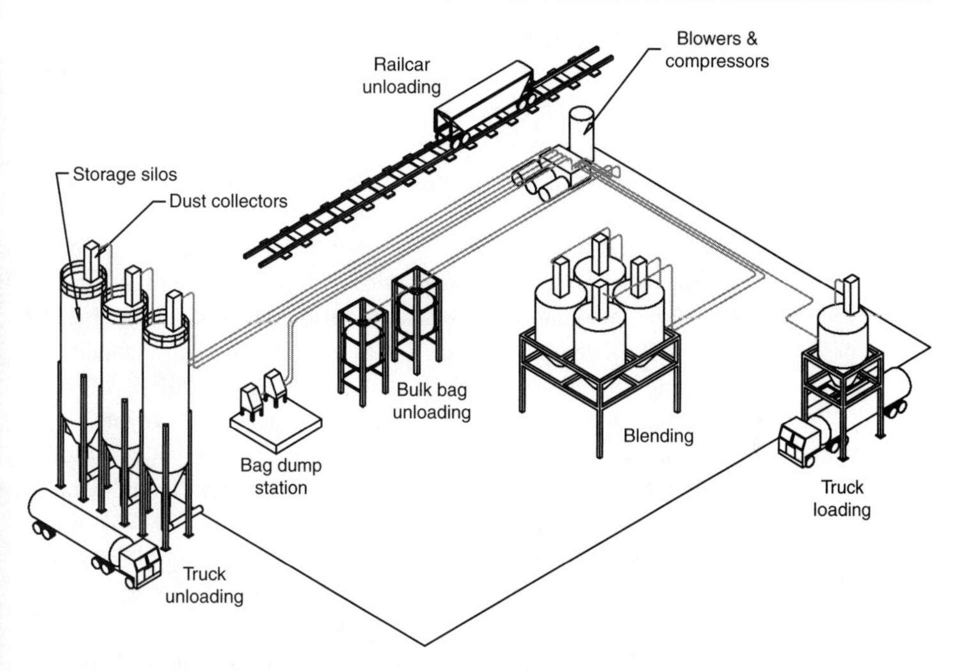

Figure 6.8 Typical pneumatic system, illustrating various functions

practice to supply them with outside air rather than drawing from the room, because room air may be heated or cooled, depending on the season, while outside air, at least in cooler months, is cool, which is desirable when it is to be compressed, because cooler inlet air results in lower temperature conveying air.

At the receiving point, there needs to be a divert valve that directs all or part of the flow to a receiver. The receiver may be on load cells and also needs a vent and filter to release displaced air without releasing dust. The receiver can serve as a loss in weight feeder to the mixer or it can discharge to another bin serving that purpose or the mixer may use gain in weight to control delivery of the bulk ingredient.

If a batch tank or mixer receives several bulk ingredients plus several liquids and some minor and micro ingredients by hand addition, access to the mixer can get crowded. There might be two or three receivers plus several liquid inlets. Minor ingredients might be delivered through a bag dump station, in which multiple bags or fractions thereof are dumped, picked up by an air stream and delivered to a receiver over the mixer. A hatch or man way is usually provided for addition of small amounts of ingredients, inspection of the mixer and cleaning of the mixer. Bakery mixers rotate on a horizontal axis for addition of hand added ingredients and for discharge of dough.

Major ingredients are generally those present in double digit percent by weight; minor ingredients are generally those between 1 and 10% by weight; and micro ingredients are those below 1%. These distinctions may vary by segments of the industry. Major ingredients often lend themselves to bulk delivery. Purchasing by bulk often saves money because there is no unit packaging. Bulk delivery does require storage facilities and, usually, a pneumatic conveying system. Some bulk solids may be handled by other mechanical conveyors, such as enclosed screw conveyors, drag conveyors and belts. They still need proper feeders and dust control. Mechanical conveyors are potentially dangerous and require care in design and operation.

Minor ingredients usually are purchased in bags, drums or intermediate bulk containers (IBC), which are large flexible bags or portable bins. Typically, the larger the container, the lower the unit cost of the ingredient, but large containers require their own special facilities for transporting, unloading and return, if they are reusable. Bags are inexpensive and convenient, but create a waste stream, which can generate dust and be attractive to rodents and birds. Empty bags are usually baled and sold for recycling. Cardboard drums are usually lined with plastic bags. The drums are often reused either in the plant or by third parties. The plastic bag liners are discarded. Examples of minor ingredients are fruits, dried vegetables, starches and cheese.

Micro ingredients are usually received in small quantities and may be fairly valuable though they are typically used in small amounts. Examples are flavors, colors, nutrients, preservatives and spices. Sometimes, for convenience, they may be premixed, often with a carrier or diluent, which may be another major or minor ingredient, such as flour or starch. When premixes are made, there needs to be another small mixer and then some way to store and dispense the premix. Alternatively, just the amounts needed for one batch can be weighed into a small tub, which does not really need to be mixed, as the entire amount is added to the batch. Premixes need to be carefully developed because there can be interaction among the minor and micro ingredients in a premix.

Having dispensed and assembled the ingredients of a mixture, it must then be made as uniform as necessary. This may involve heating to dissolve solubles, such as salt and sugar. For this reason, many batch tanks are jacketed and supplied with steam or hot water. Most batch tanks also have some form of agitation, but the agitation must suit the specific case. If a formula is intended to be relatively homogeneous, then high-speed, high shear mixing may be used. However, if the mixture is a suspension of fragile particles, such as a soup, then agitation must be more gentle, just vigorous enough to keep particles in suspension without breaking them up. High shear mixing is provided by propellers on shafts and by rotors in cages. Gentle mixing is provided by slowly rotating scrapers and helical arms. Solid/solid mixing may be agitated with horizontal ribbons or paddles or achieved by tumbling the entire vessel. Dough mixing involves heavy-duty flights on a horizontal shaft and is an integral step in the making of bread because the unique texture of bread is due to the mechanical stretching of wheat proteins during mixing. Selecting an appropriate mixer is empirical and based on testing and experience.

Continuous mixing is appropriate to long runs of the same formula. It relies on continuous measuring and feeding of each ingredient to a collection point, which may be a conveyor, pipe or vessel. The mechanism of making the mixture as homogeneous as necessary may be an in-line agitator, a static mixer in a pipe, or just the act of transporting and dumping, depending on the materials. Agitators and static mixers are appropriate for liquids. A static mixer is a series of specially shaped elements that divide and recombine a flowing stream. After the correct number of divisions, a liquid stream, even a very viscous one, is well mixed. The real issue in continuous mixing is reliable feeding. Solid feeders especially are prone to blockages and flow interruptions which then create errors in a portion of the continuously mixed stream. Continuous mixing involving solid ingredients is less common than situations with all liquid ingredients, though they do occur. Solid inclusions, such as chocolate chips and frozen fruits, are added continuously to ice cream as it discharges from the freezer. Common liquid applications include carbonated beverages, in which syrup is continuously added to water and carbon dioxide on its way to a high-speed filler.

Developing a food process involves assembling a flow sheet from the arsenal of available unit operations, recognizing the unique requirements of a given case. Knowledge of the general categories of food processes as discussed here helps apply specific information while also using the lessons and experience of well-established processes (Clark, 2005b). Tools such as modeling and simulation (Lopez-Gomez and Barbosa-Canovas, 2005) and pilot plant tests are valuable. One special feature of food process design is that it is subject to considerable regulation and constraints, which are discussed next.

Good manufacturing practices

Good manufacturing practices (GMP or sometimes cGMP, for 'current good manufacturing practices') are defined in Title 21 Part 110 of the Code of Federal Regulations (CFR). The regulations are relatively general but also are fairly extensive. For greater detail, see Imholte (1984), Clark (1993a,b,c, 1999, 2005a), Lopez-Gomez and Barbosa-Canovas (2005). Title 21 Part 110 of the CFR is mostly enforced by the US Food and Drug Administration (FDA), but the US Department of Agriculture (USDA) has regulatory responsibility for meat, poultry and eggs. Seafood has its own set of regulations. Some details of practice and enforcement differ among the agencies – a perennial topic of discussion in Washington. For example, the USDA conducts continuous on-site inspection of meat and poultry slaughtering plants and periodic inspection of other meat processors. The FDA does not routinely inspect food plants, but is entitled to inspect any plant at any time. In practice, the FDA focuses on plants that have had a problem. The USDA approves plant and equipment designs in advance, while the FDA does not. Here, we focus on the underlying principles of the regulations, from which the details are derived.

Increasingly, both the FDA and the USDA rely on the approach called HACCP, for hazard analysis critical control points. This will be discussed in more detail later, but briefly, the concept is to identify and anticipate potential hazards, identify means of preventing the hazards and document both the analysis and the performance.

The Food, Drug & Cosmetic Act, which is the basic law giving the federal government authority to regulate food for human consumption, is based on preventing adulteration. Over the years, the meaning of adulteration has been broadened and redefined to include unsafe colors and flavors, microbes and irradiation (even though irradiation does not add anything to food). As various pathogens have emerged and become subjects of concern, specific approaches to reduce their impact have also developed. As applied to the design of food plants and food processing equipment, the regulations define what is permitted in food and specify various practices that are intended to prevent inadvertent addition of physical, chemical and biological hazards to food. Recognizing the wide range of foods and food processes and that there are often options in achieving a given objective, the regulations mostly describe end results without specifying means to achieve them. Thus, a regulation may say that equipment should be made of material that is non-corrodible and easy to clean; it does not say that it must be made of stainless steel, though most food processing equipment is.

A basic principle of good food plant design is that the flow of people and material should be logical and unobstructed. In fact, one of the first decisions that must be made is the overall flow pattern – straight through, U-shaped or L-shaped are common choices. There are advantages and disadvantages to each, some of which were discussed earlier. Materials of construction and finishes were also discussed. These must be easy to clean and not sources of potential contamination. Painted surfaces are generally undesirable, but if paint must be used, it should be of very high quality on properly prepared and sealed surfaces and then carefully maintained.

Dust and dirt can accumulate on flat surfaces, so these should be avoided in food plant design. Curbs usually have sloped tops. Concrete enclosures for the bottom of columns are also usually sloped. Structural members should be enclosed because they can be difficult to clean. Perforated channel, popular for supporting electrical conduit and pipes, should not be used. Rather, solid bars or simple angle members are used. All thread rod is hard to clean and can be dangerous because of the sharp threads. Plain rods threaded just at the ends are better. The principle of being easy to clean dictates that conduit and pipe mounted on walls have about one inch (2.5 cm) clearance from the wall. Overhead piping and conduit should be minimized where food is exposed, because these can collect dirt, which can fall into the food.

Where liquids are likely to reach the floor, whether process fluids or water, the floor should be sloped to drain. Sloped floors are more expensive to install and can cause challenges in setting equipment, but it is important to prevent standing water. Microbes require moisture to grow and standing water also poses a slipping hazard. Drains may be trenches or hubs and must be designed so they can be easily cleaned. One drain per 200 square feet (18.6 m^2)

is a good rule of thumb. Because drains, especially trench drains, are wet, they can harbor microbes, which can be dispersed in aerosols by careless use of hoses during cleaning. It is common to provide special cleaning nozzles for drains and to train workers not to spray hoses directly into drains.

Rodent and insect controls are important parts of food plant operation. Correct design can make the task easier. Rodents, birds and insects can spread pathogens, foul food or ingredients with their droppings and are considered as evidence of potential adulteration. Pests are attracted by the abundant food found in a food plant. One precaution is to keep ingredients and work in process (WIP) enclosed. Rats and mice do not see well, but they use their whiskers to navigate along walls. It is common to maintain a clear path around the inside perimeter of a food plant of about 18 inches (46 cm). Rodent traps are the only objects permitted in this space. A similar path is maintained around the exterior as well, typically cleared of vegetation. Traps are placed and serviced by licensed pest control technicians. Because of the risk of food contamination, many chemical pesticides are not permitted in food plants. Insect control is by avoiding dust accumulations, treating incoming dry ingredients with pin mills to kill any insect eggs and, in some cases, using heat to kill eggs, larvae or insects. Heat treatment involves raising the temperature of bins or even the entire plant to about 140°F (60°C) and holding at that temperature for 24 hours. This requires special design of the heating system and protection of sensitive computers from the high temperature.

Rats and mice can enter through very small openings, so care must be taken to seal under doors to the outside. While less common today, some plants have rails entering the plant, which can provide tempting entrances to rodents if not carefully sealed. Cracks in walls and penetrations for pipes and conduits must be properly filled and sealed. Birds are attracted by edible wastes and so these must be properly enclosed and removed regularly.

Potential contaminants such as wood, glass, mercury and cleaning chemicals should not be used where food is exposed. This may require transferring ingredients from wooden pallets to plastic or corrugated paper pallets for handling inside the plant. Mercury in glass thermometers may still be required as standards for retorts used in canning, but they should be protected against accidental breakage. Modern temperature measuring instruments are accurate and preclude the need for mercury in glass thermometers. It is good practice to isolate dirty raw materials from areas where food is exposed. Bags and drums can be opened in a separate area and contents transferred to reusable totes or containers. Dust can be controlled and wood and paper are kept from food contact. Cleaning chemicals such as caustic, acid and detergents are often received in bulk and stored in tanks. Only the quantities needed are delivered to use points during cleaning-in-place (CIP) and sanitation. Workers must be trained in the proper use of chemicals for their own safety and to prevent food contamination.

Dry process plants can be prone to dust explosions. Flour, sugar, starch and some other fine particle food ingredients can become entrained in air and, if an ignition source exists, can ignite and explode. A common occurrence is for an initial explosion to raise a larger dust cloud, which then causes damage and injury. Precautions include good dust control by collecting dust at the source – bag dump stations, for instance, and other open transfer points. Dust should be removed from surfaces by vacuum cleaning, not by blowing with compressed air, as is unfortunately common practice. Potential ignition sources should be eliminated, by grounding metal pipes and chutes, by enclosing wires in conduit, by using correctly designed motors, by using low voltage control wiring and by avoiding tools which can spark if dropped. Bucket elevators, frequently used to transfer grains and powders, can accumulate dust because they are usually enclosed in panels and can create their own ignition source by metal against metal wear. The solution is frequent inspection, cleaning and good maintenance.

Fire protection is usually governed by local codes and regulation, but because many jurisdictions are not familiar with food plants, the regulations may not always be appropriate. The designer and owner of a food plant must know the potential hazards and include correct protections. For example, a central refrigeration system may have a substantial inventory of ammonia. Alarms and controls are necessary to detect leaks and to minimize harm to people, the environment and products. Food plants with large fryers must guard against ignition of hot oil. Process areas with ceilings need sprinklers inside and outside of the ceiling, which is one reason ceilings are avoided unless necessary. The upper surface of flat ceilings is rarely inspected and can become covered in dirt and dust, offering harborage for insects and potential contamination from dropping dirt. If a ceiling is necessary, for temperature control or protection against leaks, then access for inspection and cleaning should be provided.

In summary, design for GMP should create spaces that are easy to maintain for cleanliness, prevent contamination of food and be safe for workers.

Personnel practices

Good manufacturing practices also include personnel practices that are intended to prevent inadvertent contamination of food. Companies often modify the minimum requirements with their own concerns. Workers in food plants cannot have communicable diseases or infections if they come in direct contact with food. Some companies also require passing of tests for illegal drugs, on the grounds that impaired performance poses a hazard. Workers with bandages or open sores are not permitted near exposed food. Provisions may be made to reassign workers with chronic conditions so they perform tasks, such as driving fork trucks, that do not endanger food but allow workers to retain a job. Workers, and often visitors, wear uniforms or smocks in place of or over street clothes. Normally, a company provides uniforms and arranges for them to be cleaned regularly. Most plants require hairnets, to prevent hair from falling into food. Beards should also be covered. Some plants require hard hats and sometimes safety shoes. In very wet plants, rubber boots may be issued.

Uniforms and smocks usually close with snaps rather than buttons, which can come off. Jewelry and items in shirt pockets are removed, again to prevent loss into food. Uniforms and smocks usually do not even have pockets except below the waist. Uniforms can be color-coded to identify areas where workers are intended to be. This can help prevent cross-contamination by identifying workers moving from raw material handling to where finished goods are exposed. Care must be taken with visitors and maintenance people, who may move among several areas of the plant. Sometimes there are enclosed visitor galleries to protect both the food and the visitors. This architectural feature may add to initial cost, but it pays off in reduced risk of injury and makes a good impression on visiting customers.

Good practice is to require workers and visitors to wash their hands before entering the plant. When this is required, foot operated sinks and soap dispensers must be provided at entrances. Some plants also use footbaths to sterilize footgear and tires of moving equipment. Common practice is to issue photo identification badges, which may also serve as electronic keys for entrance to closed areas. Employees usually escort visitors. Employees are trained to challenge undocumented strangers or employees who seem out of place. This is to enforce the precautions against cross-contamination but also as a first line of security. In addition to the hazard of accidental contamination of food, there is growing concern about deliberate sabotage. Disgruntled employees have often caused past incidents of deliberate contamination.

Food plant employees need to understand the processes going on in the plant and must be trained in safe behavior for their own sake and for that of their co-workers. Plants need an evacuation plan and must designate those responsible for shutting down and securing the facility when necessary. Visitors need to be briefed on how to behave in an emergency. Workers need to be trained in ergonomic work behavior, such as how to lift heavy objects without causing injury. Some food processing tasks are repetitive and have caused injury in the past. Examples are hand packing of cookies and cutting meat from larger pieces. Precautions against repetitive motion injuries are to limit the time spent on such tasks by providing frequent relief and cross-training so workers can do different tasks. Lifting devices are provided so workers do not have to lift more than 40 pounds (18 kg) vertically. Such devices include vacuum hoists and scissor lifts so that bags of ingredients can be moved horizontally. Tasks that were performed manually might be done by programmable robots, such as stacking cases on pallets.

Eating, drinking and smoking are not permitted in a food plant. There are designated areas for breaks and meals. Locker rooms and rest rooms are always provided and often there is a nurse's station. Materials not needed to perform a given task are not permitted in the plant. Tools must be appropriate and properly accounted for and only those people authorized to do so should touch or modify equipment.

Maintenance is a skill in its own right and needs to be scheduled and performed competently. Traditionally, maintenance has been reactive, responding to machine failures. This is repair, not maintenance. Since failures usually occur during operation, waiting for failure is costly, because it causes down time, lost production and wasted labor hours. Properly done, maintenance occurs before a failure, is done at a convenient time and does not impact production. Scheduling maintenance requires data on the needs of each type of equipment, strict discipline in adhering to the established schedule and cooperation and understanding from all parties. Scheduled maintenance also permits the timely ordering of replacement parts, as compared with emergency deliveries. Failures will still occur and so some flexibility is required to respond and to maintain production, but once well established, a preventive maintenance program experiences fewer emergencies. Maintenance technicians are better utilized, because most of their work is predetermined rather than in response to sudden calls.

The personnel practices used in food plants are intended to help prevent accidental or deliberate contamination of food while promoting safety of workers and visitors. Most conform to common sense, but may come as a surprise when encountered for the first time. After visiting or working in several food plants, the subtle differences among their practices become noticeable. While law or regulation does not dictate the details, one might wonder why every plant does not issue smocks to visitors or require workers to wash their hands before entering a plant.

Regulatory issues

The fact of regulation for food plants has been mentioned already and some of the implications discussed. Here we review the agencies and how they influence food plant design and operation. Food safety is a changing arena, as the public demands improvements because of widely publicized recalls and cases of food-borne illness. In particular, there have been calls for regulation by a single agency with the authority to order recalls of contaminated food. As of 2007, no agency has the authority to force a recall of food, though they do have some powerful leverage.

The Food and Drug Administration (FDA) is supposed to be responsible for the safety of all food made or consumed in the USA. Most countries have a similar agency or authority. In the USA, the Department of Agriculture (USDA) has responsibility for meat, poultry and eggs. The FDA exercises its responsibility by approving food additives, such as colors and flavors. These need persuasive scientific evidence that they are safe in the proposed use and quantities. Typically, feeding tests are conducted on a new compound using two species of animal (mice and dogs are common) and administering quantities sufficient to induce some effect. Feeding tests are conducted for at least the average normal lifetime and may include allowing reproduction in some tests to detect possible birth defects. If a level is found at which some effect occurs, then a level several orders of magnitude less may be permitted in food use. Toxicology is a complex science in part because there are so many possible effects of consuming a chemical. Further, the biochemistry of animals is different from that of humans. Well-meaning experts can differ on the seriousness of effects observed in feeding tests and thus on whether a proposed additive is safe or not. The FDA often relies on panels of experts to evaluate data and issue recommendations to administrators.

Many food additives achieve a status as 'generally recognized as safe' (GRAS) either by long use in the diet with no ill effects or by scientific consensus. The Institute of Food Technologists and other organizations publish lists of GRAS substances and their allowed uses. It is the responsibility of a food company in formulating foods to use GRAS substances or to obtain approval for any proposed ingredient. Failure to do so results in an adulterated food, which cannot be sold or must be recalled.

While the FDA cannot force a recall, except in the case of infant formula, because of the vulnerability of that class of consumer, it can strongly suggest that a company conduct a recall under threat of negative publicity. The USDA has a stronger lever in its threat to remove inspectors from a facility, making it illegal for the company to continue operations. One proposed change to food regulations in the USA is to grant authority to force a recall when necessary. This is generally opposed by industry organizations because of the perceived risk of abuse.

The USDA regulates its industry segments by providing continuous inspection services at meat and poultry slaughter plants and periodic inspection at meat, poultry and egg processing plants. Veterinarians who are specifically looking for evidence of disease in animals being slaughtered for food often perform meat inspection. Animals intended for food are supposed to be healthy and alive before they are killed. That is, they cannot be used if they die of other causes or if inspection reveals signs of disease. One criticism of the meat inspection approach is that it cannot detect microbial contamination by visual inspection. But, microbial contamination by such organisms as *Escherichia coli O157:H7* and *Listeria monocytogenes* is the most common cause of food-borne illness and of product recalls. Microbial contamination occurs by contact of meat with skin or fecal matter. Some approaches to prevention include greater care in skin removal, surface pasteurization with steam and surface washing with mild acids or other agents.

The USDA traditionally approved plant and equipment designs in advance of construction. The agency required special drawings showing equipment layout, material flow, location of people and location of hand washing stations. Equipment was approved for being easy to inspect, easy to assemble and disassemble with minimal use of tools and construction from non-corrodible materials. The FDA does not pre-approve designs or equipment, nor does it provide routine inspections.

Both agencies now promote the HACCP (hazard analysis and critical control points) approach and, in some cases, require it. Seafood and juice manufacturers are required to have HACCP plans on file and can be audited for them. The HACCP approach relies on anticipation and prevention as distinct from reaction and after the fact testing. There are seven principles of HACCP:

1. Hazard analysis. A flow chart is prepared describing the specific process and then potential biological, chemical and physical hazards are identified. Only hazards to human health are considered; quality and economic issues are addressed in other ways.
2. Identification of critical control points. A critical control point (CCP) is a step, point or procedure in a process where a hazard can be prevented, eliminated or reduced to an acceptable level. Some examples are cooking, metal detection and cooling. There are many control points in a process, but only a few are critical in the sense that they occur near the end of a company's control of the product.
3. Establishment of critical limits. A critical limit is the maximum or minimum value to which a parameter must be controlled at a CCP. Typical parameters are time, temperature, dimensions, pH, moisture and salt content. Ranges must be established that recognize the natural variability of the process and satisfy regulations and scientific evidence.
4. Establishment of monitoring procedures. Monitoring is a series of observations or measurements designed to assess whether a process is under control and to produce an accurate record of performance. Monitoring can be continuous or non-continuous. Because there is a cost associated with measuring and recording observations, it is important to limit

the number of CCP to those that are truly critical. A common error is to have too many CCP and then become overwhelmed with data.

5. Establishment of corrective actions. A HACCP plan includes the specific actions that must be taken if there is deviation from the target range of a CCP. These are written in advance and must be followed and documented.
6. Establishment of verification procedures. The HACCP must be validated, meaning it is carefully analyzed to ensure that limits on CCP are adequate, that the correct CCP are identified and that monitoring and record keeping procedures work. Verification involves observing the HACCP plan in action, ongoing calibration of instruments and reviewing records for completeness and accuracy. The HACCP plan should be reassessed at least annually and whenever there is a significant process or ingredient change and the plan changed as necessary. Finally, the appropriate regulatory agency must be satisfied that the plan works as intended.
7. Establishment of effective record keeping. The HACCP plan must be written and records kept of all observations and corrective actions. Typically, some of these records are chart recordings of temperatures, observations of ingredients at receiving and final product observations. Regulatory agencies look first at the documentation when inspecting a plant or investigating an incident. Another reason for taking special care in preparing a HACCP plan and in choosing CCP is to make record keeping as simple as possible so that the plan will be followed and so that it can be audited and reviewed efficiently.

Another federal agency that can be involved in food processing is the Occupational Safety and Health Administration (OSHA), which is concerned about worker safety and health. Food processing can be surprisingly hazardous for workers, primarily because of repetitive motion injuries, muscle strains and slips and falls. As previously mentioned, ergonomic lifting assists should now be routine to help prevent injuries from lifting heavy bags. This also addressees the issue of giving women equal access to jobs requiring physical strength. Wet and oily floors can pose slipping hazards, which are reduced by good drainage and cleaning spills. Some floor finishes have sand or fine stone embedded to improve traction.

All too common hazards in food plants are the many conveyors used to move materials around. Schultz (2000) has written one of the few texts addressing conveyor safety. He emphasizes that owners and managers are ultimately responsible for safety in designing and operating a plant, beginning with the layout and selection of equipment. Because conveyors have moving parts and easily reached pinch points, they are the occasion of many accidents. Screw conveyors are especially dangerous and are found in many meat processors, because they are effective at moving ground meat without smearing the fat pieces. Conveyors need interlocks that prevent them from starting if protective covers or hatches are open and should have covers over drive belts. Conveyors should be high enough off the ground that people can walk under easily or so close to the ground that stiles or small bridges can be provided for crossing.

OSHA can perform unannounced inspections but rarely do unless there has been an accident or complaint. The agency can punish violators with substantial fines, and some food companies have had that experience, for repetitive motion injuries and for inadequate emergency exits, among other violations.

Finally, in many states there is a public health department, which may regulate some food plants. For example, many milk and dairy plants are regulated by states using the standardized Pasteurized Milk Order (PMO). This shifts the burden from the FDA.

Discussion questions or assignments

1. Select a food product other than those used as examples in this book. Prepare three versions of a flow diagram, starting with a block flow diagram, then a schematic process flow (using proper symbols, see Appendix III), then one with key process parameters such as flow rates, temperatures and pressures.
2. Using the data presented earlier for time and temperature combinations of milk pasteurization, derive the decimal reduction time, D, at reference temperature 180°F (82°C), assuming the standard was a 5 log reduction in initial load. Using the same data, derive the value of z, the temperature change required to change D by a factor of 10. Repeat assuming the target is a 10 log reduction.

3. It has been suggested that microbial death rates from heating can be modeled as a first-order reaction. How would this change the way the data in the previous exercise are analyzed? Hint: D values are the reciprocal of rate constants and rate constants vary with the reciprocal of absolute temperature. Compare the two approaches. Discuss possible reasons for deviations from either model.
4. The simple process of size reduction and size separation can quickly become quite complex. Draw three different flow sheets using a simple binary separation and recycle of overs to produce a medium sized product from a large sized feed. Assign a simple performance characteristic to each step, letting F_{ij} be the fraction of size range i, where $i = 1$ is large, $i = 2$ is medium and $i = 3$ is fines, from each stage j. (Note: only two values can be set independently because the fractions must add to 1.0.) Write the equations for yield of medium product. Before assigning values, can you distinguish among the processes? Assign some values and evaluate.
5. Using the ingredient and nutritional label from any ready to eat (RTE) breakfast cereal, estimate the recipe. What is the approximate cost of raw materials? (Consult the *Wall Street Journal* for commodity prices; if you cannot find prices of vitamins, minerals and flavors, try using $1/lb (0.45 kg) and $10/lb.) Estimate the cost of the package. Discuss your results.
6. Select a piece of food process equipment, such as a slicer, mixer, oven or pump. List the maintenance tasks that might be appropriate and give an estimate for the frequency. Hint: think of parts that might wear.
7. Research floor and wall finishes that might be used in a food plant. (See any of the trade magazines for ads by vendors.) List the options and discuss advantages and disadvantages.
8. Exchange a flow sheet with a classmate or colleague, or find one in the literature. Critique it with the following questions.
   a. Is it clear and easy to follow?
   b. Are all materials accounted for? In particular, where do the wastes go?
   c. Can you tell what equipment is intended or probably used?
   d. Are critical control points identified? If not, can you find them?
9. What agencies regulate food plants in your state?

7 Equipment selection

Food processes are composed of relatively standard equipment, such as tanks, pumps, pipe, valves and heat exchangers, some with special features, combined with proprietary equipment that is specifically designed for unique purposes. The study of process equipment and unit operations using such equipment is at the heart of chemical, food and mechanical engineering curricula. The objective of this chapter is to give general and useful guidance to the selection of process equipment relying on other texts for the details of each unit operation (McCabe and Smith, 1976; Geankoplis, 1993; Valentas et al., 1997; Singh and Heldman, 2001; Barbosa-Canovas, 2005, among many others).

Food processing equipment must conform to and support good manufacturing practices. This means that it should not contribute to adulteration and should help to prevent it. In turn, those requirements mean that food processing equipment must not offer places where dirt or microbes can hide, must not corrode, must be easy to clean and must be easy to inspect for cleanliness. In practice, these characteristics mean that many pieces of equipment are made from stainless steel, often have highly polished surfaces and are designed to be disassembled easily, preferably with simple tools. Some industries establish and maintain voluntary standards for equipment design. Examples are BISSC (baking) and 3A (dairy). The published listings of approved equipment are revised frequently and can be obtained from the respective associations. Some common design features include:

- Rounded joints, where surfaces intersect, for easier cleaning
- Ground and polished welds, to remove crevices

Practical Design, Construction and Operation of Food Facilities
ISBN: 978-0-12-374204-9

- Widely spaced threads with square profile, for easier cleaning than closely spaced, sharp threads
- O-ring gaskets at flanges
- Wing nuts to close flanges
- Valves that disassemble quickly and easily
- Clamped pipe fittings (more properly, tube fittings, as sanitary piping is usually made of stainless steel tube. Tube differs from pipe in that, for the same nominal diameter, the outside diameter of tubing is close to nominal while the inside diameter of pipe is close to nominal. Nominal diameter is that size by which the pipe or tube is identified, for example 1 inch or 25 mm. Tube usually has a thinner wall than does corresponding pipe)
- Avoidance of painted surfaces.

Often, the motors on powered food processing equipment are designed to resist damage from water, because it is expected that most such equipment will get washed deliberately or inadvertently. Equipment for use in dusty environments must have electrical equipment appropriate to that use, meaning the equipment is sealed against sparking and is properly grounded. Lubricants used on food equipment must be approved for food use, because there is always a risk that the lubricant may contact food.

Many plastics or polymers are acceptable for food contact and are used as scrapers on agitators, as conveyor belts and buckets, as gaskets and in other services. Because they may wear in certain services and get added accidentally to food, polymers in food equipment must be approved.

Beyond the design features, food process equipment must be sized correctly for its intended service. Conventional engineering wisdom is to oversize most equipment as a safety margin for errors in estimating and as an opportunity to discover increased capacity in the future. This is not always a good idea in food processing. For example, if the heat transfer surface provided in a continuous thermal processing unit (pasteurizer or aseptic processor) is too large, there may be more residence time than needed or intended, leading to overcooking and poor quality. It is better practice to size most food processing equipment as closely as possible – recognizing the limits of available data and models. If a wide range of possible rates is required – that is, a wide turn down ratio – then provisions to add or remove rate-limiting features should be provided. It is not good practice, normally, to design for a worst case, say highest flow rate and highest viscosity. When doing so, it is commonly assumed that if the most challenging case is covered then all other cases are as well. In food processing, this may not be true.

Another illustration of the challenge of properly designing food processes is pumping. Centrifugal pumps are commonly used in many process industries because they are inexpensive, durable and flexible. However, they can impart significant shear to fluids, especially if flow is restricted, because they simply keep turning while retaining fluid in the case. Many foods are shear sensitive and such treatment can affect texture and composition. For example, cream could be churned to separate butter if subjected to excessive shear. More common in food processing are positive displacement pumps, such as a rotary lobe design, which use lower speeds and less shear. They are also designed to be easy to open for cleaning.

These common design features for food process equipment can distinguish even relatively standard equipment from their counterparts used in other industries.

Relatively standard equipment

Tanks used in food processing may be single walled or double walled, that is jacketed for heating or cooling (Figure 7.1). They are almost always made of stainless steel, though carbon steel is acceptable for storage of oils and corn syrup and epoxy coated carbon steel tanks are used in bulk aseptic storage tanks. All tanks should be designed for complete draining, which means flat-bottomed tanks are sloped to a drain at the perimeter. Storage tanks usually have dished or cone-shaped bottoms with drains at the center. Storage tanks may be vertical or horizontal. Tanks to hold liquids have welded seams that are ground smooth. Wall thickness must be sufficient to withstand the hydrostatic pressure of a full tank plus any additional pressure that may be applied, as by purging headspace with inert gas to reduce oxidation. Headspace of storage tanks should be vented and the vent protected with a filter to prevent contamination. Because condensation of moisture can occur in the headspace of storage tanks, drops of water can fall into the surface of syrups, reducing local concentration and creating conditions in which mold could grow. To prevent this, ultraviolet lights may be installed over syrup

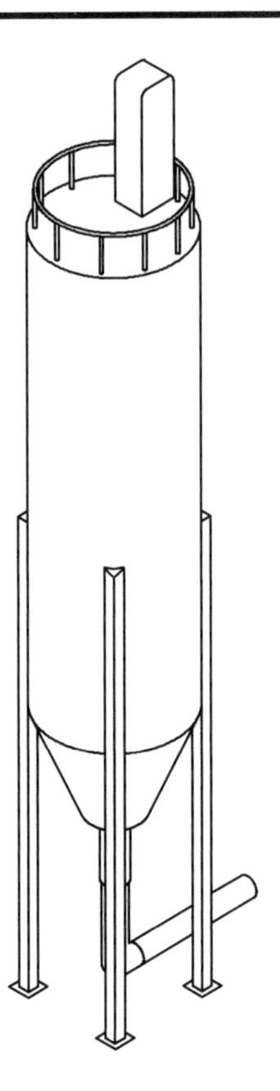

Figure 7.1 Storage tank

surfaces. Milk storage tanks often are equipped with air injection to agitate the contents and prevent separation. It is common practice to label tanks, and other equipment, with an identifying number and an indication of its function, such as 'corn syrup storage'.

Solids storage tanks may be made of bolted panels or welded. Solids flow from tanks or silos is more difficult to initiate and control than is the flow of liquids. There are special inserts for solids storage tanks that can reduce bridging and rat holing, common flow issues. Bridging means the creation of an arch of solids over an opening so that solids flow is interrupted. This occurs when solids are cohesive. Rat holing means the creation of a passage through a bed of solids so that most of the solids are stagnant along the walls. Newly added solids fall straight through the hole and, after a while, the accumulated material falls down into the center hole. This occurs when the bin or tank is not designed for mass flow of solids. The sudden collapse of built up solids from along a tank wall can create enough force to rupture the tank. Exits for solids should be as large as practical and often have vibrators or air injection to facilitate flow. Most solids storage tanks have conical bottoms, which should have as steep an angle as can fit in the allowable space.

Storage tanks are limited to about 11 feet (3.3 m) in diameter for shipping from a shop over land, but larger tanks can be assembled on site. It is usually better to have multiple, smaller tanks than one large storage tank, because it is common to clean tanks periodically. Cleaning is usually done by spraying all interior surfaces with nozzles or perforated balls permanently installed. The design and operation of a clean-in-place (CIP) system is a specialized skill. Normally, a tank fabricator will install cleaning nozzles and piping if requested (Seiberling, 1997).

If the temperature of the contents of a storage tank must be controlled, the tank may be jacketed or a single wall tank may be installed in a temperature controlled room. Some tanks have coils or panels inside for heating or cooling, but these can be difficult to clean and heat transfer may be poor.

Mixing and processing tanks are more complex than storage tanks (Figure 7.2). Usually they are jacketed and often they have one or more agitators. Because many foods are viscous but also must be treated gently, agitators may be scrapers that conform to the interior surface and rotate slowly. A separately driven high shear agitator might be also provided for dispersing powders or oils. Some mixing tanks may have lids and these are often divided and hinged, so they can be partially opened for inspection or addition of ingredients. Tanks used for cooking should have hoods to remove vapors that otherwise might condense on cold surfaces in the plant. Some smaller tanks are mounted on horizontal shafts so they can be tilted and contents poured out. Usually, contents are drained from the center of a rounded bottom. Multiple tanks of various sizes may be installed in a kitchen or preparation area of a food plant, with work platforms arranged for access to the tank tops.

Properly maintained, tanks should last a long time and often are a good value in the used equipment market, because there is little that can wear or fail on them. The drives and bearings of agitators are wear parts and need maintenance. Jackets that have been subjected to thermal shock, as by switching from steam heating to cooling quickly, may have leaks and failing welds. While the same

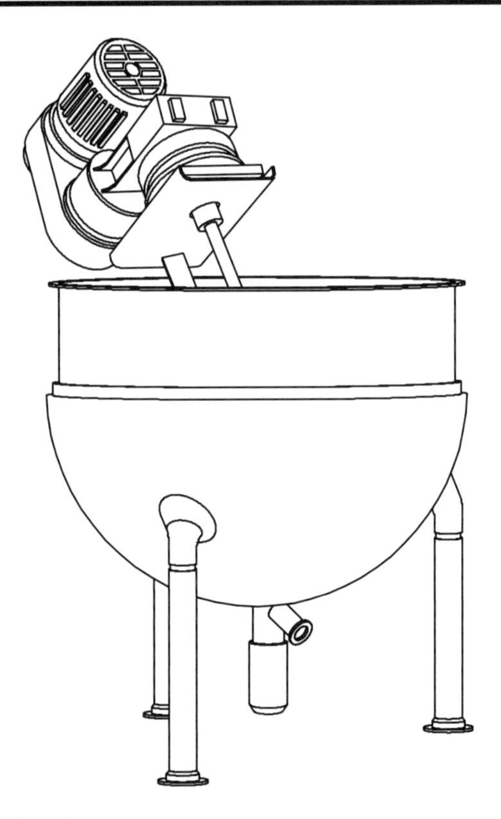

Figure 7.2 Mix tank

jacket can be used for heating and cooling, it is better practice to use separate tanks for each function if possible, and thus avoid the potential damage to the tank.

Pumps are used to transfer fluids from place to place and to recirculate the contents of tanks for mixing. Pumps are sized by the rate of fluid flow and the pressure or head that must be provided. The power that is required can be calculated from the change in potential energy that is delivered and the efficiency that is assumed. Manufacturers' data must be consulted to select a particular model once a type of pump is chosen. Pumps are either centrifugal or positive displacement. Centrifugal pumps create pressure by increasing the velocity of a fluid as it is rapidly rotated by a specially designed rotor inside a circular casing. Fluid enters at the center of the casing and exits at the perimeter. Centrifugal pumps can operate safely against a dead end or closed line, because the trapped liquid simply keeps spinning around. As mentioned previously,

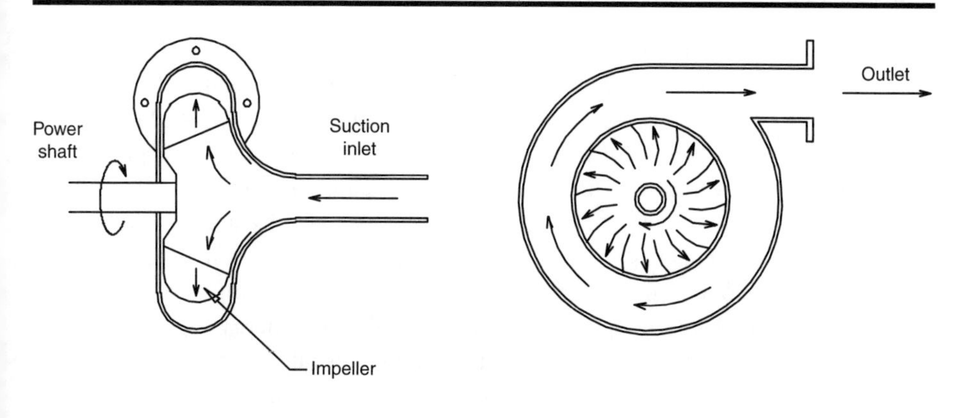

Figure 7.3 Centrifugal pump

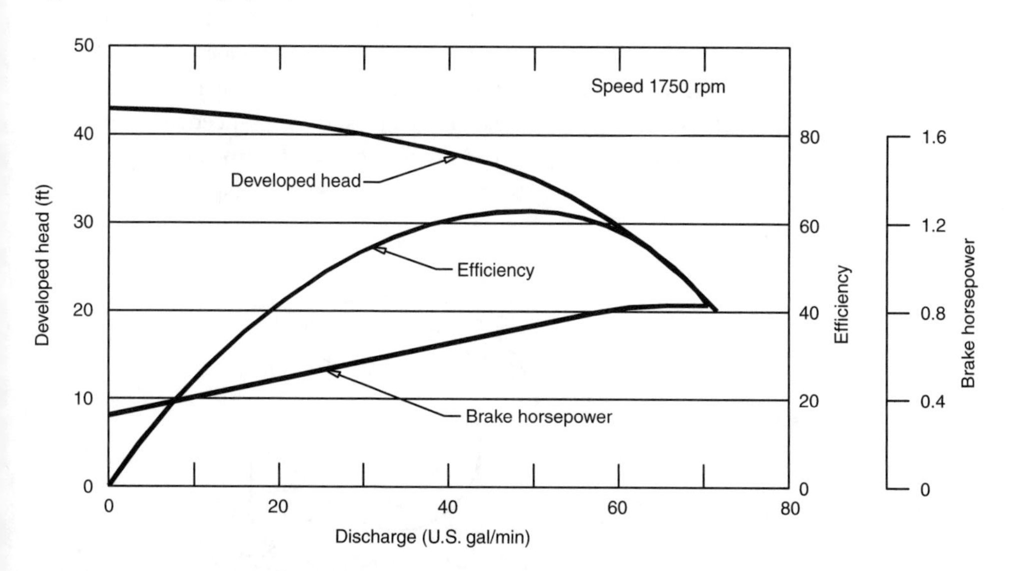

Figure 7.4 Centrifugal pump head curve

this may be harmful to some foods, because of the added shear and heat generated by friction. However, for many fluids, there is no harm, so such pumps are commonly used to move water, oil and syrups. Centrifugal pumps (Figure 7.3) can generate high fluid velocities, which are needed in CIP of piping systems. Centrifugal pumps are characterized by a head curve (Figures 7.3 and 7.4). The curve (Figure 7.4) shows that flow rate is inversely proportional to pressure or head; that is, as flow rate increases, the output pressure declines. However, as flow through a pipe or equipment increases, the back pressure or resistance to flow increases also. This creates the criteria for selecting a particular size and model of pump. The flow and pressure must match the required conditions. Over-sizing a centrifugal pump for most fluids is generally a good idea, within limits, so as to have a range of operating conditions available. Cost is one limit – a larger pump costs more. Operating cost is another – an excessively over-sized pump will waste energy.

Positive displacement (PD) pumps operate by pressurizing a finite volume of fluid by moving a piston or rotating a tightly fitting rotor in a casing. Usually piston pumps have several pistons – at least two and often more – to minimize the slight fluctuations in delivery rate caused by their cyclic operation. Rotary lobe pumps have two rotors that are machined to fit closely together and close to the perimeter of an oval casing. Fluid enters one end of the casing and exits the other (Figure 7.5). For a given model, output is proportional to speed of the pump and is not very sensitive to the resistance to flow. Positive displacement pumps cannot be safely operated against a dead end because they generate as much pressure as is needed. A pressure relief valve and bypass is usually provided to protect the pump and system against excessive pressure. Positive displacement pumps

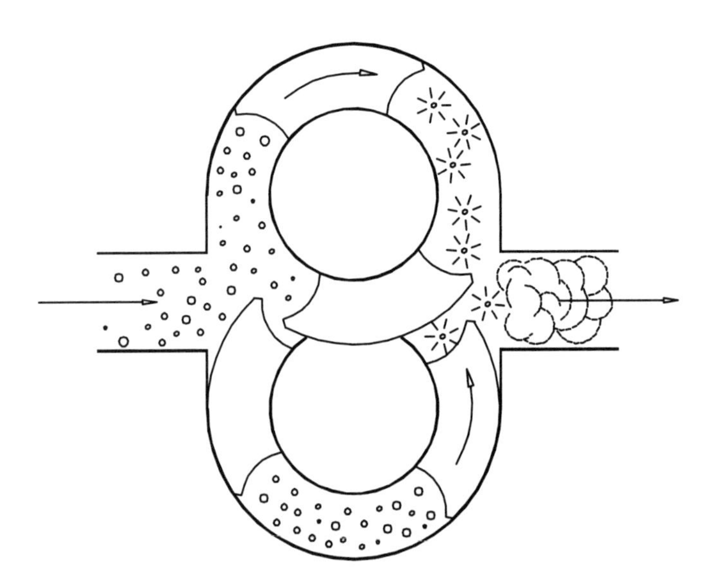

Figure 7.5 Rotary lobe positive displacement pump

do have an upper pressure limit, usually set by the capability of the seals on the rotating shaft from the motor. Efficiency in a PD pump declines slightly as output pressure increases because the higher pressure causes backflow past the rotor and casing or past the piston and cylinder. Backflow is sensitive to viscosity, with high-viscosity fluids showing less effect of pressure on efficiency.

In addition to piston and rotary lobe pumps, other types of positive displacement pumps include gear pumps and progressing cavity pumps. Gear pumps use intermeshing gears in a close tolerance casing to move viscous fluids very precisely. However, they are more difficult to disassemble and clean than other designs and are not common in food applications. Progressing cavity pumps have a spiral shaped rotor made of stainless steel within a matching polymer sleeve. Fluid enters at one end and exits at the other. Speed can be low and the relatively soft stator (the sleeve) allows the pump to handle particles and abrasive slurries, if material for the sleeve is properly chosen.

The operating range of PD pumps can be more limited than that of centrifugal pumps. In many cases, it is necessary to remove a PD pump from the system and insert a different unit for CIP. This can be done by valve arrangements. CIP of piping systems requires fluid velocities that may be several times higher than the velocity of process fluids. US practice is a minimum velocity during cleaning of 5 ft/s (1.5 m/s).

It is important to understand the fundamental characteristics of centrifugal and positive displacement pumps in order to select the appropriate type for a given application. Vendors provide the detailed performance characteristics to enable selection of the correct model, but the broader decision is which type to use in the first place. Each type has its useful place and often both are found in a food process. Pumps are often mounted together with their drive motors on a small platform on casters to permit moving them around and rapid replacement if a unit needs servicing.

Maintenance on pumps includes regular replacement of shaft seals, lubrication of bearings and checking rotors and casings for wear. In a rotary lobe PD pump, the clearance between the rotors and casing starts very small, but can increase slowly with use. As it does, the pump efficiency declines, so speed must increase to maintain flow rate and pressure. Good practice is to monitor performance, to note when required speed increases and to replace worn parts before the pump fails and shuts down the process.

Many companies try to standardize on one supplier of pumps and other types of equipment in order to simplify spare parts management. Maintaining the right amount of parts can be a challenge. Too few or the wrong ones and there are delays in repairing failed units. Too many parts tie up precious cash. Speed and quality of service from a vendor should be one of the selection criteria when choosing a supplier. Modern preventive maintenance anticipates the need for spare parts and orders them as needed, keeping only the minimum of critical parts for occasional emergencies. Proactive preventive maintenance not only uses maintenance resources more efficiently, but also improves manufacturing efficiency by avoiding unanticipated shutdowns.

Heat exchangers are used for heating and cooling foods and process fluids, such as cooling water and hot water. Some common types are:

- Shell and tube
- Double pipe
- Triple tube
- Plate
- Swept surface (also called wiped surface, scraped surface).

How to perform energy balances and to size heat exchangers are treated at length in many other texts and are treated briefly in Appendix I (McCabe and Smith, 1976; Geankoplis, 1993; Singh and Heldman, 2001, and many others). Briefly, the heat transfer rate depends upon the area, the temperature driving force and the heat transfer coefficient, which in turn, depends upon fluid properties, velocity and the geometry of the equipment. The important fluid properties are density, viscosity and thermal conductivity. The temperature driving force may be limited by constraints such as available heat source (pressure of steam, for example), burning or fouling, especially in foods, and phase changes, such as freezing or vaporization (except when those are intended). The usual design exercise is to estimate the required heat transfer area for a given duty. The duty is determined by the flow rate, the starting temperature and the target or end temperature. The heat transfer duty is the change in enthalpy of the stream between the two temperatures or conditions, if there is change in phase. The change in enthalpy is determined from thermodynamics, itself a topic of many other texts. For fluids not undergoing a phase change (boiling or freezing), the enthalpy change is determined by the temperature change and the heat capacity, a fluid property.

Types of heat exchangers are illustrated in Figures 7.6–7.10. Shell and tube heat exchangers are common in other industries and have many variations, including multiple passes, baffles and arrangements of tubes designed to maximize heat transfer surface.

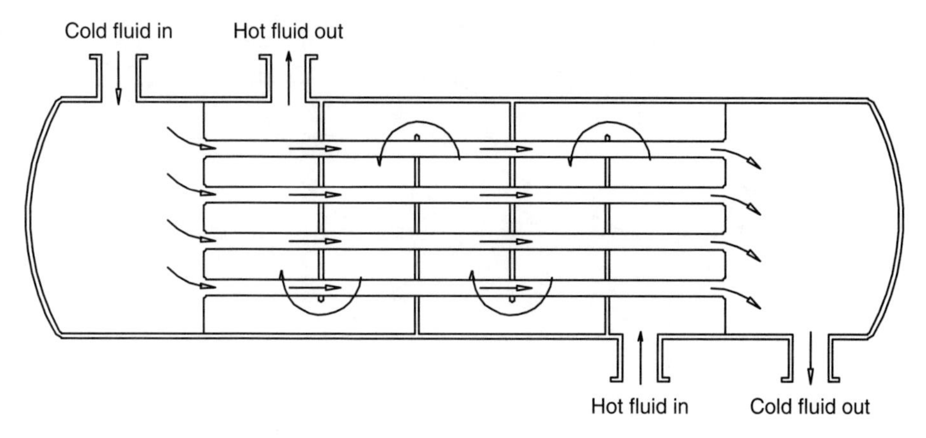

Figure 7.6 Shell and tube heat exchanger

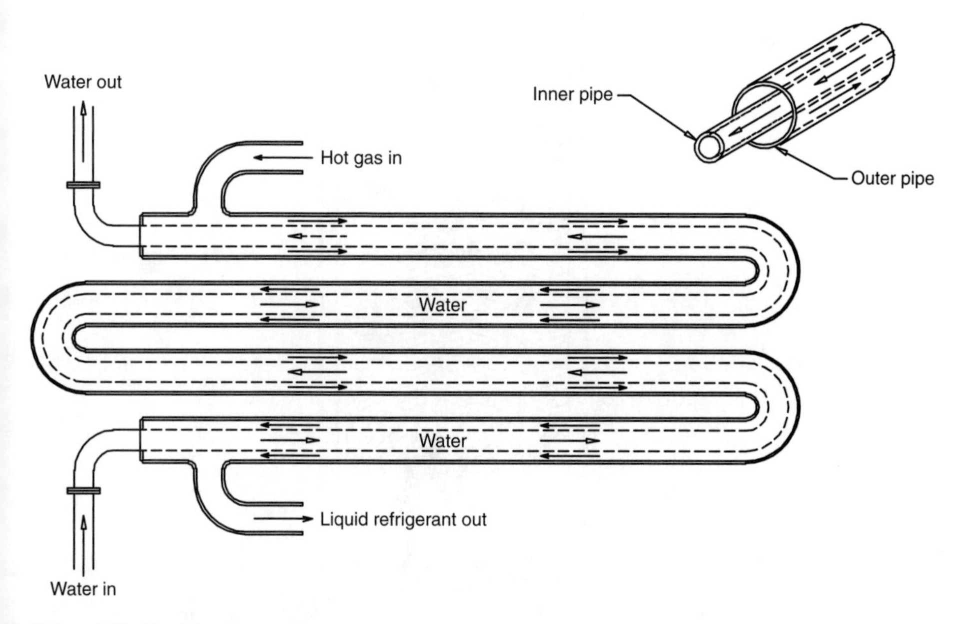

Figure 7.7 Double pipe condenser

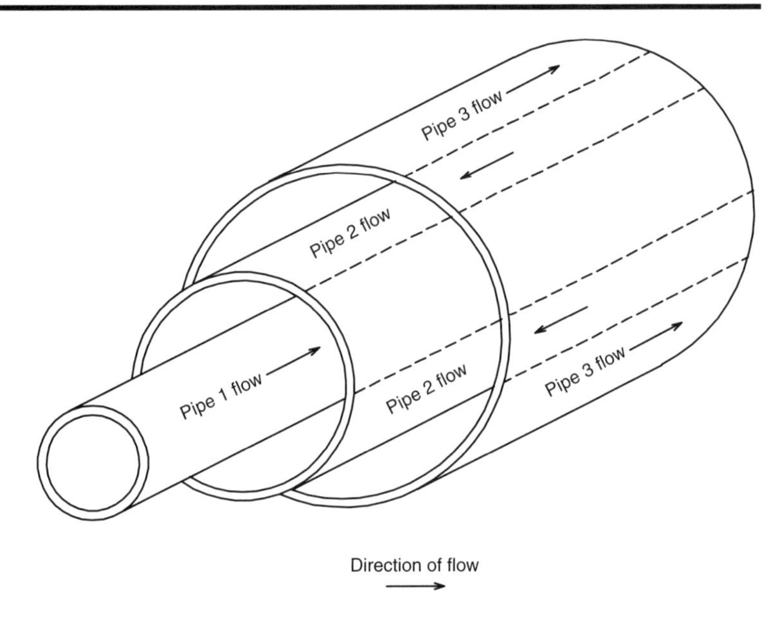

Figure 7.8 Triple tube heat exchanger

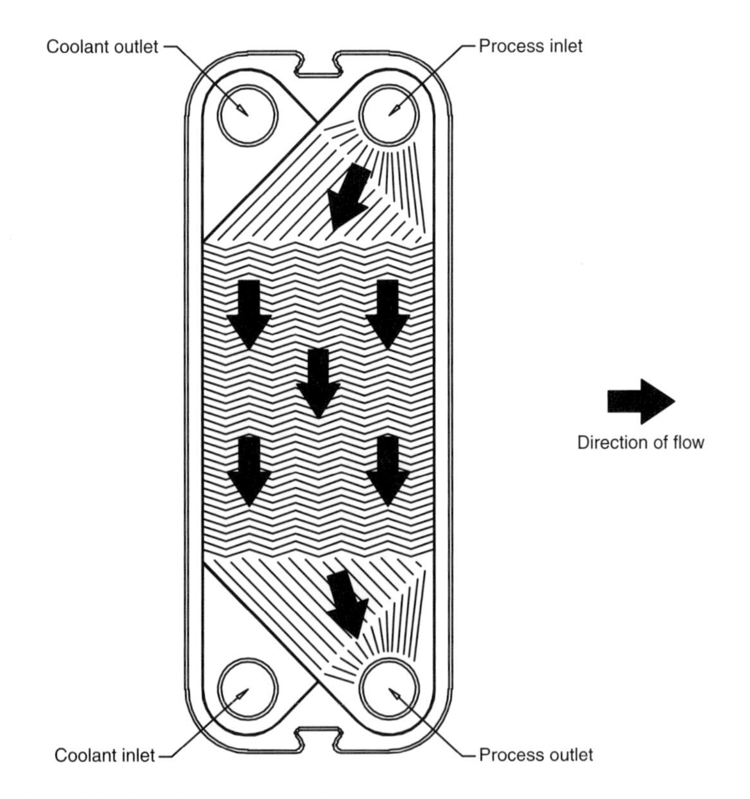

Figure 7.9 Plate for plate heat exchanger

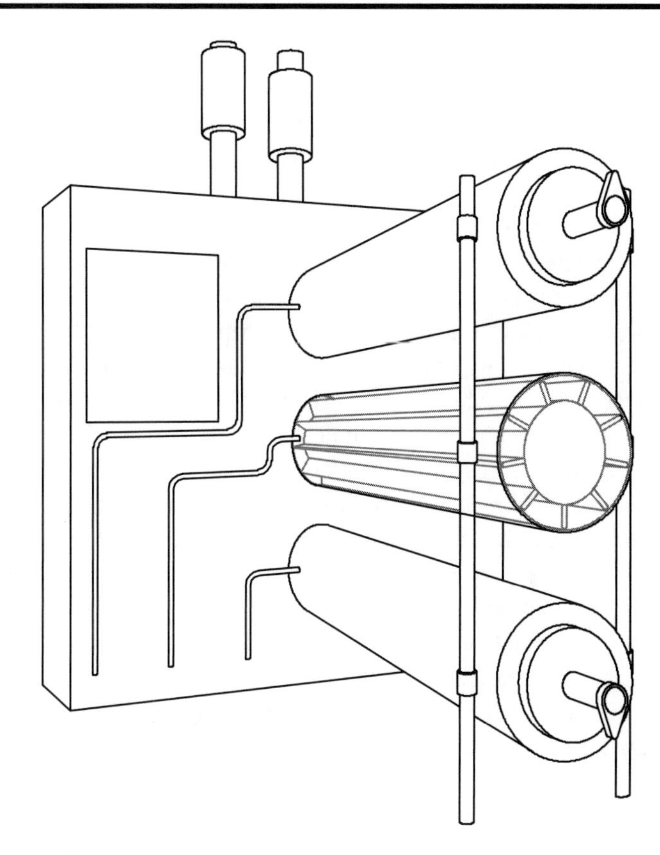

Figure 7.10 Swept surface heat exchanger used as ice cream freezer

They can be found in food plants where circulating water or oil are heated by steam, where circulating water or glycol solutions are cooled by refrigerants and where cleaning solutions are heated for cleaning in place (CIP). Rarely are they found where foods are heated or cooled, because they can be difficult to clean and inspect. Also, many foods are viscous and have suspended particles, making even distribution among tubes questionable and increasing the risk of plugging of tubes. This is a good example of a case where the constraints of Good Manufacturing Practices on equipment design almost eliminate an entire family of equipment.

The double pipe heat exchanger is one of the simplest designs – one pipe or tube inside another. Heating or cooling medium flows in the annular space between the two pipes and process fluid flows in the inner pipe. Normally, the pipes are straight and as many sections are connected with U-bends as are needed for the given service. The pipes can also be coiled, but this makes it more difficult to inspect after cleaning. Also, a helical double pipe heat exchanger is usually fixed in its dimensions, reducing flexibility to add or remove heat transfer surface, when that is desired. In food processing, the pipe or tubes transporting process fluids are usually one inch in diameter or larger, because this reduces the resistance to flow of viscous foods.

Recognizing that heat transfer to the center of a one-inch diameter (25 mm) (or larger) tube could be slow, a variation on the double pipe heat exchanger was developed – the triple tube heat exchanger. In this design, heating or cooling medium flows in the outer annulus and innermost pipe while the process fluid flows in the annular space between the inner pipe and the middle pipe. Sometimes the surfaces of the pipes are corrugated or otherwise deformed to improve heat transfer rates. There are many proprietary designs of heat transfer surfaces, which are said to improve efficiency, but at an increased cost. Double pipe and triple tube heat exchangers typically come in standard length modules which are connected together as needed and mounted on racks. One advantage of the modular construction is that heat exchange area can be added or removed as needed. In aseptic processing and pasteurization, where such exchangers are common, this capability can be important when flow rates may change dramatically. If excess heat transfer area is used for a reduced flow rate, the product may be overcooked.

Plate heat exchangers are common in food processing because they can provide a large heat transfer area in a rather compact space, the area can be easily expanded or reduced as needed, and they can be easily disassembled for inspection. Such heat exchangers are routinely used in pasteurizers, evaporators and many other services. The clearance between plates is relatively small and so pressure drop through such a unit can be high. Various patterns are embossed on the plates to maximize heat transfer rates. The gaskets sealing the edges of the plates must be of food grade polymer and must be heat resistant. The gaskets may need periodic replacement, especially if the plate heat exchanger is routinely opened for inspection or modification. Many plate heat exchangers are not opened often and so require relatively little maintenance.

Swept surface heat exchangers use a rotating shaft inside a double tube to improve heat transfer especially of viscous fluids. Ice cream freezers are often swept surface heat exchangers. The fluid flows in a helical path in the annulus between the shaft and the tube surface. The shaft has blades, which have a small clearance between the tip and the tube surface. Both the blade tip and the tube can wear with use and need periodic repair. It is common to resurface the tube every year. The shaft also has bearings and seals, which wear out and need to be replaced. Because of the wear parts and the need for regular maintenance, swept surface heat exchangers have a higher operating cost than other designs but, in some services, they are uniquely effective. Swept surface heat exchangers come in standard sizes and are routinely linked together to provide sufficient heat transfer surface. Heat transfer rates for heating are usually higher than for cooling, in part because temperature driving forces can be larger for heating and viscosity (which influences heat transfer coefficient) decreases as temperature increases. For these reasons, it is common to have twice as many coolers as heaters in an aseptic process using modular heat exchangers, such as swept surface exchangers.

Almost all heat exchangers used in food processing have stainless steel food contact surfaces. It is not strictly necessary for the parts contacted by water, steam or oil to be stainless steel, but it is common for them to be. The tips of swept surface agitators are often high density polyethylene, which is acceptable for food contact and reduces wear on the tube surface.

In selecting heat exchangers, the major consideration is that there be sufficient heat transfer area for the intended flow rate. If the same equipment is to be used for various flow rates and various fluids, then some provision for adapting to changed conditions must be provided. Modular units lend themselves to providing this flexibility. Pressure drop though the units connected in series at the highest flow rate and with the highest viscosity must be estimated and the feed pump chosen accordingly. If the pressure drop seems too high, such that it exceeds the pressure rating of fittings, for example, then it might be necessary to connect some heat exchanger modules in parallel rather than all in series. A parallel arrangement has many advantages, but care must be taken to ensure balanced flow to the parallel branches. Two or three branches are usually sufficient to manage pressure drop while providing adequate heat transfer surface.

The different types of heat exchangers may have different heat transfer coefficients for the same fluid and flow rate, which means that different heat transfer surface areas may be required, depending on the design. The various designs also have different unit costs. It is often true that the designs with the highest heat transfer coefficients also have the highest unit costs, so they may require somewhat less heat transfer surface than does a design with a lower unit cost. The net effect may be that there is not much difference in the initial cost of heat exchanger systems of various designs for the same flow rate and fluid. If that is true, then the selection might be based on other considerations, such as ease of modification for changes in flow rate or fluid, space occupied, cost of operation and cost of maintenance. As a general rule, heat exchangers with moving parts are more expensive to maintain than those without moving parts. Heat exchangers with straight modules are easier to inspect and modify than those wound in coils. Plate heat exchangers are compact, have no moving parts and are easy to modify, but may have high pressure drop for a given flow rate. Choosing among the available designs requires careful analysis and consideration of more than the heat transfer duty.

Mixers are pieces of equipment that help disperse solids in liquids, mix several solids together, disperse gases in liquids, form emulsions of oils and aqueous solutions, and improve heat transfer in jacketed vessels (Figure 7.11). For each service, there are units specially

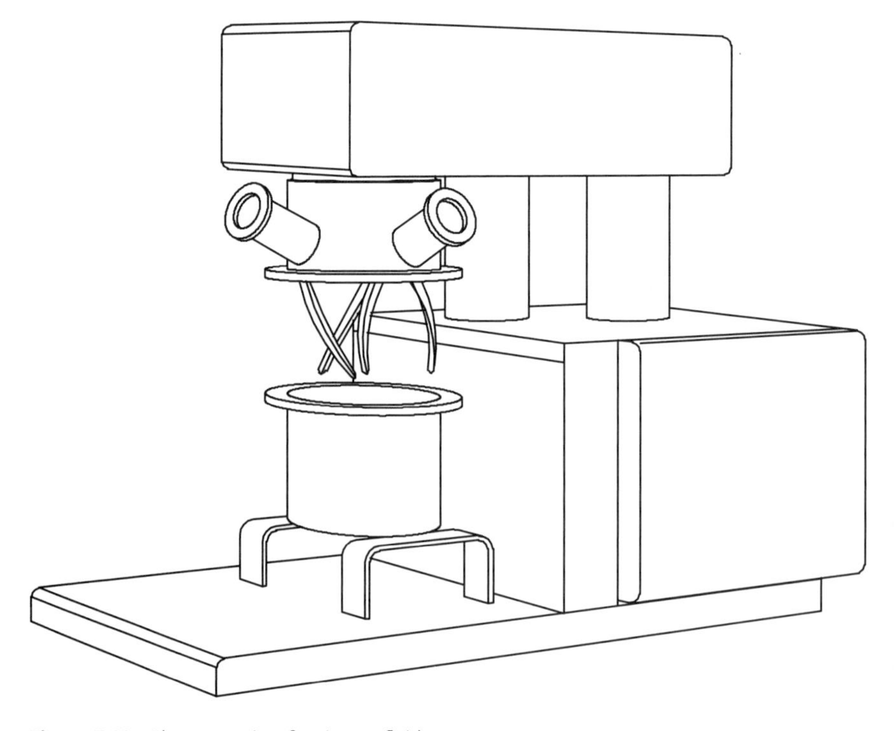

Figure 7.11 Planetary mixer for viscous fluids

designed. Mixer sizes are determined by the time it takes to achieve a given result, which often must be established experimentally. All mixers rely on creating movement in the bulk material, whether liquid or a bed of solids. Typically, this is accomplished by some means of agitation, such as a rotating propeller on a shaft in a tank of fluid. The propeller creates circulation in the fluid, which improves mass transfer from a solid that is being dissolved or suspends particles. Propellers used for simple mixing of fluids may look like airfoils or may be flat blades fixed on a disk. Different designs create different flow patterns and consume different amounts of energy in being driven. The density and viscosity of the fluid contribute to the challenge of fluid mixing, with high viscosity consuming more energy. Air entrainment may be desired or not, which may dictate whether a vortex (a whirlpool-like region in the fluid) should be allowed to form. Baffles in the vessel can break up a vortex and reduce air entrainment. Agitators that create high local shear but do not cause bulk circulation also minimize vortices.

Agitators for mixing may enter a tank from the top, the sides or the bottom (Figure 7.12). One issue is keeping the propeller submerged as liquid level changes. The propeller should be a distance from the tank bottom so as to allow room for liquid to circulate. A tall mixing tank may require a shaft so long that it whips or deflects when rotated. A thicker shaft reduces deflection but also makes the agitator heavier. Side or bottom entering shafts can be shorter but then require mechanical seals to prevent leaks. Such seals require maintenance because they wear and are sensitive to suspended solids. They may also be difficult to clean.

Close fitting rotors in stationary cages provide high local shear without bulk circulation and are used to homogenize emulsions and disperse solids such as starch and gums which are prone to 'fish eyes', clumps of solids that are wet on the outside but remain dry in the center because the wet shell prevents further dispersion. High local shear breaks up the lumps.

Solids are mixed with other solids and small quantities of liquids in horizontal vessels with rotating shafts that may have paddles or a helical ribbon to agitate the contents (Figure 7.13). Such mixers can only be filled a little above the shaft so that the contents have room to circulate. Other solids mixers are cone or V-shaped vessels that tumble about a horizontal axis. These also may only be filled to about 50% of total volume. Dough mixers have heavy-duty shafts that can deliver energy to a viscous paste or dough. Often such vessels tilt on their horizontal axis to empty the contents.

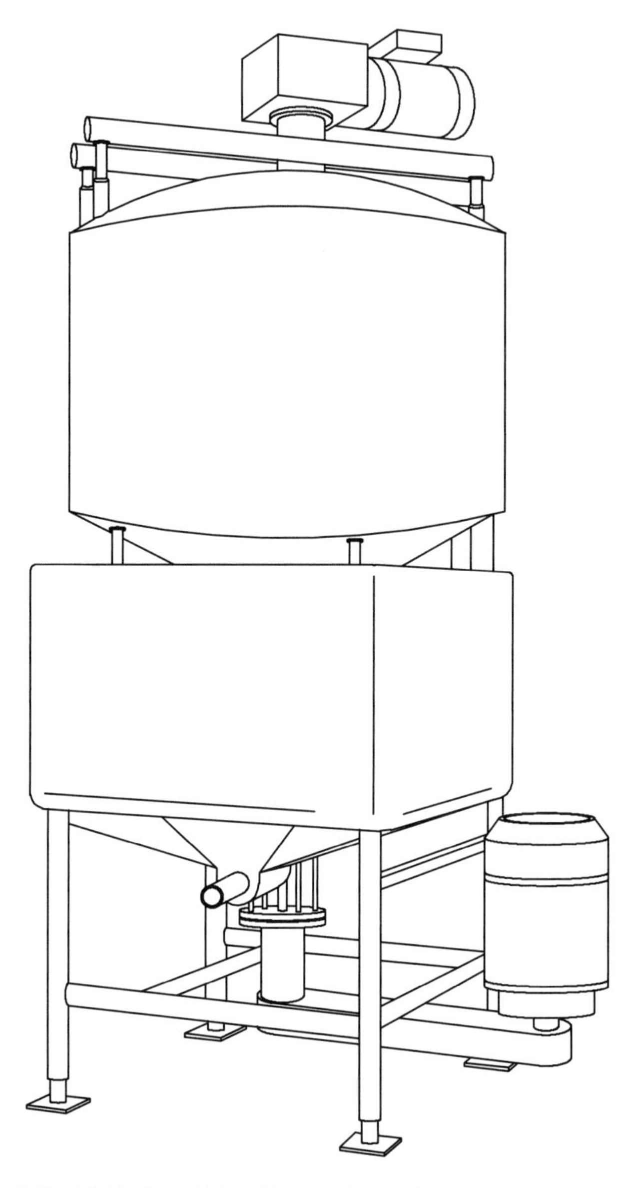

Figure 7.12 Multi mixer with batching vessel over mixer

Most mixing is done in batches, but continuous mixing is possible. Liquids are mixed with other liquids by metering separate streams together and then passing through a static mixer, which is a series of metal elements in a pipe or tube that repeatedly divide

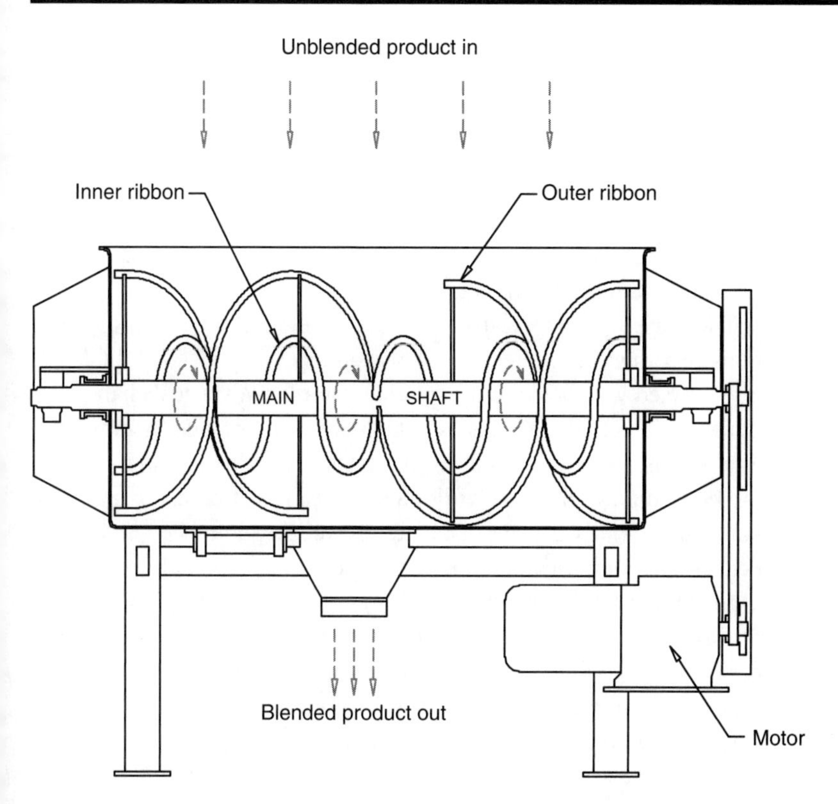

Figure 7.13 Ribbon mixer for solids

a flowing stream and recombine the portions until it is well mixed. Juices are reconstituted from concentrate with water in such systems. There are no moving parts and only slight resistance to flow, expressed as increase in back pressure. Properly designed, the elements can be cleaned in place. Solids may be mixed with solids by combining separate streams on a conveyor or in a pneumatic tube.

In continuous mixing, the real issue is reliable feeding of each component. Liquids may be fed volumetrically or by detecting mass flow and controlling a valve or the speed of a pump. Solids are more difficult to feed reliably because they are liable to have flow interruptions or to flood if they are aerated. Typically, solids are fed volumetrically through star or screw feeders or by using vibrating chutes. Because feeders are usually governed by controllers that detect a value, compare it to a set point and then make some correction, such as opening or closing a valve, changing the speed of a pump, or changing the speed of a feeder, they are almost always slightly in error. This means that a continuous mix is almost always deviating from its target composition. The deviation must be within acceptable limits for continuous mixing to deliver a correct result. The only way to determine whether this is so is to conduct tests at realistic volumes with the exact materials involved. Such testing can be expensive and difficult to conduct. Controllers may need to be finely tuned to obtain the desired accuracy, and so continuous mixing, especially of solids, tends to be applied in dedicated lines making one product or a small family of similar products.

There are many specialized mixers developed for specific conditions that then find other uses. For example, very viscous fluids are often mixed with heavy-duty spiral agitators on a vertical shaft using replaceable cylindrical vessels, which are then emptied by dumping. Tanks of liquids or solids are sometimes mixed by blowing air from the bottom or, in the case of liquids, by recirculating using an external pump. Solids can be dispersed by feeding into the center of a centrifugal pump recirculating the liquid around a vessel.

In selecting mixers, one must know the properties of the materials involved, must decide whether the mixer is for one purpose only or must be flexible, and should compare various potential choices on cost, maintenance and sanitary design. Mixing takes energy and some designs are more efficient at using energy than others, but the first concern is whether the mixer does the right job.

Proprietary equipment

Proprietary equipment describes units that, at least originally, had unique designs, as distinct from the previously discussed categories in which units from various manufacturers may be quite similar. When purchasing standard equipment, once performance parameters are established (volume, horsepower, area, or whatever is appropriate), a choice can be made largely on price and service. With proprietary equipment, as used here, comparison among suppliers may be more difficult because while an end result might be comparable, the means to achieve it may be very different. Size reduction is an example, where the target might be an average particle size or size distribution, but the means might be a hammer mill, a roller mill, an attrition mill, or a paddle finisher, all very different from each other. Each type has its appropriate applications and each type usually has multiple suppliers. Selection of a piece of equipment for a given purpose then becomes an exercise in selecting an approach and then a vendor. This section discusses a representative sample of categories of equipment in which there are widely differing types of choices.

Ovens are heat transfer devices used for many different purposes, including drying, baking, roasting and texturizing. Ovens are sized by the necessary residence time and the throughput capacity, which is a function of belt dimensions, product density and bed depth. Ovens may be batch chambers, often used for drying, freeze drying and baking, or continuous, using conveyor belts to transport product or containers, such as loaf pans. Ovens used in the food industry are usually heated by burning natural gas, but they may also use steam, hot water or oil, or electricity. Most ovens operate at atmospheric pressure, but batch chambers can use vacuum to reduce the temperature of drying and to improve the rate of water removal. It is difficult to move solids into and out of a vacuum, but it can be done, using double door locks, which cycle between atmospheric and vacuum conditions.

Continuous tunnel conveyor ovens or dryers often have multiple passes, meaning several belts arranged one above the other with product transferring at the end of each pass. This permits rearranging a bed of product to promote more uniform exposure to the heat source. Product must be robust enough to withstand the fall from one level to another. Ovens and dryers also often have multiple temperature zones regulated and controlled separately. This is somewhat more challenging to arrange with a multipass configuration. Products that cannot stand a transfer must be handled in a single pass. Cookies and crackers are baked in a single, closely packed layer on very long belts. Bread and other products baked in pans go through multipass ovens. Multipass ovens or dryers can occupy less floor space than a single pass oven with the same capacity (Figure 7.14).

Heat transfer in ovens is usually by convection, with heated air and combustion products being circulated at high velocity over and sometimes through the bed of product, or around pans, if those are used. Higher circulation rate improves the heat transfer rate to the surface of the product but, in many cases, the limiting rate may be internal heat transfer, which is not affected by air velocity. Impingement ovens use jets of hot air directed perpendicular to the surface being heated dramatically to improve heat transfer rates. Impingement ovens are used in small ovens to cook pizzas quickly in restaurants. Heat transfer can also be by infrared radiation from

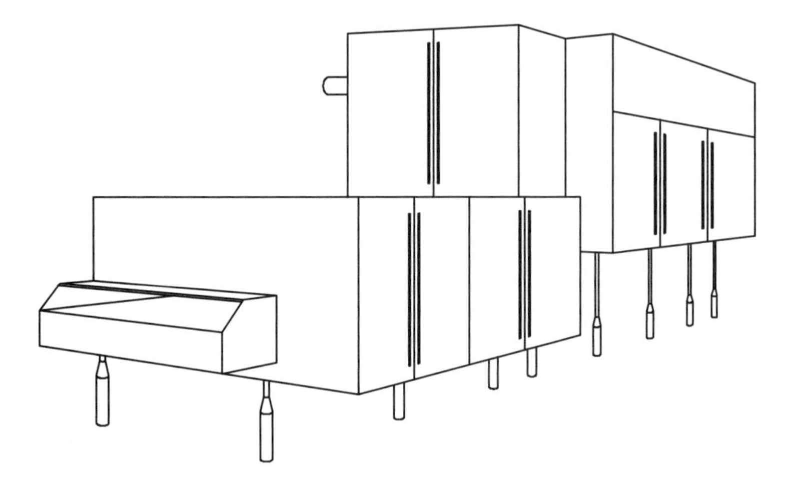

Figure 7.14 Multipass dryer

special burners or electric resistance heaters. In this case, only the surface of product that is exposed to the radiation receives energy, so product either is in a single layer or must be turned over periodically for uniform heating. Microwave energy can be applied on an industrial level either in a batch chamber or continuous tunnel. One application is thawing of frozen meat blocks. There is some conduction heating in a belt oven because the metal belt gets hot and delivers energy by contact, especially at the entrance of such an oven. Belts can be solid or porous, either perforated or woven. A porous belt can leave a distinct pattern on the surface in contact with the belt if the entering product is soft, such as cookie or cracker dough.

Most of the heated air in a convection oven or dryer is recirculated to save energy, but some must be discharged to remove the water lost from the product. The balance between recirculation and discharge is controlled by dampers and a stack that goes outside the plant. The temperature of discharge gas must be above the dew point or condensation temperature at the stack wall to prevent condensation on the stack, which could cause corrosion and could drip back into the oven or dryer. Keeping that constraint in mind, some heat can be recovered from the discharge gas for use in space heating or for heating hot water. The discharge from most ovens and dryers is safe to release to the atmosphere, but the gas from baking ovens contains a small amount of ethanol from the fermentation of bread. This is considered a volatile organic carbon (VOC) which can contribute to the formation of smog and so must be controlled. Some methods of control of VOC include incineration using natural gas (burning up the ethanol), catalytic oxidation (burning the ethanol over a solid catalyst, not using additional fuel) and cryogenic condensation (condensing the ethanol and water using a heat exchanger cooled by liquid nitrogen or carbon dioxide). The condensate from the last approach is discharged as liquid waste. The simplest and most reliable approach seems to be incineration using fuel, but there is a cost.

Ovens for food use are usually constructed of stainless steel for ease of cleaning but, in some applications, it is not necessary for the shell to be made of stainless steel. The challenge of cleaning is somewhat reduced when the product is in pans, but can be quite significant when the product is handled as a deep bed. It is common for product to fall off belts and collect in the bottom of a tunnel and between the levels of belts. Access doors are usually provided along the sides of a tunnel to permit cleaning and maintenance of burners and the drums over which the belt moves. In laying out a tunnel oven or dryer, it is important to allow room for the access doors to open. Belts expand when heated and so a conveyor oven or dryer needs a mechanism for maintaining tension on the belt and for keeping it tracking straight. Some systems also include a means of cleaning the belt on its return, with a rotating brush or even a brief wash.

Drying or baking rates can be determined in batch experiments and the results used to design a proper continuous unit. The temperature profile and bed depth must be established and maintained between the experiment and the commercial unit. Turn down ratio and flexibility can be an issue if the oven is to be used for multiple products. For instance, the bake time for different varieties of bread can be different, even for the same size loaf. Ovens that handle pans may need the ability to change pan size, which can be tedious because there typically are hundreds of pans in an industrial sized baking oven. Robots and specially designed pan handling systems have helped reduce the labor intensive task, but these add cost and demand additional space.

Some ovens and dryers include a cooling section, which usually uses ambient air to reduce product temperature before discharge. Since ambient air may change properties with the season, the performance of the cooling section may be variable unless some provision is made to control the cooling air. This is not common, but probably ought to be more so.

Temperature control in the heating sections has often been manual, with operators adjusting burners individually. Modern equipment has automatic control of temperature by section, but temperature distribution across a belt may not be uniform because of heat loss through the walls and poor distribution of fuel. Observation of the color of product can reveal temperature distribution issues if they exist. There are temperature recording instruments that can be sent through a tunnel oven to measure temperature profiles. When this has been done for commercial baking ovens, surprisingly wide variations have been found (Altomare, 1994).

In choosing a continuous oven or dryer for a food application, the flexibility, the ease and precision of control, the quality of fabrication and the ease of cleaning should be major considerations.

Homogenizers are specialized pieces of equipment designed to disperse finely droplets of oil in water or of water in oil, that is to make emulsions or to break up and disperse particles of solids in liquids (Figure 7.15). There are several types, including high-pressure pumps that force a feed stream through a restrictive orifice and high shear shaft mixers that can be immersed in a tank.

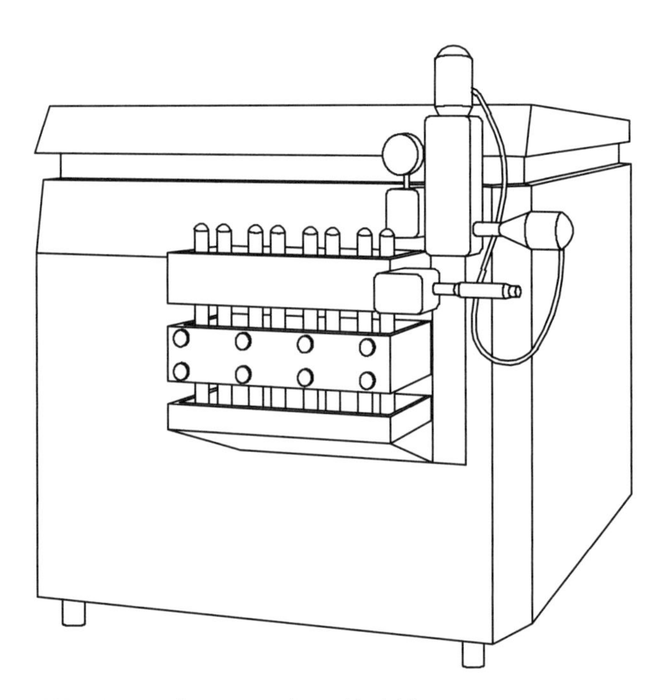

Figure 7.15 Homogenizer commonly used in dairies

The pump types can be sized by knowing the required flow rate. Often these are used in a pasteurizer both to maintain proper pressure when regeneration occurs and to protect milk, cream and ice cream mixes from separating into cream and skim milk. In milk pasteurization, homogenization is made easier when the milk is hot because of the lower viscosity at elevated temperatures. A homogenizing pump can also be used to feed a spray dryer.

A colloid mill has two plates that rotate with a very small clearance between them through which passes an oil and water mix, such as a salad dressing formula, creating a smooth and uniform emulsion. Smooth peanut butter, face creams and other mixtures of oil and aqueous solutions are often processed with a colloid mill. High shear shaft mixers used as homogenizers are generally sized empirically on the basis of delivered power per unit volume (Figure 7.16).

Presses are one form of batch filter and special types are used to express liquids from solids, such as juices and oils from fruits and oil seeds. They usually consist of a sturdy structure on which can be mounted alternating plates that are either solid or hollow

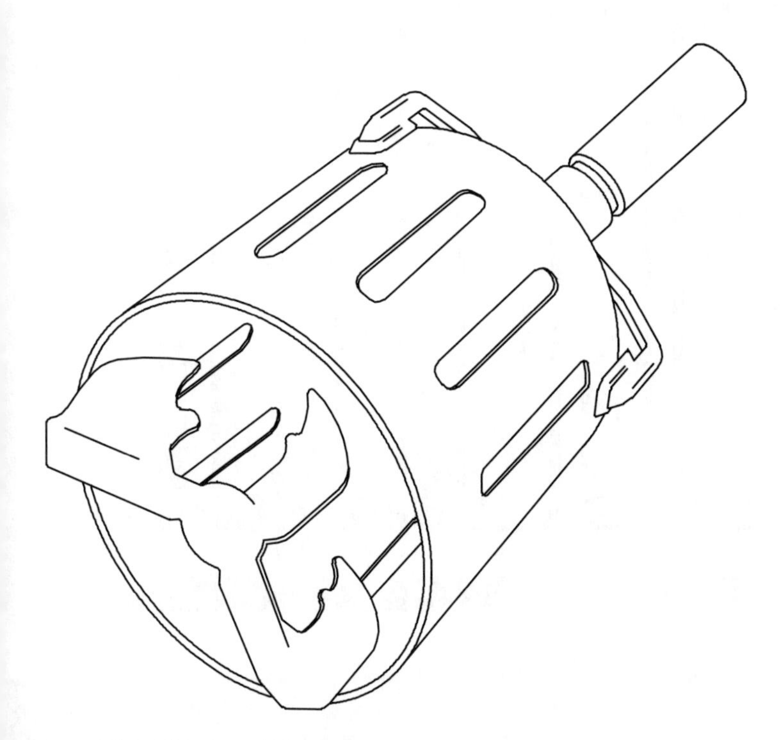

Figure 7.16 High shear shaft mixer

frames. For a filter, a heavy cloth is draped over the hollow frames and a slurry is pumped into the frames. Clear liquid passes through the cloth and is removed through channels in the solid plate or may just drip into a trough or drain under the structure. The assembly is pressed together by a screw or hydraulic device. Solids collected in the hollow frames are called press cake and may be washed by passing water or another liquid through the same path as the slurry used. Sometimes solids are partially dried by blowing air through the cake as well. These plate and frame filter presses can be labor intensive to operate because the assembly and disassembly is usually manual and the filter cloths are usually washed in an industrial washing machine after each use (Figure 7.17). Cocoa solids are

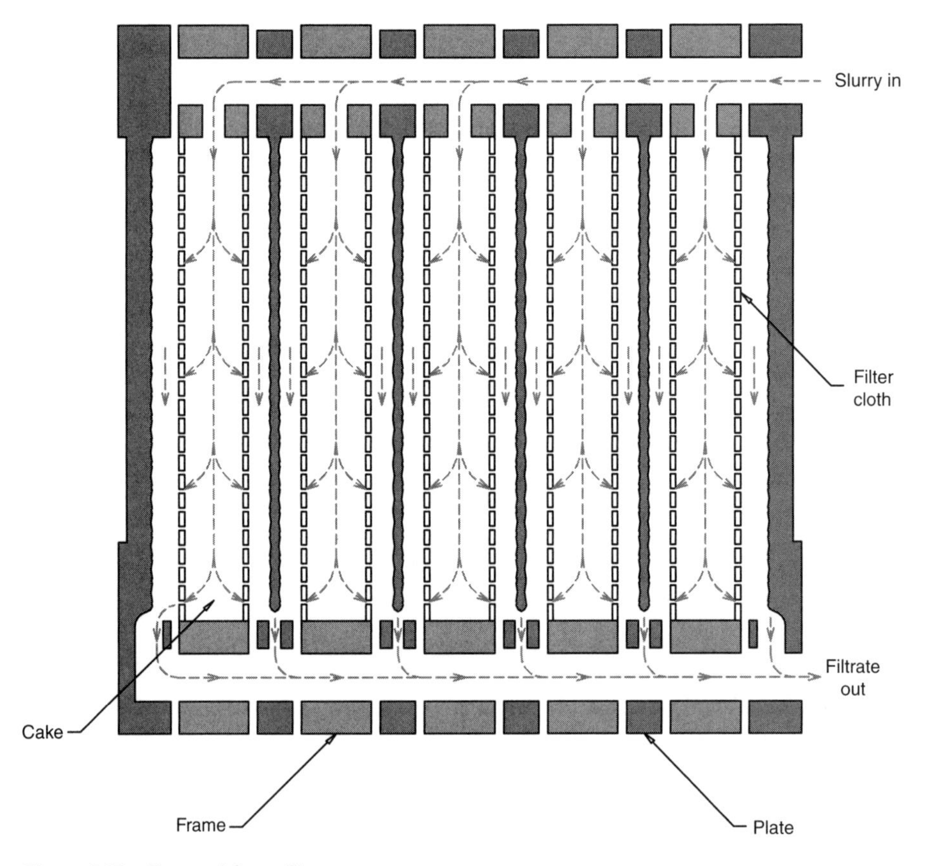

Figure 7.17 Plate and frame filter

recovered from cocoa liquor with cocoa butter the clear liquid in such machines.

Fruit and vegetable juices are pressed from ground raw material in similar arrangements, where the hollow frames are usually stacked vertically (instead of horizontally) and the fruit or vegetable pulp is wrapped in cloths and a number of frames are placed one on top of the other. The pile is pressed hydraulically and the juice runs out the sides and is collected in a trough. Because fruit and vegetable pulp can blind the cloth, sometimes a filter aid is used to create a porous press cake. Rice hulls and cellulose fiber are often added for such use. If the juice is subsequently concentrated, the pulp may be washed with water to recover additional soluble solids and sometimes hydrolytic enzymes are used to release more juice. Juice that is not concentrated cannot use pulp or press cake washing because of the dilution with wash water.

Other presses use air inflated rubber bladders to press fruit pulp against a fine mesh screen or cloth. A different fruit juice press uses cloth tubes that look like fire hoses and air pressure to force clear juice through the tube while retaining solids on the outside. Presses and filters can be sized from small-scale tests using the same raw material and filter medium. They are modular, so larger capacity is achieved by adding more area. Usually, filtration rate increases with pressure, but at too high a pressure, the cake can compress and become more resistant to the flow of the filtrate, so there is usually an optimum pressure. Cycle time for a batch operation needs to include the time for assembly, disassembly and cleaning, which may be greater than the time actually spent pressing. Filtration rate declines with time as the cake builds up and so filtering stops when the rates become negligible, which is determined by observation and experience.

Forming equipment includes size reduction equipment, molds, rolls, sheeters, mills, cutters, dicers and slicers (Figure 7.18). Some require a feed that is relatively soft, such as dough, while others rely on the hardness or brittleness of the material to help make small pieces from larger ones. The objective for some foods is to create uniform pieces or shapes, while for others a more random appearance is desired. Sizing this category of equipment is almost always empirical because the rate depends on the exact size of piece formed, the physical properties of the material and the power supplied by the equipment. Often there are wear parts, such as knives, whose replacement contributes to the annual operating cost. It is wise to

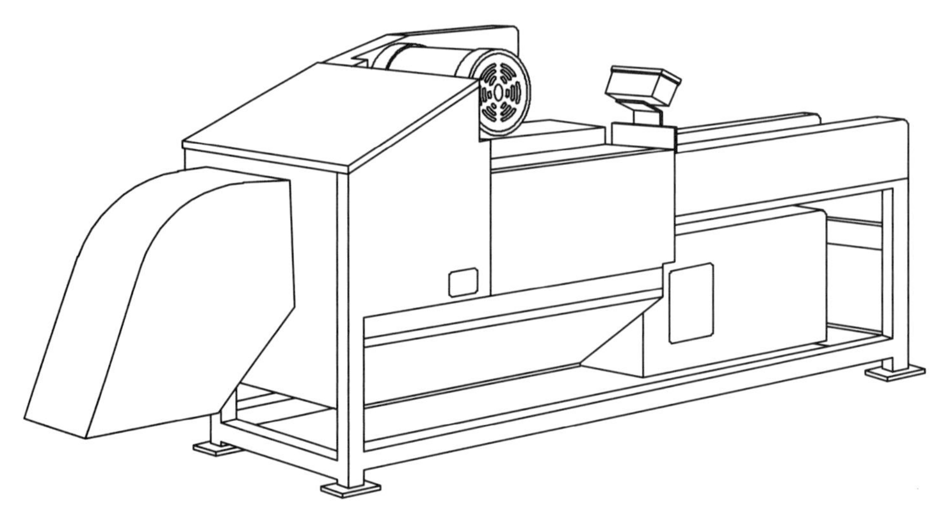

Figure 7.18 Dicer

protect this type of equipment with magnets and screens to prevent metal or stone contaminants from damaging it. Because of the sharp and moving parts, size reduction and forming equipment can be dangerous and must be properly guarded. It should never be operated without protective shields in place, which is usually assured by interlocks.

Mills operating on hard materials can create dust, which can be an explosion hazard as well as a contamination risk. Sometimes mills must be in blast-hardened enclosures with blowout panels, which release the force of an explosion to the outside, preventing damage to the rest of the plant. Size reduction often creates a size distribution, which may require sorting or separation to produce the desired particle size range. This can be done with screens, with over-sized pieces being recycled and undersized pieces discarded or used for another purpose (Figure 7.19). Equipment should be chosen that maximizes yield of the desired size, and this is usually discovered by experiment. Roller mills are known to give a tighter size distribution than some other types of mills.

A rotary molder presses a soft material, such as dough, into cavities shaped to produce a desired form (Figure 7.20). A small piston or a puff of air dislodges the pieces. Some cookies and crackers are formed with such machines.

Extruders are a special class of versatile equipment in which foods are mixed, cooked, transported, shaped and partially dried

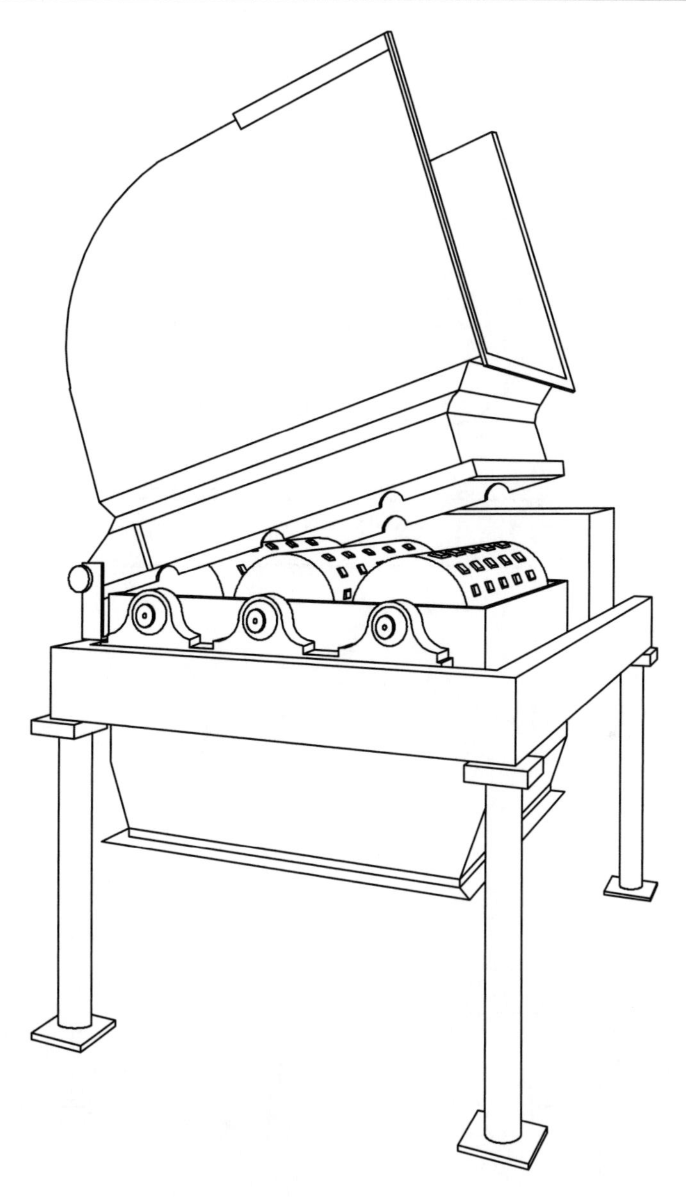

Figure 7.19 Pre-breaker

(Figure 7.21). They are commonly used in pet foods, snacks and ready to eat breakfast cereals. There are single screw and twin screw extruders and they can be heated and cooled by jackets or by electrical resistance heating. Extrusion processes are often characterized by specific mechanical energy (SME) (Valentas et al., 1991), the energy

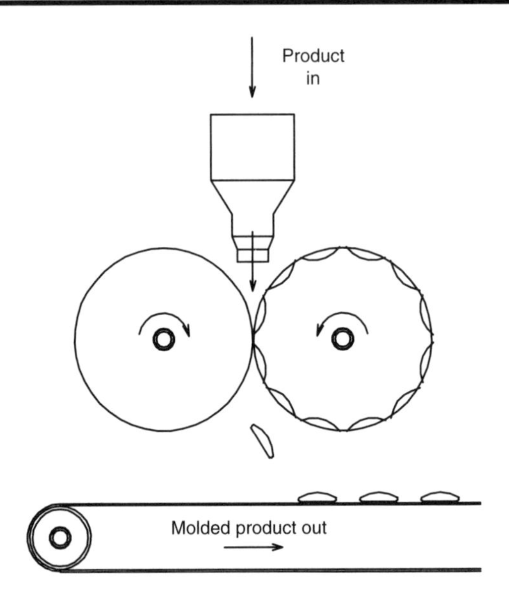

Figure 7.20 Double roll mold

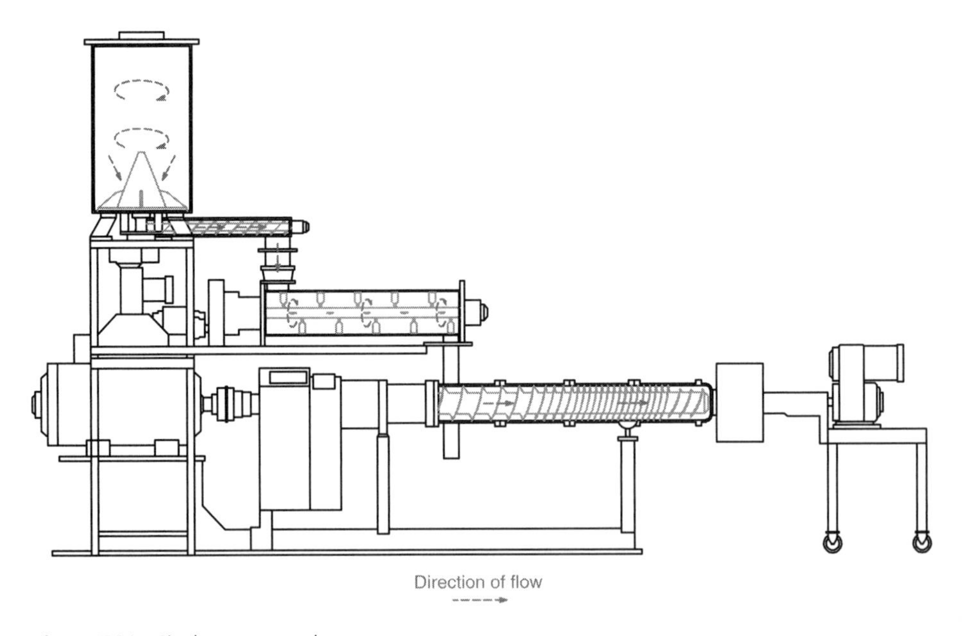

Figure 7.21 Single screw extruder

delivered per pound of product. For a viscous material, the delivered energy can be sufficient to heat the product significantly. Extruders operate by transporting a powder or dough with one or two rotating shafts in a barrel. The shaft or shafts are machined with a constant or varying screw pitch (distance between flights) and may have varying channel depths. A twin screw extruder usually has intermeshing screws, but there are designs with parallel screws in separate barrels. As the pitch and channel depth change, the material is compressed and pressure is increased. A die plate at the end of the screw restricts flow. Holes are machined in the die plate, which give shape to the exiting stream. As pressure is released, the exiting stream expands, in part due to release of strain and in part due to release of steam created by heating moisture in the material. This can cause considerable puffing, giving texture and reducing the density of the pieces. Individual pieces are created by cutting the exiting stream with rotating knives.

Variables include the rotational speed of the shafts; the length of the barrel; the configuration of the screws; the size, shape and number of holes in the die plate; the temperature of the barrel, which can be heated or cooled in sections; the composition of the feed, with moisture content being very important because it influences rheological properties; and the presence or absence of special features such as kneading sections on the screws and back pressure regulating valves. With so many parameters, predicting the behavior of an extruder from theory is difficult. It is common to develop a process on a small scale, using a vendor's or a university's facility. Experience teaches that such experiments should be done on relatively large machines to obtain reliable data.

Selecting and buying equipment

The first step in buying new or used process equipment is truly to understand what it must do. Usually this requires that a process line or the specific piece of equipment be designed, a classic engineering task. For someone who is not an engineer, this means that all the pieces of equipment in a line must be identified, including those pieces, such as conveyors, that connect various operations. Sometimes a line is similar to others in the company, but often the line is a new arrangement intended to make a product that is unfamiliar. This situation calls for creativity in assembling the unit operations, choosing from among alternative approaches and understanding how the performance of each step is characterized. There are many texts devoted to the details of various unit operations, but relatively little discussion about the practical aspects of actually buying equipment.

In the course of designing a line, a critical step is the preparation of material and energy balances. These are fairly simple but essential calculations that account accurately for all material and energy entering and leaving each step or unit operation. For example, an evaporator might have a feed rate of 10 000 pounds (4536 kg) per hour of fruit juice and a product rate of 2500 pounds (1134 kg) per hour. The difference between those two rates – 7500 pounds (3402 kg) per hour – is the water removal rate, which often characterizes an evaporator, along with the pressure at which it operates and the configuration of its heat transfer surface. Roughly 7913 mega Joules (7.5 million British thermal units (BTU)) per hour must be provided and removed in this example. In the case of evaporators, there are many possible choices, involving trade offs between capital and operating costs, which we will not deal with in detail here. Briefly, a multi-effect evaporator reduces operating cost by adding chambers in which the vapor from a previous vessel is used again to drive off more vapor. The initial cost of a multi-effect evaporator is higher than the cost of a single effect evaporator, but the operating costs are greatly reduced and, in practice, several effects are most often used. An alternate approach is the use of mechanical recompression to achieve much the same result – a significant reduction in operating cost by investing more capital. An engineer, either in the company, a consultant, or an equipment vendor, makes some detailed calculations and determines the desired heat transfer area, material of construction and mode of operation.

For other types of equipment, there are appropriate parameters. For instance, a pump is described by its mode of operation – centrifugal or positive displacement – the size of its drive motor and its performance curve, which shows flow rate against various pressures. It is an over simplification to think of a pump only in terms of its nominal capacity – 30 gallons per minute (GPM), for example. Heat exchangers are described by their heat transfer area and the details of their construction – plate, shell and tube, triple tube, swept surface – and dimensions, such as plate clearance. Tanks and vessels are described by their capacity, material of construction, dimensions and other features, such as jackets, agitators and number of nozzles for adding and removing streams.

Equipment with more specialized functions and designs are often described by their nominal capacity – so many pounds per hour – or, in the case of packaging equipment, so many packages per minute. Mass flow rates – pounds or kilograms per hour – should be converted to volumetric rates as well – cubic feet per minute, cubic meters per second or gallons per minute – because equipment sizes and capability are often more dependent on volume than on mass. This obviously requires knowledge of the bulk density of various streams. Many fluid streams found in food plants are mostly water and so can be approximated with the properties of water, but solids, such as powders and grains, are not only more variable in density but also their density can change in the process due to aeration, attrition (particle breakage) and moisture pick-up or loss.

The material of construction for much food equipment is stainless steel, but this is not dictated by law. Rather, the requirement of good manufacturing practices (GMP) is that food contact surfaces be non-corrodible, easy to clean and easy to inspect. Stainless steel satisfies the requirement, but so also do good quality epoxy coatings, approved polymers and even carbon steel in certain services, such as for holding oils and syrups.

Buying new equipment

Vendors of new food processing equipment can be categorized as multiline suppliers or as more specialized suppliers. Through consolidation, many formerly specialized suppliers have become parts of larger organizations offering a diverse catalog of equipment. International firms manufacture much food equipment and even US-based firms may fabricate many of their offerings overseas. This can be a factor in a purchasing decision, because international designs may be in metric dimensions and the supply of parts and service may be challenging with international sources. Most foreign firms have substantial representation in the USA because it is such a large market. A multiproduct firm may be able to provide most, if not all, of a line, which can be convenient, but not necessarily the most economical nor the highest quality approach. It is rare that every offering in a large catalog is the best in class.

In an effort to simplify maintenance, training and parts inventory, many companies establish lists of preferred vendors, especially for such common units as controls, pumps and valves. If one is responsible for purchasing a piece of equipment in one of these categories, the choices may be limited to those on the list. However, in other cases, it may be necessary to find qualified suppliers. The Internet is a great help, of course, as are directories such as *Food Master*, published annually by BNP Media, Bensenville, IL.

Having identified potential sources, how does one make a choice? The more completely described or specified a need is, the more likely it will be filled satisfactorily. That is, the more information that can be provided, the better job a supplier will likely do. There needs to be a balance, however, between defining specific needs and allowing some flexibility in response. Some types of equipment are custom fabricated exactly to order, while others are standardized, although the range of options can be very broad. It is important to know what parameters are critical and which are less so.

Cost, of course, is always important, but it should not be the only determining factor. Competition is healthy and is expected – almost every type of equipment can be obtained from more than one source. Specifications and requests for quotations can be sent to three or four possible suppliers with a deadline for reply. More bids are rarely necessary and only add to the effort of evaluation; sending fewer requests risks not having much choice, as some candidates may decline to reply. The quality of communication, timeliness and amount of detail provided in a bid should influence the evaluation of a bidder. If a buyer does not have direct experience with a supplier, he or she should seek references and directly inspect samples of the supplier's work. Total costs over the life of a piece of equipment, including purchase cost, shipping cost to site, cost of installation, sales tax, operating cost, maintenance costs, salvage costs and reliability should be estimated and compared.

Used equipment can be a good value

Used process equipment can range from 'new in box' – never used – to little better than scrap. Used equipment dealers obtain their stock by buying complete plants or individual items from food, chemical and pharmaceutical companies. If they can, they leave the equipment in place, to save the cost of moving it twice. They also maintain large yards where they store pieces they own.

Buying used equipment has its risks, but companies in this business rely heavily on repeat customers, so they make special efforts to ensure satisfaction. It is risky to buy a piece of used equipment sight unseen, but some dealers have a return policy, allowing customers to return and exchange equipment under certain circumstances. The buyer pays shipping costs.

Used equipment with moving parts, such as pumps, centrifuges, swept surface heat exchangers and agitators are most likely to require some rehabilitation. Equipment such as tanks, vessels and heat exchangers are likely to be in fairly good condition, even after years of use. Buying used equipment to construct a line or to fill a specific need may require some compromise of the detailed specifications that should have been prepared. It is important to understand how such compromises can be made. Normally, using a larger tank than called for is acceptable; using a smaller heat exchanger than is required may restrict operating rate.

Used equipment is sold 'as is, where is' unless a different arrangement is made, so the buyer is responsible for determining acceptability and suitability. Look beyond surface dirt and realize that good quality stainless steel equipment can be cleaned up and made serviceable fairly easily. Prices can be negotiable when multiple units are involved. Some used equipment dealers are prepared to renovate equipment and also newly fabricate certain types, such as mixers.

The big advantage of used equipment is the short lead time compared to that of new equipment, which can easily approach 9–12 months.

Other factors in evaluating equipment

In addition to being correctly sized for its intended function, process equipment must be reasonably priced, durable, safe to operate and maintain and economical to operate. The purchase cost of many types of equipment is often proportional to its weight, because metal is the main raw material used in fabrication. Prices fluctuate with the cost of stainless steel, as well as with relative demand. Since many types of food process equipment are imported to the USA, costs are also sensitive to the exchange rate of the US dollar. Costs of relatively standard types of equipment tend to be more competitive than those of proprietary types, because there are more potential suppliers. It is normal to solicit bids or proposals from at least three suppliers when purchasing equipment. To do so, precise specifications must be prepared.

Durability is related to quality of construction, which can be challenging to evaluate. One indication is the quality of surface finishes, especially at welds. Welds that are rough, discontinuous and irregular suggest deficient skills at a fundamental level. It is not essential that surfaces be highly polished, but they should be smooth and uniform in color, because visual inspection is one way to ensure that equipment is clean. The sturdiness of shafts, bearings, seals, motors and controls are indicators of quality. Generally, heavier duty choices in these areas are a good investment. Ease of access for maintenance is important and may require inspection by a trained mechanic to evaluate. As an example, it is convenient for seals to be installed external to vessels and pumps, if possible, so they can be inspected and maintained without requiring access to the inside of the vessel or the casing of the pump. Shaft seals in potentially abrasive service are often rinsed with a small stream of water to reduce wear. The thickness of walls in vessels must be sufficient to withstand internal pressure when filled and should resist dents and punctures. Using thicker walls than strictly necessary may increase cost, but it will also prolong the life of a tank or vessel.

Safe operation always includes guards over belts and chains, lids on screw conveyors, insulation on hot or cold surfaces and interlocks that prevent operation when a guard is out of place. Some equipment, such as slicers and mills, can be very dangerous intrinsically and are usually covered in intimidating warning signs in several languages. Equipment with parts that rotate at high speeds can lose pieces if not properly attached or due to failure of welds. Guards and enclosures usually prevent such pieces from going far. The rollers on belt conveyors are pinch points that can cause injury and are hard to guard completely. Good practice is to place conveyors overhead or close to the floor so it is more difficult accidentally to become entangled. Line layout can introduce safety hazards by creating obstacles for people, who are then tempted to step over or under conveyors. Stiles are short steps and bridges on which people can safely cross conveyors. Equipment that tempts workers to step on parts to reach an area for maintenance should be provided with access platforms or movable pulpit stairs as a safer alternative.

Electrical gear should be designed for the expected environment if it may be wet or dusty. Electrical boxes should be made of stainless steel even though they do not contact food, because the boxes are prone to corrosion in a typical food processing environment. Electrical wiring should be protected by conduit or cable trays and should be properly insulated to prevent sparking or short circuits. Pipe that is under pressure, such as those that carry compressed air, steam or hydraulic power supplies, should be designed for the service and protected with pressure relief valves. Pressure relief valves must discharge in a way that does not endanger people.

The cost to operate equipment is affected by its consumption of utilities, such as electricity, natural gas and steam and by the cost of maintenance. Electrical motors can differ in efficiency, with higher efficiency motors being a good investment. Ovens, dryers and heat exchangers are usually insulated to increase thermal efficiency and thicker insulation is probably a wise choice. Wear parts, such as knives, bearings and seals may be relatively standard commodities or they may be proprietary designs of the manufacturer. In the latter case, they will probably be more expensive than similar parts available from an industrial supply house. Sometimes such special parts are of high quality, and their use may be required under terms of a warranty. In other cases, the use of such parts is a ploy by the manufacturer to gain a steady income from parts replacement. Try to select equipment that uses easily found and inexpensive parts, if possible.

Finally, evaluate the service and support available from a supplier. Most international suppliers have a network of technicians all over the world and many have well-staffed offices in the USA, but others do not. Smaller and more specialized firms may have only a few employees who know their equipment well and getting their attention in an emergency may be difficult. If training is offered in operation and maintenance of a complex piece of equipment, take advantage and be sure more than one person attends. Relatively standard equipment is also relatively easy to operate and maintain and most plant maintenance people already know what they need to do. The greater challenge is with more complex and specialized units. Not only is the mechanism more complex, but also the control system is likely to be computer based and demand a high skill level. Many companies insist that even equipment supplied by European firms uses US electronics, to the chagrin of the suppliers, who believe their choices to be superior. However, the US customer prefers having one family of controllers and electronics in all his factories, for ease of training, data collection and upgrading when necessary. That is a matter of strategic choice, but should be a factor in an evaluation.

Discussion questions or assignments

1. Prepare a process flow diagram for a food not discussed elsewhere in this text.
2. List all of the equipment needed.
3. Identify two vendors for each piece of equipment listed.
4. Obtain a diagram of one relatively standard piece of equipment, as defined in this chapter. Identify the parts and places you would examine when evaluating it for purchase. Identify the potential safety hazards, if any.
5. Repeat the exercise of item 4 for a more complex or specialized unit, such as packaging equipment, an extruder or other choice.

8

Project management and execution

There are many books and texts on project management in many fields (Martin, 1976; Burstein and Stasiowiski, 1982 are two examples, among many others). There are few, if any, that specifically relate to the process of seeing a food facility to completion. Earlier chapters discussed design and selection of equipment. This chapter describes the construction phase and the next chapter addresses some aspects of operation. Leadership in both phases requires skills that are best acquired by experience, but these chapters, written with the perspective of such experience, should provide the foundation on which subsequent experience can build.

The typical phases of a project

Most projects, large or small, go through the following phases in one form or another. Some projects may expand or contract some phases, but it is not wise to skip any of them. Each will be discussed.

- Feasibility study
- Appropriation request
- Funds granted

Practical Design, Construction and Operation of Food Facilities
ISBN: 978-0-12-374204-9

- Design (itself in several phases)
- Construction
- Commissioning
- Production

Feasibility

Determining the feasibility of an idea is, in many ways, among the most difficult of tasks, because so much information is needed and so little is available. There are also almost always time pressures such that analysis and estimates must be made quickly and, usually, with too few resources. These conditions are just reality. While, in theory, changes can later occur in scope, schedule and budget, in fact, most of these parameters are set during the feasibility study and are actually difficult to change later. That fact makes this phase especially important. The cost to perform a feasibility study is usually relatively small – perhaps 1–5% of the ultimate cost of the project – but it is money well spent, if spent wisely.

The feasibility study itself has two significant parts – first, determining and defining the scope, budget and schedule; and second, comparing the economic value of the defined project to some corporate standard or to other options for investment (Valle-Riestra, 1983). Some of the elements of scope include (Clark, 1999):

- Process description
- Process flow diagram
- Raw ingredient utilization and procurement
- Operations and production parameters
- Packaging and filling
- Degree of automation
- Packaging material utilization
- Materials handling methods
- Finished product storage
- Utility requirements
- Site parameters (size, configuration, owner's style).

Neither the building nor the facility is designed in detail at this phase, but the definition needs to be sufficient to support the economic evaluation. Feasibility studies are best performed by multidisciplinary teams with representatives from the owner's various concerned departments and outside consulting assistance.

Departments that should be involved include engineering, operations, research, purchasing and finance. Marketing, human resources, information technology and quality departments should be informed but rarely have direct contributions to make. Outside consultants may include architects, process engineers and construction managers. Often, feasibility studies are performed entirely by corporate personnel, with selection of outside consultants deferred until later. Selection of a consultant at this phase does not commit an owner to using that same consultant for the entire project, though the consultant would probably wish that were not so. There are consulting firms that are especially good at feasibility or preliminary studies and may be less qualified or efficient at later phases. The reverse can also be true – that is, there are consulting firms whose strength is in detailed design or construction more than in early phase studies.

There are consulting firms that specialize in one or more disciplines and others who focus on just one or two disciplines, for example, there are architectural firms that only do architecture, while other firms have all the disciplines for a major project under one roof, even to the extent of having construction workers on staff. An owner may have preferences for specific firms or for certain types of firms – that is, for specialized or multidisciplinary, for large or small, etc. In selecting consulting firms, their experience with an owner and with the type of project should be a major qualification. Financial strength, ability to absorb risk and reputation should also be factors.

The economic evaluation phase of the feasibility study needs to determine and define:

- Present and historical sales of the product(s) (if relevant)
- Projected future sales (volume and selling price)
- Costs of raw materials
- Costs of utilities
- Costs of labor and other factors
- Capital cost of equipment and facility
- Net present value of future cash flows, return on investment and other financial parameters as preferred by the owner
- Sensitivity of projections and estimates to various factors, such as delays, price changes in selling or raw materials, or shortfalls in projected volume (Maroulis and Saravacos, 2007).

Much of the difficulty in performing feasibility studies arises from the economic evaluation, as compared with the project definition phase, because so much of the evaluation relies on estimates and snapshots in time. All costs are subject to change often due to events that are beyond anyone's control. Time and resources available limit the degree of detail that can be determined in the equipment and building specifications and therefore constrain the accuracy of cost estimates. Most professionals believe that cost estimates at the feasibility phase deserve contingency allowances of at least 30% of the total cost (Clark, 1997a). However, many corporations dictate that contingency can only be 10%, a level of accuracy that is rarely achieved in reality at any phase (Merrow et al., 1981). This dilemma is routinely resolved by inflating other line item estimates, which results in there eventually being contingencies on contingencies in the estimate. If estimates are too greatly inflated, the project may appear economically unfeasible when, in fact, it may be attractive. This is the reason for sensitivity analysis – if the project is marginal, it will be very sensitive to small variations in cost estimates. If it is robust, it will be less sensitive.

A feasibility study results in a report, which should be concise but complete, because one that is well done can serve as a road map for the balance of the project. It can be helpful to give the project a code name, in part for some security against competitors, but also to begin establishing an identity for the team associated with the project. While the consultants, if any, may or may not continue with the project, at least some of the owner's employees should continue to maintain continuity and corporate memory. The report documents the assumptions and reasoning, but it is difficult to record every discussion, so retaining some of the people who were involved can be quite useful. If a project involves a new facility, some successful firms identify the future plant manager and make him or her the project manager during design and construction. This creates a sense of ownership and responsibility.

The report must have an executive summary of about three pages in which all the significant results are conveyed, especially the economic analysis. The bare facts of what the facility is to do, but not necessarily how or why, must be included in the executive summary. The report must be dated and all the participants identified.

The body of the report includes the drawings, estimates, schedule and a narrative that describes the operation. All the significant assumptions, compromises and supporting data must be included either in the body of the report or in appendices. A rendering or perspective drawing is not strictly necessary, but can be very effective in communicating with executives who are not adept in reading plan and elevation drawings. Such a drawing shows what a facility will look like from the outside. Modern drafting software can also produce three dimension-appearing drawings that are more accessible to non-engineers than conventional drawings (which are flat and two dimensional). The relatively small cost of such communication aids is justified by the improvement in understanding at the levels of management that must approve investments. Emphasis in a feasibility study is on the economic value of a proposed project. The project must be clearly defined, but the technical details are less important than the potential value and its risks and sensitivity.

Even if the result of a feasibility study is that a proposed project is not attractive, the study should be equally well documented as if it were attractive, because circumstances could change. It is important to understand why a proposed concept fails – perhaps there is a need for research in a new direction or maybe making the same product with a co-manufacturer instead of building a new facility would be wise. Understanding what it costs to make something is helpful when negotiating with a co-manufacturer and that is one result of a feasibility study.

Appropriation request

Most companies have a procedure for budgeting and spending capital and expense money. For major projects, this procedure often is a capital appropriation request (CAR), which is a specific document that is routed for approval and signature through the executive ranks and departments. The focus in a CAR is on the economic evaluation, with very concise descriptions of the project scope and schedule. Most of the data for a CAR are developed in the feasibility study, but they may need to be recast to fit the format of the CAR. The CAR may need to be expedited by the responsible project manager, because it is just one of many issues competing for the attention of busy executives. By conveying the document personally to the parties who need to approve the project, the project manager is also available to answer questions and to add detail if that is required. Sometimes a group of executives can be educated at one time by making a brief presentation to a staff meeting or to the board of directors. Brief is the operative word. It should take no more than 5–10 minutes and three slides – what, why and how much – what the project is, how much it adds to the corporate value and how much it costs. If the group wants to know more, they will surely ask.

There should be a sense of urgency about the CAR. Projects can be time sensitive. New construction may have a limited window for the start of outside work. There may have already been commitments made for a product introduction or rollout. The sooner a project is completed, the sooner it starts earning a return. Most executives understand the time value of money, but there are many demands on their attention and even an important project can get put aside in a perceived emergency. One way or another, get the CAR through the system and get it approved. For this purpose, and for others, it is critical to have an executive sponsor for the project. He or she has access and can probably make demands for attention that even a senior project manager may not wish to make. The executive sponsor may be from engineering or operations, but should be one who has an interest in the success of the project and should be kept well informed throughout the project life.

Funds granted

The requested appropriation may be approved as described, or it may be modified, usually by being reduced, or by being split into spending phases to control cash flow. Changes may or may not be negotiable. If they are so draconian as to imperil the project, then that should be communicated. If the scope needs to be changed to comply with a reduced budget, then that should be done. The consequences should be made known. If the CAR and supporting study were well done and the budget was not overly inflated, then it should be clear that the same capacity or economic return cannot be achieved with a drastically reduced budget. Some skeptical executives believe, often with good reason from past experience, that every request is fat and can be arbitrarily cut with no serious consequences except to the complacency of the requestor. It only confirms such skepticism when managers accept cuts and then make significant compromises in an attempt to do the near impossible. The outcome is rarely happy, but it is usually blamed on incompetence, rather than on inadequate matching of budget and scope.

This issue of arbitrary budget cuts and the games playing that has evolved over the years is one reason why trust and integrity are the single most important characteristics of a successful project manager. He or she must be accurate and honest in making and communicating the estimates and, when confronted with inadequate funds, he or she must associate the cuts with corresponding changes in scope. This requires diplomacy, discipline and courage. If all else fails, document all the facts, do the best you can and prepare a clean résumé.

One way or another, the funds are in hand, with whatever constraints and limitations may have accumulated. The scope has been modified, if necessary. Some scope changes are less onerous than others, and those can be made without protest, such as choosing alternative materials of construction that are still acceptable, but perhaps require higher maintenance. Most corporations permit up to a 10% overrun with no dire consequences, but may require board of directors' approval for more. Good project managers aim for the budget target, but rely on this small cushion to cover the inevitable extra costs that arise. It is not wise to attempt the impossible, but a good project manager with the facts on his or her side should be able to get the budget and scope synchronized. The owner will control how funds are dispersed, usually against invoices submitted by consultants, contractors and vendors. The project manager approves invoices and monitors the budget, but the accounting department issues checks. It is important to use consistent coding systems for the line items in a budget and the accounting system. It is common to identify equipment with the same type of number that accounting uses for asset records so a conversion does not need to be made in the future.

Detailed design

Detailed design may have several phases, involving increasing levels of detail, but permitting modification and evolution of the design to occur with minimal cost ramifications. The earlier in a design that potential issues are raised and resolved, the easier it is to include the solutions with fewer consequences to other disciplines. The major divisions of a design are process, utilities, site and facility (or architectural). Within these there are various disciplines, such as electrical, mechanical, structural, fire protection and piping. Drawings that are prepared include:

- Schematics
- Equipment arrangements

- Piping details
- Building plans and elevations
- Site layout
- Architectural details.

One of the early tasks is a listing of all the drawings that each discipline expects to produce, in part because the cost of the engineering correlates somewhat with the number of drawings. The other major products of design are written specifications for all the systems. The act of listing the expected drawings and specifications also is the occasion for creating a numbering system for each document. Some owners have established systems for identifying documents while others rely on whatever approach various consultants employ. When there are several independent consultants, such as architects, process engineers and mechanical engineers, the overall project manager must dictate the documentation system and conventions. A common approach is to have a project number, a discipline letter identifier and a drawing sequence number – 2008-1–ST–100 would indicate a structural drawing for the first project in 2008.

Because there is a cost associated with each document, there is a temptation to minimize the number of documents either by doing without or by compressing too much information on one sheet. This is a mistake. Clarity and understanding should be the prime criteria. Good sense will usually prevail and there are customary practices in most disciplines that suggest which drawings are commonly prepared. For a food plant, it is good practice to have schematic drawings of all the mechanical systems, even though that may not be customary. (Schematic drawings are not to scale, but show the relationship of equipment and operations to each other. A process flow diagram is a schematic drawing.) Refrigeration systems are complex processes, but the mechanical engineers who design them do not always prepare schematics. They probably should.

One of the major challenges in the detailed design phase is the avoidance of physical interferences of process piping with HVAC ducts and electrical conduit, and of equipment units with elements of the building. Even within the building, interferences can occur through miscommunication, such as a structural member running where a door was meant to be. Interferences occur because most of the disciplines work in parallel rather than in sequence. That is, once there is a background drawing giving the dimensions and shape of the footprint of a building, each group of engineers tries to design and place the systems for which they are responsible as logically as they can. But they do not usually know what their counterparts are doing and so each often reaches for the same area or place in the building. This is normal, but if allowed to persist into construction, it can become very expensive to correct.

Modern computerized drafting software often has tools to identify potential interferences, but it takes human intervention to resolve them. One approach is to assign paths or chases for certain functions, such as process piping, utility piping, electrical conduits and HVAC ducts. Functions that are relatively flexible, such as lighting, can be assigned after the less flexible functions are located. The constraints of sanitary design complicate the challenge, because it is preferred not to have piping and equipment over places where food is exposed, so that limits available areas for these uses. Some project managers assign one or more people just to find and resolve interferences and still interferences occur. Allowing sufficient room for access to equipment is another challenge. On a drawing of an oven or dryer in a layout, it may not be clear that there are doors along the side that are opened for cleaning and inspection, so another discipline may run a line too close or someone may place another unit closer to the oven or dryer than it should be.

Detailed design begins with a broad view and narrows as agreement is reached on the larger issues, such as overall layout, material flow and process concepts. In a food plant design, the process is the major function and architectural form follows function. The process is laid out in the most efficient manner possible, given the constraints of site, existing space, other processes, etc. The architect defines the new or existing space and shows required elements, such as exit doors, structural supports, floor drains (if existing) and other features that might affect what the various disciplines can do. If the project involves a new building, the issue of bay spacing must be resolved. (Bay spacing refers to how far vertical supports or columns that hold up the roof are spaced apart. Bays can be square but do not have to be.)

Structural engineers like relatively close spacing of vertical supports because that permits a lighter roof structure, which is less expensive. A process engineer would prefer that there be no vertical supports, because they inevitably interfere with where equipment might like to go and limit flexibility to make changes in the future. In a food plant, it is usually decided to make one dimension of the structural bays at least 40 feet (12 m), while the other dimension can be less, say 25–30 feet (7.6–9 m). The exact dimensions usually depend on the overall building size and shape. In an effort to use common and uniform structural members – the columns and beams – bays are usually the same size, but they do not have to be uniform. Making bays overly customized reduces future flexibility and increases cost by requiring custom-made members.

The material of construction is another early decision, because it dictates many other choices. The cleanest form of construction for a food plant is pre-cast concrete, because it does not have to be painted and can have very large bay spacing. (Pre-cast concrete uses custom-made concrete beams and columns that are made off-site in a special factory. A version, often used in California, called tilt-up, casts concrete panels on site and lifts them into place after curing.) A pre-cast roof supported by steel columns also works well. Many existing buildings have steel columns supporting a steel bar joist roof, which is hard to clean and usually is painted, requiring regular maintenance. Buildings with bar joist roofs may need to have ceilings over the process area to protect the food from contamination.

Detailed design may occur over several months, with each discipline on a different schedule, because the volume of work for each varies. The project manager needs to monitor the budget of each department, or each firm, if the work is being done by separate consultants. It is important to have frequent meetings to resolve interferences, to identify missing information, to monitor schedule and budget and to transmit decisions. Minutes must be kept of all meetings and promptly distributed in order to document decisions. Fundamental changes in concept and scope should not occur during detailed design, but it is normal for relatively minor changes to occur because of new information. Such changes might modify the capital cost estimate, which was based on assumptions made before the design was started. It is important to resist cost creep, which occurs as engineers and architects get good ideas during the course of design. Sometimes a cost increase can be accepted because it accompanies a significant improvement in efficiency or another benefit but, generally, even good ideas that cost more must be resisted, or the approved budget will be in jeopardy before construction even begins. The time for creative thinking was during the feasibility study, when assumptions were being made that dictated the estimated cost. Once the budget is approved, it is very hard to change. All those assumptions are part of the scope.

Cost reductions, on the other hand, are generally welcomed if acceptable quality is not compromised. Having a construction manager involved during detailed design can introduce potential economies, because of his or her knowledge of local practices or of developments in the supply community. Sometimes cost reductions can offset cost increases for improvements that are desired but precluded by budget discipline.

Construction

There are many different contractual approaches to the construction phase of a project. The choice of one depends on local customs and practices, corporate culture and the skill and availability of corporate personnel. The critical issues in the construction phase are control of the budget, schedule and quality of construction. Different approaches are all intended to address these issues while distributing the risks and rewards fairly. Ultimately, the owner bears almost all the risk of departures from the budget and schedule, but he or she may try to distribute some of the risk by the form of contracting.

The owner can act as his or her own general contractor by engaging individual sub-contractors in the various trades needed, such as structural, electrical, mechanical and architectural. In this case, the owner must appoint a project manager with the authority to commit financial resources and to hire and discharge contractors and personnel. The individual sub-contractors follow their sections of the detailed design documents and the owner's representative/project manager is responsible for resolving ambiguities and conflicts, usually with the continuing help of the design team. It is a sad fact of life that, no matter how hard all parties try, design documents are rarely perfect. If the schedule for design was tight and if costs were unwisely cut during that phase, there will be more errors and ambiguities. It is a rare owner who has on staff people with the experience and skill to manage a significant construction project, because such an activity is relatively rare in the course of most manufacturing careers. Thus, acting as one's own general contractor may not be the wisest course. When this path is chosen, it may be because the owner believes this approach will save money. That is rarely true.

A more conventional approach is to engage a general contractor (GC), who is in the business of building facilities. It is wise to select a contractor who has experience with the type of facility being built, that is with food plants, distribution centers or laboratories. Contractors whose primary experience is with general purpose warehouses, light manufacturing or commercial offices or stores are not likely to understand the challenges of sanitary construction. The normal approach to selecting a qualified general contractor is to issue the complete design documents – drawings and specifications – to at least three previously screened firms and to request proposals within a specified time frame, usually about two weeks. Firms are pre-screened by requesting expressions of interest and qualifications using a general description of the scale and type of project. Interested firms submit descriptions of past projects, describe their project approach and may include references and testimonials from past clients. It is wise for the owner to interview firms in person and to visit representative past projects, if possible.

General contractors make their money by charging a fee on top of the passed-through costs of sub-contractors. Some GCs have certain trades on staff and may perform some of the work themselves, while others focus on managing the work of others. Each GC usually has a list of sub-contactors with whom they are comfortable and to whom they routinely turn for the respective skills. One consequence of this practice is that the owner has no control or influence over the sub-contractors; they only report to the GC. The GC is responsible for regular payments to the sub-contractors, for which he invoices the owner. Sub-contractors are entitled to file liens against the project to protect themselves and GCs request waivers of liens from the sub-contractors on the owner's behalf. A common issue is dispute over performance of a sub-contractor, leading to withholding of payment and possible litigation, ultimately against the owner. The GC is supposed to protect the owner against such conflicts, but a wise owner obtains his own insurance for the project just the same. One common variation is design/build, in which the architect works for the GC, or the architect provides a construction manager, instead of the architect working directly for the owner.

Under a GC approach, the owner does not have access to all cost information. The GC generally quotes a fixed price for the original scope and includes unit prices for work beyond the original scope. The GC has the potential for extra profit beyond the included fee if sub-contractors' prices are less than estimated or if all of the included contingency allowance is not used. The GC also faces some risk if costs escalate or some other event causes costs to increase. The risk absorbed by the GC and the opportunity for additional profit to the GC are supposed to insulate the owner from some of the risk of increased cost, but it is not wise to rely heavily on this protection. Most GCs will find a way to blame increases on a cause beyond their control and will look to the owner for a change order and increased price.

In the design/build approach, sometimes the owner can request that the GC engage an architect suggested by the owner, perhaps because the owner believes the selected architect to be better qualified than the one the builder might otherwise choose. Most builders will agree, though with some reluctance, because they often get 'free' services from their favored architect, with the implied promise that the architect will be engaged for future design/build projects. Unless the owner is satisfied with the qualifications of the architect 'favored' by the design/builder, the owner should insist on his or her own choice or revert to a more conventional approach to contracting. The conventional approach is often called design/bid/build to distinguish it from design/build. The architect works for the owner in this case. It is believed by many that the conventional approach takes more time than does design/build. However, the owner does have more control and total costs should not be much different among the various approaches.

The most common source of blame for increased cost is incorrect or inadequate design. The accusation may or may not be well founded. Designers are human and not perfect. Designs are created under stressful circumstances. Scope may be imperfectly defined and inadequately understood. For all these reasons, care during the design phase is especially important, and even with great care, a wise owner budgets for some extra contingency. A wise owner also monitors the performance of a GC and sub-contractors during construction and scrutinizes all invoices and progress reports for early signs of trouble. Data such as daily head count on site, yards of concrete poured, feet of pipe installed and number of pieces of equipment installed are good indicators of progress.

An increasingly common approach to construction is to engage a construction manager (CM) who acts as a consultant to the owner, does not perform any of the work himself and advises the owner on the hiring of sub-contractors. The CM monitors the budget, schedule and quality for the owner. A CM charges a lower fee, usually, than does a GC, because the CM accepts none of the risk of cost increases, nor does he normally have the potential for an extra profit. The owner holds all of the cost risk. Some CMs negotiate incentive contracts in which they can share in cost savings and may agree, reluctantly, to penalties for schedule delays. Owners should be cautious with such incentives, because the search for cost savings may lead to cutting corners and compromises on quality. The time for value engineering is during design; once scope is defined and specifications are written, the construction should proceed according to the design, unless extraordinary circumstances occur.

GCs and CMs are often part of firms that also perform design and offer services as a package, called design/build. There can be efficiencies in communication among designers and constructors when they have common ownership, but this is not always realized in practice, because there are cultural differences among designers and builders, no matter how they are organized. Design/build can save some time because there is less need to seek bids, but there is increased need for trust by the owner, because there can be less transparency. Owners are often concerned that a design/builder can somehow conceal his errors and make compromises without the checks and balances of a third party manager. A wise owner may engage an independent CM or assign an experienced employee as his site representative, no matter the contractual arrangement, as an extra pair of eyes to monitor progress and quality.

During construction, the GC, CM or owner's representative have certain routine tasks. The overall goal is coordination among the various trades that are on site. Each sub-contractor is responsible for his own staff and usually has a trailer for his site leader. Each sub-contractor is motivated to complete his tasks as soon as possible, but there is a certain sequence in which order the tasks must occur. There are issues of access, use of power, use of common equipment, release of equipment and parts and allowance for concrete to cure and paint to dry. The site manager resolves these issues at daily meetings with sub-contractor site supervisors. Often an owner will select and assign the future plant manager as the owner's site representative, which gives that person an early sense of ownership and responsibility.

Union issues can complicate construction. Laws and practices vary among states and regions. Some sites permit union and non-union firms to work on the same project, often by using two gates. Site representatives must be sensitive to labor laws and practices to avoid work stoppages and other interferences.

Sub-contractors are responsible for ordering their supplies, but these must be received on site, protected and released as needed. Major equipment is often purchased directly by the owner, to avoid the fee of including it in a general contract and because the owner should be responsible for the process. Equipment vendors and specialized sub-contractors may be involved in installation and start-up of process equipment and support systems. These activities must be coordinated with the progress of the facility construction. For example, under floor piping must be installed before a floor is poured and both must be complete before equipment can be set in place.

As work is completed, it is inspected and certified so that payment can be made. It is normal to retain a portion of each payment against correction of defects that are documented on a 'punch list'. The punch list and 'as built' corrections to drawings are maintained throughout the project. As costs are incurred, the budget is adjusted and projections made for cost to complete. The owner must be almost continuously informed of the budget status. Other documents such as operating manuals, warranties, permits and certificates are collected and maintained by the site manager. It is critical to maintain an accurate record of any deviations from the design, any disputes and any other issues that may arise, because resolution may take some time after the event and memories can be unreliable.

Construction of a major facility is a complex and challenging task, requiring experience, skill and diplomacy. Assignment as an assistant site representative can be a great learning experience for a young engineer, even if his or her career path is in design or operations, because it is in construction that designs come to life and the ease or difficulty of manufacturing is fixed.

Commissioning

Commissioning refers to the time period between completion of construction and operation at rated capacity. This can only occur after all process and utility equipment is installed. Usually the sub-contractor installing equipment is responsible for making sure that motors turn over correctly, that controls work as intended and that instruments read correctly. These tests are typically done individually and in isolation. Commissioning then involves testing an entire line as a unit. This may require coordination of speeds, alignment of conveyors and integration of controls. Vendors of process and packaging equipment routinely provide assistance in this phase. Operators are trained in safe operation and maintenance of the line. Realistic raw materials are used in an attempt to produce acceptable product. Design efficiencies are not expected and any acceptable product is seen as a dividend.

Each unit operation is assessed over its expected range of operation and compared with process design and equipment specifications. Deficiencies, if any, must be corrected or otherwise accommodated, perhaps by lowering expectations. The limiting components of the system must be identified. These may be different than those intended or expected in design. Ideally, at the end of commissioning, the new process line is operating at expected design rate and efficiencies, the operators are trained and self-sufficient, the vendor technicians have departed and the plant is ready to accept orders routinely.

Close out and production

Completion of a project is like graduation from college – it is the end of one phase and the beginning of another. It is important to have a formal completion conference among the owner, the constructor, the designer and major vendors to transfer remaining documents, resolve any outstanding invoices and transfer accumulated knowledge and experience. Sometimes this can correspond in time with dedication of a new facility and could involve some modest ceremony. On other occasions, it can be a simple business meeting, but it is important to mark the official end of a project somehow.

The completion of the design and construction project marks the beginning of the production phase. If the plant manager and some of his or her staff have been involved all along, they move smoothly into operation of the plant. If the operating team is new to the project, they must learn their way around, which presumably started to happen during commissioning. Production requires its own skill set and is discussed in a later chapter. Raw materials and packaging materials are procured in a timely fashion, stored properly and dispensed as needed. Packaging of raw materials is properly disposed of. Operators are hired, trained and scheduled as needed. Orders are received and line time scheduled. Products are made, checked for quality, stored and shipped. Equipment is maintained on a regular schedule, in advance of the need for repair. Almost as soon as production is started, plans are considered for improvement, expansion and increases in capacity. The cycle begins again.

Roles and responsibilities during design and construction

Large and small projects require a multidisciplinary team from within and outside the corporation, because no single discipline or person maintains all the skills needed. Most of the skills are technical, but equally important to the success of a complex project are marketing, finance, human resources and general management. Leadership of a facility project may fall to the engineering department, if there is one, but it may range from the CEO to any available manager, depending on the scale and the company's resources. Leadership of a major project is not to be taken lightly. Large amounts of money can be at stake, not to mention a company's future.

Typical members of a company team contemplating a new or expanded facility include: engineering, research, marketing, operations, finance, human resources and general management. Other departments and individuals may be interested and many others may need to be informed, but the core team should be limited to those with direct contributions to make and direct stakes in the success of the project. Too large a group has difficulty meeting and making decisions.

Outside resources that may be involved include: architects, engineers, construction managers and vendors of key equipment. It is delicate to involve outside consultants early in a project because there may be an understandable presumption that they have been engaged for the life of the project when, in fact, that decision may not have been made. Many consultants contribute their services early in a project at a low or zero fee in the hope that they will be selected for the more lucrative later phases. It is more professional to engage services for an equitable fee as needed, with no guarantees of subsequent involvement. Vendors are accustomed to contributing advice and information as part of their normal sales effort.

Consultants who are engaged early have the advantage of learning about the project and the owner and the opportunity of making a good impression. Not all consultants are equally skilled at all phases of a project – some are especially good at feasibility studies, others at design and still others at construction. Some companies have established relationships with consultants and routinely involve them as appropriate. It is wise to develop such relationships when possible, because consultants perform better with familiar clients about whom they know the personalities, culture and technologies.

Individual consultants and consulting firms have networks of others who have compatible skills and can often be relied upon to assemble a team of experts to supplement a company's own team for executing a project. No matter how the team is assembled, nor from where the participants come, the single most important person is the leader. This must be a responsible executive with the authority to make significant decisions, the ability to communicate with the disparate parties and the confidence of the CEO and board of directors. One of the single greatest challenges and needed skills of the leader is the willingness and ability to make decisions when required. No one makes perfect decisions but, in the context of moving a complex project forward, making a decision is almost always better than not making one, even in the absence of complete information. Once a good leader is identified, it is crucial that he or she continue through to the end of the project.

Issues

Broadly, the issues faced by a project team are always the same: scope, budget, schedule and quality. Scope refers to what the project is to accomplish and how it will do so. This includes capacity, location, technology, packaging and provisions for the future. Great effort, time and attention go into defining the scope and, once defined, it should be considered almost sacred in its inviolability. Common sense, of course, must prevail. Circumstances do change, new technologies are discovered, markets change. When such events occur, the scope should be adjusted as necessary. But care and wisdom must be applied; change for its own sake is rarely useful. The leader is the custodian of the scope and demands very persuasive arguments before approving changes.

The budget flows directly from the scope, but is more prone to change with time, as details are added. The total budget rarely changes dramatically, as previously discussed, because once a budget is approved, companies are reluctant to increase project budgets. However, the amount allocated to contingency, as a reflection of uncertainty in estimates, does change with time. When properly managed, the careful adjustment of contingency allowances can partially compensate for the inevitable upward creep of line items in project budgets.

The schedule is similar in that it is subject to the development of more detail with time, but the overall schedule may be relatively fixed, once it has been approved. This can become a problem if critical decisions are deferred. That is one reason why it is so important that the leader be decisive – he or she should not be the cause of delay. Others may be causes of delay and the leader must do what is possible to reduce the impact of such obstacles to progress.

Quality is a continuing issue through the life of a project because of the perceived impact on cost. As costs creep up, there is pressure to cut corners and compromise specifications to reduce cost. Wisdom and discipline are needed to maintain the required standard of quality while also controlling costs. It is common in early phases to set relatively high standards for finishes, for instance, only to realize later that costs are prohibitive. 'Green' construction standards are a current example, where many companies would like to use sustainable building materials and environmentally benign methods, but find that conventional materials and methods are still less expensive. This situation may change as more suppliers offer green materials and methods, but cost competitiveness has not yet occurred in this area.

Tools of project management

The Internet and intranets within companies are powerful tools for improving the speed and accuracy of communication among a team that may be physically dispersed widely. Communication of information, issues and decisions is the vital lifeblood of a team. Frequent meetings, in person, by phone or over the network, are important because of the nuances of communication that are often lost in writing. Drawings are the medium of communication for engineers and architects, but not all team members are comfortable reading drawings, which have arcane symbols and conventions. It is common to maintain a common electronic file of all drawings so that only one version is ever used. This also permits ongoing resolution of interferences.

Likewise, meeting minutes must be prepared promptly, distributed and readily available. Minutes and memos should document decisions as they are made. Roles and responsibilities are established at the beginning of a project and as much continuity as possible maintained. That is, people should not be added or removed from a team unless that is unavoidable, because institutional memory is carried in people. Every new person requires orientation and some time to learn the project.

Discussion questions or assignments

1. Draw the organization chart of a project team for a large and a small project in the context of your firm or one you select. Who would fill the various roles? How do the charts differ?
2. Identify some outside consultants you might use for a new food plant project. What are their strengths and weaknesses?
3. Locate the appropriations request form used in your company or from another source. Could you complete it for a project? If not, where would you get the information you need?

9 Plant operations

Food engineers often become responsible for plant operations, even if their careers begin in research or engineering. Supervision and management are aspects of leadership; they require people skills in addition to technical knowledge. Integrity and clarity in communication are the foundation of success in leadership. Integrity means that people can trust a leader and believe what he or she says. Clarity in communication means that people can understand what the leader says. In plant operations, there are numerous, often conflicting, issues that the leader must resolve, using his or her people skills (see Schonberger, 1986; Walters, 1987; Kotter, 1988; Wheatley, 1992, among many other references on the topic).

First among the many challenges is quality, both in the sense of food safety and in the sense of meeting the requirements and standards for the product. Without a safe and desirable product, there is no business. The consequences of unsafe foods appear in the newspapers almost daily. Companies have disappeared because of one massive recall and the deaths and sicknesses of consumers resulting from unsafe products. Much of this text has been concerned with the design of plant and equipment capable of producing safe food, but it falls to the management of the plant to ensure that operations are, in fact, producing safe food. Human error has often been responsible for food contamination. Human error is prevented, at least in part, by competent leadership. The essence is making people who work in the plant care about the safety of the product and, ultimately, about the survival of the firm and their own jobs.

Practical Design, Construction and Operation of Food Facilities
ISBN: 978-0-12-374204-9

Human safety is a second high priority. Food processing can be a surprisingly hazardous occupation, primarily because of repetitive motion injuries, which result when workers are required to perform the same task for long periods of time. Hand packing of cookies is an example. Meat packing workers experience injuries from cuts, slips and falls as well as repetitive motion injuries. It is common to issue protective gear, such as metal mesh gloves, aprons and steel toed boots in meat packing plants, but still the injuries occur, in part because of high turnover in the meat industry and the constant need for training. Reducing turnover is one approach to reducing injuries. Rotating workers through various tasks helps prevent repetitive motion injuries, but this requires cross-training. The variety and stimulation of doing new things can improve morale as well as help to reduce injuries.

Paying attention to hazards such as low conveyors, unguarded belts and gears and uncovered screw conveyors can improve the safety of workers. Ultimately, workers must be responsible for themselves, but they must be given the training, tools and motivation to observe rules, reduce hazards and care for each other. Leadership sets the example by observing plant regulations, preaching the need for safe operations and rewarding safe conduct, such as long stretches of time without lost time accidents. There is financial motivation for the company also, as workers' compensation insurance and liability insurance rates decline when a plant's safety record is especially good. Teaching and practicing safe operations is never ending, because of turnover and the natural complacency that grows with time.

Demands from corporate management for excessive overtime and unusual scheduling practices should be resisted by plant management because these can lead to worker fatigue, which then leads to accidents. A plant manager should be protective of the staff and insist on the proper resources and time to achieve results. Common sense and diplomacy are critical in balancing corporate demands with local responsibilities.

Security is related to safety and quality in the sense that workers need to be protected against potential violence and consumers need to be protected against potential sabotage. There have been enough incidents of deliberate and inadvertent contamination of food to justify improvement in the control of access to plants and of people to the food in process. Certain security measures are common and routine:

- Perimeter fencing with controlled access for vehicles and people

- Photo identification badges for employees and distinctive badges for visitors
- Visitors are always accompanied by employees
- Color-coded uniforms for employees identifying work areas and permitted access. (Maintenance employees present a special challenge, as they commonly cross boundaries between work areas)
- Controlled access to areas of plant by electronic badge or key pad
- Workers are trained to challenge unrecognized people and unauthorized activities.

Workers know who should be present and what they should be doing. They have as much at stake as anyone in protecting their employer and their jobs. One of the more common sources of sabotage has been a disgruntled employee, who is especially dangerous because he or she knows how the plant operates and has a familiar face. Fellow employees are the best defense – they know who is unhappy and they know what is and what is not permitted behavior.

It should be difficult for a stranger to enter a food plant and do deliberate harm, but the risk exists. Employees need to be conscious of the risk and to be vigilant against it occurring.

Every food plant is under almost constant pressure to increase capacity because unit fixed costs decrease as capacity increases. Capacity increases are achieved in small, incremental improvements in operation, which are identified and implemented with experience, usually by operators, who are deeply familiar with the equipment. Depending on local practices, there usually is spare capacity in working extra hours during the week – few plants are scheduled 24/7. However, without adding extra staff, few plants can work many hours of overtime without stressing staff and machinery. The best source of increased capacity is improved efficiency – greater yield from raw material, less waste, less down time. This is achieved by strict attention to statistics reporting losses, causes of down time and accounting for waste and by performing diligent preventive maintenance. Leadership that understands the process can motivate the staff to focus on all the little things that add up to improved efficiency. It is not glamorous. The objective is to improve every day (see Harmon and Peterson, 1990).

Some would have put cost as the first on the list of concerns, but when it is, some of the more critical issues tend to be neglected, with the result that costs increase. Costs for food processing are heavily dependent on the costs of raw materials and packaging materials – labor, energy and other costs are usually only about 30%. Costs of raw materials are rarely under the control of plant leadership. Thus, pressure is always applied against labor costs, even though these are relatively minor in the grand scope of the financial picture. Plant leadership must be sure that staffing levels are correct for the needs of production, that staff is not so stressed that hazards are increased and that production is not impacted by insufficient staff. Union and local regulations can affect leadership's flexibility in responding to changing needs. It is wise to learn and observe such restrictions as early as possible. There have been instances in which reducing labor beyond a certain point actually reduced yield and cost much more than it appeared to save. Restoring jobs improved yield and profit. Likewise, it is often true that operating lines more slowly improves efficiency so that net capacity actually increases. Making waste faster makes little sense.

Leadership and organization

The organization of manufacturing plants has become flatter than it was traditionally, with fewer layers of supervision today. This is best exemplified in the team approach, where members of a group are held responsible for various tasks with less supervision than they might have received previously. They schedule and discipline themselves. Intermediate levels of management in plants have largely disappeared and younger (or less experienced) workers may not even know how things used to be. A flatter organization generally means that everyone carries more responsibility and that there is less opportunity to point a finger at someone else for a failing. Workers trusted with greater responsibility and the authority to implement changes have accomplished great improvements in operations because of their intimate knowledge of the equipment and their innate creativity. Workers familiar with equipment who are motivated to improve operations can make valuable suggestions and implement modifications that are significant improvements. As one example, a team servicing a packaging machine suggested replacing stainless steel panels on their machine with clear plastic so they could more easily inspect interior parts, saving the time of removing and replacing the panels. Simple, but cost effective. Few managers would have thought of that modification, but it dramatically increased time on stream for that machine.

Workers must be cross-trained so they can relieve each other and often they are expected to perform their own maintenance on their machines. Maintenance requires additional training, but having operators perform at least some maintenance has the benefit of giving the operators a better understanding of how equipment works. When workers accept the system, the results can be extraordinary.

Leadership involves motivation more than discipline; inspiration more than control. The foundation of successful leadership is mutual respect. Leaders respect their staff and, in turn, earn respect. Workers need to be more talented, because of the greater sophistication of modern controls and computers and are thus in greater demand, than they used to be. Every effort should be focused on retaining skilled employees and in motivating them to perform.

Troubleshooting

Is it human or mechanical? That is the question when seeking the source of a problem in food manufacturing. It could be either, but if the plant and equipment have been designed and constructed with a view to food safety and sanitation, then there must be a suspicion of human error. Humans are not perfect and they do make mistakes. It is not constructive to punish for any but deliberate errors, but the opportunity to make errors should be reduced as much as possible. Automation and the integration of information go a long way towards reducing errors in data introduction and use.

It might be observed that this book has almost no equations, though it is written by an engineer. There are plenty of books that discuss the mathematical modeling of processes and equipment. This book has tried to demonstrate that the practical design, construction and operation of food facilities depend heavily on leadership, communication and qualitative evaluation skills. These are rarely documented and difficult to teach. Perhaps this book will become a resource for those wanting to acquire some of these skills.

Discussion questions or assignments

1. If you are associated with a plant, evaluate its security arrangements. If you can arrange a field trip to an operating plant, evaluate the security practices. How would you breach them? How could they be improved?
2. Consider your plant or one you visit. Describe its organization. Does it elicit the best performance from each employee?

Appendix I: Basic heat transfer

The heat added or removed from a stream is equal to its change in enthalpy, a thermodynamic term that is dependent on the change in temperature or the change in phase, if any. *For no change in phase*,

$$Q = mC_p\Delta T \qquad (1)$$

where,
Q is heat added or removed, Watts (=0.293 BTU/h)
M is mass flow rate, kg/h (=0.454 lb/h)
C_p is heat capacity, kJ/(kg K) (=4.187 BTU/(lb F))
ΔT is temperature change, (Δ, Greek delta, symbolizes change or difference)
K is degrees Kelvin (=1.8° Fahrenheit).

The heat capacity of water is 4.187 kJ/(kg K). Many food liquids have physical properties similar to those of water because water is such a large component of food liquids.

If there is a phase change, such as evaporation of a liquid or freezing of a liquid to solid, then

$$Q = m\Delta H \qquad (2)$$

where,
ΔH is the change in enthalpy upon phase change, kJ/kg (=2.326 BTU/lb).
The enthalpy of evaporation for water is 2326 kJ/kg. The enthalpy of freezing for water is 330 kJ/kg.

Practical Design, Construction and Operation of Food Facilities
ISBN: 978-0-12-374204-9

The heat added or removed to a stream, calculated by either Eq. (1) or (2), must be transferred according to Eq. (3):

$$Q = UA\Delta T_{LM} \tag{3}$$

where,
U is heat transfer coefficient, $W/(m^2\ K)$ (=5.678 BTU/(h ft^2 F))
A is heat transfer area, m^2 (=0.093 ft^2)
ΔT_{LM} is log mean temperature difference, K (=F/1.8).

The log mean temperature difference is the average driving force for heat transfer between a hot stream and a colder stream. The process fluid may be either the hot or cold stream and the other stream may be steam, hot or cold water, a refrigerant, hot oil or cold glycol solution. Heat flows from hot stream to cold stream at a rate proportional to the difference in temperature. If the temperature difference at the inlet for the process fluid is ΔT_{IN} and the temperature difference at the outlet is ΔT_{OUT} , then the ΔT_{LM} is defined in Eq. (4):

$$\Delta T_{LM} = (\Delta T_{IN} - \Delta T_{OUT})/\ln(\Delta T_{IN}/\Delta T_{OUT}) \tag{4}$$

where,
ln is natural logarithm.

For the case where the temperature driving force is equal at each end, Eq. (4) is indeterminate, but the temperature driving force difference is obviously whatever that value is.

Heat transfer coefficients depend on the properties of the fluids, the configuration of the heat exchanger and the velocity of the fluids. The actual value can vary widely. Where possible, it should be measured with real fluids under realistic conditions. This is not always practical. Equipment vendors have models for estimating heat transfer coefficients and should be consulted. However, they need to know what fluids are involved and the relevant physical properties. For steam heating, values range from 1000 to 3000 $W/(m^2 K)$ and for viscous liquid foods, from 200 to 1000 (Maroulis and Saravacos, 2007).

The typical heat transfer problem is to estimate the required size of a heat exchanger, meaning A in Eq. (3) is the only unknown. The temperature change for the process fluid is usually specified and the temperature change for the heating or cooling medium is chosen or specified (perhaps because it is an existing system).

Experience suggests that a good rule of thumb is to have a heating or cooling stream that does not change phase flow at about three times the rate of the process stream. The trade off in specifying a heating or cooling circuit is between the cost of pumping and the size of heat exchangers. The amount of energy exchanged is set by the temperature change of the process fluid. The smaller the flow rate of the heating or cooling fluid, the smaller the temperature driving force for heat transfer and the larger the heat exchangers must be. The smaller the flow, the lower the pressure drop through the lines and exchangers and so the smaller the circulating pump and the less energy it consumes. In a circulating system, there are two exchangers – one between the primary heat or cooling source, such as steam or ammonia refrigerant, and the other between the heating or cooling fluid and the process fluid. One might ask why add the complexity of a circulating system?

Steam and refrigerants can be exchanged against process fluids and often are. However, intermediate fluids for heating or cooling can be less hazardous than steam or refrigerant, both of which are under elevated pressure. Temperature control may be more precise with a circulating fluid. Also, there may be less risk of fouling when temperatures are lower than they would be with steam.

In cooling systems, there is the opportunity to conserve energy by using an ice building system, where an ammonia refrigeration system runs at a constant rate to freeze water into ice, which accumulates in a vessel. When cooling is needed, a glycol solution is exchanged against the ice, melting it and cooling the glycol, which then is exchanged against the process fluid. Since the ammonia compressor runs constantly, including during times when electricity rates are typically lower (because of low demand at night), the compressor can be smaller than it would be if it were sized for the peak demand for cooling and it uses lower cost power.

Appendix II: Residence time in hold tubes

The objective of a hold tube in a continuous thermal fluid process is to provide enough time at a given temperature to achieve the desired reduction in target microorganisms or other effect. The required time must be achieved for the fastest moving portion of the fluid. Fluids flowing in a tube have a velocity profile such that the velocity is highest at the center of the tube and is usually assumed to be zero at the wall of the tube. For Newtonian fluids, in which the viscosity is not a function of shear rate, that is, the viscosity is constant at a given temperature, the flow regime is defined by the Reynolds number, $N_{Re.}$

$$N_{Re} = \rho Du/\mu \tag{5}$$

where,
ρ is density, kg/m^3 (=16.02 lb/ft^3)
D is tube diameter, m (=0.305 ft)
u is average velocity, m/s (=0.0051 ft/min)
μ is viscosity, Pa s (Pascal seconds) (=0.001 centipoise)
(Pa s has units of kg/(m s)).

Laminar flow is defined as having $N_{Re} < 2100$ and turbulent flow is defined as having $N_{Re} > 4000$ (Steffe and Singh, 1997). The flow regime between laminar and turbulent is called the transition regime. For purposes of calculating residence times, it is conservative but safe to use the procedures for laminar flow. Laminar flow

Practical Design, Construction and Operation of Food Facilities
ISBN: 978-0-12-374204-9

is so called because flow occurs in smooth, concentric layers with the velocity changing smoothly from zero at the wall to a maximum value in the center. In turbulent flow, flow is in eddies and chaotic, so that the velocity profile is relatively flat.

Viscosity is obviously a strong determinant of flow regime. Typically, it is measured in a laboratory using one of a variety of instruments. Values for some familiar foods, expressed in centipoise (cP) are 1.0 for water, 2 for orange juice, 45 for sugar syrup (65% solids) and 36 for olive oil at 40°C.

Many foods have viscosities that change with shear applied and are adequately described by the power law.

$$\mu_a = K\gamma^{(n-1)} \tag{6}$$

where,
μ_a is apparent viscosity, Pa s
K is consistency coefficient, Pa s^n
γ is shear rate, s^{-1}
n is flow behavior index, no units.

Values of K and n are measured in the laboratory by determining a flow curve, which shows the force required to rotate a spindle at a range of speeds. They are also reported for many foods in such sources as Steffe and Singh (1997). Values of K and n can vary widely and even among samples of the same food, so it is best to determine the values experimentally for a given case.

The value of Reynolds number for a power law fluid is given by Eq. (7):

$$N_{GRe} = [(D^n u^{2-n} \rho)/(K\, 8^{n-1})][4n/(3n+1)]^n \tag{7}$$

Laminar flow for power law fluids is defined as those having N_{RePL} less than a critical value that varies with n, reaching a maximum of about 2400 at n = 0.4.

For Newtonian fluids in laminar flow, the maximum velocity at the center of the tube is twice the average velocity. For power law fluids, the ratio is a function of n and is given by Eq. (8):

$$u_{max} / u_{avg} = (1+3n)/(1+n) \tag{8}$$

$$u_{avg} = V/(\pi R^2) \tag{9}$$

where,
V is volumetric flow rate, m^3/s (=0.0005 ft^3/min)
R is tube radius, m (=0.305 ft).

Hold tube length is determined by establishing the desired hold time for the fastest moving portion of fluid, say 30 seconds. The required volume to give an average hold time is calculated and then adjusted for the flow regime using the flow rate, say 20 gallons per minute (GPM).

$$V_T = V\,\theta \tag{10}$$

where,
V_T is tube volume, m^3 (=0.003785 gallons)
θ is average residence time, s.

Using the example values,

$$\begin{aligned} V_T &= 20\text{ GPM }(0.000063\ (m^3/s)/\text{GPM})\ 30\text{ s} \\ &= 0.03785\ m^3 \end{aligned}$$

The actual volume required is twice this or 0.0757 m^3 if laminar flow is assumed.

The length is calculated by dividing the volume by the cross-sectional area for various tube sizes.

Outside diameter (Inches)	Inside diameter (mm)	Area (m^2)	Length (m)
1.0	22.9	0.000412	184
1.5	35.6	0.000995	76
2.0	47.5	0.00177	42.7
3.0	72.9	0.00417	18.2
4.0	97.5	0.00746	10.1

It should be noted that sanitary tubing in metric sizes has slightly different dimensions than those in US units, which were used in this example. Hold tubes are often about 3 inches in diameter to reduce the length and the accompanying pressure drop, not to mention the additional space required. Checking the N_{Re}, the value for tomato juice is about 11 000, clearly turbulent, which means the hold tube could be safely shortened by a factor of 2, since the required volume was previously doubled under the assumption of laminar flow.

For fluids in turbulent flow, the average velocity is very close to the maximum value and hold tubes are designed accordingly. It is important to check assumptions if the same equipment is to be used for multiple materials and varying flow rates. As previously discussed, if flow rates vary widely, for heat sensitive products it would be wise to have the capability to use varying lengths of hold tube as well as varying amounts of heat transfer area.

Hold tubes are often constructed of parallel, horizontal lengths of tube linked by 180° turns. Vertical runs are not counted for hold tubes because the velocity profile is harder to predict reliably.

Appendix III: Flow chart symbols

Practical Design, Construction and Operation of Food Facilities
ISBN: 978-0-12-374204-9

Storage tank	Conveyor belt	Process vessel	Compressor
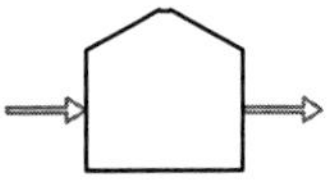	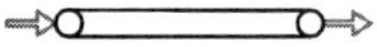	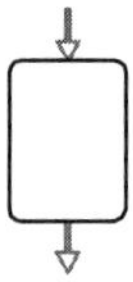	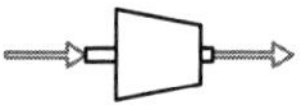
Pump	Fan	Agitated jacketed tank	Belt dryer
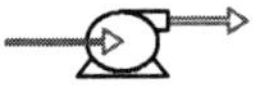	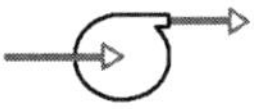	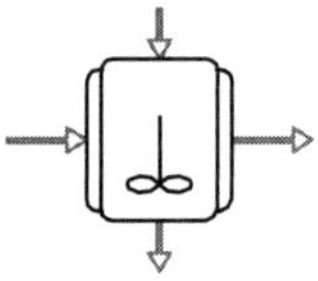	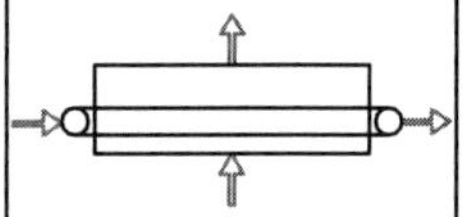
Centrifuge	Extruder	Packaging equipment	Forced circulation evaporator
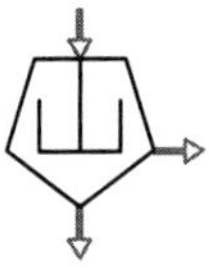	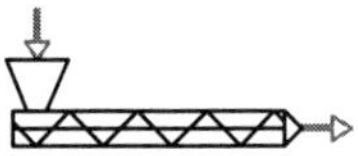	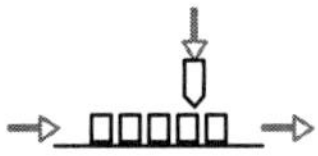	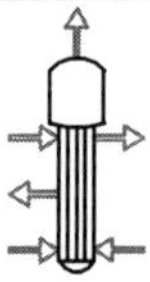
Plate filter	Vibrating screen	Plate heat exchanger	Rotary dryer
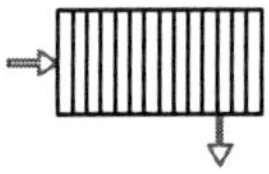	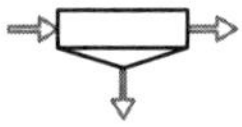	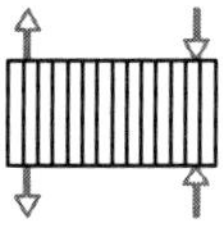	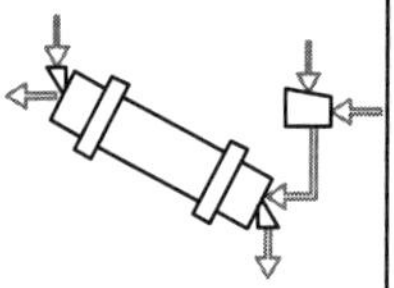
	Heat exchanger	Valve	
	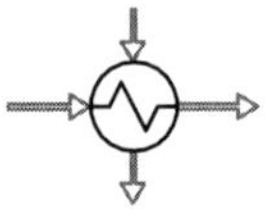	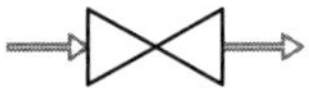	

Appendix IV: Glossary of some terms used

Aerobic bacteria: microorganisms that require air to grow as distinct from anaerobic bacteria, which can grow in the absence of air.

Air break: separation of plant drain lines from sewer lines, occurring in catch basin.

Annulus: the space between two concentric tubes; shaped like a donut.

Aseptic: refers to a food process in which foods and containers are sterilized separately and then combined in a sterile environment.

Bay spacing: in facility design, the distance between vertical supports defining a regular rectangle or square.

Bridging (of solids): cohesive particulate solids forming an arch over a discharge point and interrupting flow.

Catch basin: an underground vessel connected to drain lines from the plant and to sewer lines going to treatment. The basin serves to separate the plant from the sewer, preventing back flow. It also helps to remove fats, oil and grease as well as heavy solids.

Chase: in facility design, a designated space for a certain function, such as a passage allocated exclusively for pipes.

Cohesive powder: particulate material which tends to stick together under mild pressure.

Practical Design, Construction and Operation of Food Facilities
ISBN: 978-0-12-374204-9

Cooling tower: equipment in which warm water loses heat to ambient air by partial evaporation of the water, allowing reuse of the water for cooling in the process.

Dew point: the temperature of humid air at which moisture begins to condense. It is a measure of relative humidity.

Enthalpy: thermodynamic term referring to the energy change in a material due to a temperature change or to a change in phase, as from liquid to vapor or liquid to solid, or the reverse.

Fermentation media: nutrient solution in which microorganisms are grown.

Fermentation reactors (fermentors): equipment in which microorganisms are deliberately grown by providing nutrients, controlling temperature and providing air when needed.

Fryer: equipment holding large quantities of edible oil with provisions for heating the oil, immersing food for a given time and draining oil from food.

Good manufacturing practices: regulations for the operation of food plants, defined in the Code of Federal Regulations title 21 Part 110.

HACCP: Hazard analysis critical control points, a seven-point approach to ensuring food safety.

Headspace: the portion of a vessel or container above the contents.

Heat transfer coefficient: parameter in equation by which heat transfer area is calculated; it is a function of geometry, fluid properties and fluid velocity.

Hermetically sealed: gas tight; refers to containers that are closed so that gas cannot enter or leave; food containers that can maintain a vacuum inside.

Hydrostatic pressure: the force per unit area exerted on the walls of a vessel from the height of fluid or solids contained in the vessel. Water exerts about 0.5 psi per foot of height.

Interlock: electrical control, which prevents a motor from operating if a lid is open or a guard out of place.

Intermediate bulk container: large bag, cardboard box or metal bin, which is portable and used to hold quantities of liquids or solids.

Internal heat transfer: movement of energy from high temperature region to lower temperature region by conduction through material as distinct from movement of portions of gas or liquid, known as convection.

Irradiation: the act of exposing a material to ionizing radiation, usually for the purpose of sterilizing the material.

Microflora: the mixture of microbes residing in a food or on the surface of equipment.

Potential energy (of a fluid): the change in height, pressure and friction loss that must be provided by a pump to move a fluid from one point to another.

Press cake: the mass of solids removed from a slurry in a filter.

Pressure relief valve: control device, which opens when a given pressure is exceeded as a safety precaution to prevent damage to equipment or injury.

Punch list: in construction project management, a dynamic 'to do' list that identifies defects, omissions and other issues that must rectified along with responsibility, date added and date resolved.

Rat holing (of solids): solids in a vessel adhering to the walls leaving only a narrow passage down the center of the vessel.

Rendering: architectural drawing, usually freehand, which shows appearance of a facility in perspective or as it would look from the outside.

Retort: a pressure vessel into which containers are placed for high temperature cooking.

Rheological property: referring to fluid flow, the viscosity or the parameters that correlate the apparent viscosity.

Schematic drawing: diagram not to scale of equipment pieces in relation to one another.

Screw feeder: device for metering and controlling the flow of particulate solids from a vessel by using a horizontal screw fed by a slot to remove a measured amount of solids with each revolution of the screw.

Shear: in fluid flow, the movement of portions of a fluid mass with respect to other portions.

Star feeder: device for metering particulate solids by rotating a cylinder with vanes in a horizontal cylindrical casing with openings at top and bottom such that a portion of solid is captured in the space between vanes and discharged while preventing gas from passing into the solids storage vessel.

Static mixer: series of specially shaped elements inserted in a pipe to divide and recombine a flowing stream in order to make it homogeneous.

Sterile: the absence of microorganisms.

Sterilize: to remove all microorganisms using heat or chemicals.

Stochastic process: an operation in which chance or probability helps to determine results.

Temperature driving force: temperature difference in heat exchangers between hot fluid and cold fluid.

Vortex: whirlpool-like motion of fluid being agitated in a vessel.

Appendix V: Short Discussions of Various Topics, based on the Processing Column in *Food Technology*, published by the Institute of Food Technologists 2002–2006

Practical Design, Construction and Operation of Food Facilities
ISBN: 978-0-12-374204-9

Topics concerning design and commercialization

Pilot plants

Pilot plants are generally relatively small-scale operations in which new processes and products are tested and developed as a step in scale-up and commercialization, but they can also be used for teaching, research and demonstration. Each of these missions has certain implications for designing and equipping a pilot plant.

When more than one mission exists, some confusion can result.

How food companies use them

Many food companies have had pilot plants for years and certain traditions tend to accrete around them. For example, a company that processes seasonal crops, such as tomatoes, may have a tradition of processing each new crop on a small scale into a range of products, such as juice, sauce, and paste. The stated purpose is to identify any issues that the manufacturing plants might encounter in the new season. The pilot products are evaluated for solids, acid, taste, color and texture.

One might ask if the same scouting purpose might equally be accomplished by fundamental measurements on the raw material. Is it necessary to demonstrate every manufacturing step and produce a final product? One answer might be that yes, it is necessary to uncover unknown or non-obvious consequences of weather, variety changes or cultivation. Another answer might be that more fundamental measurements in the laboratory, combined with years of experience, could suffice.

Pilot plants can be expensive to build, equip and operate, so such questions are being asked more often, especially with consolidations that lead to closing of older laboratories and pilot plants and the question of what, if anything, to build in replacement.

For academic purposes, maximum flexibility is important, while in an industrial setting, less flexibility may be required. A consequence of flexibility is the influence on design, especially of utility systems. Where equipment is relatively fixed in location and function, electric power, steam, water, gas and air may be hard-piped or -wired. Controls can be centralized and maybe even automated. In a more flexible pilot plant, utility connections are provided in clusters evenly distributed around the perimeter of the room.

Likewise, floor drains should be evenly distributed where wet processes may occur, while with more fixed equipment, drains can be tailored to the need and even eliminated in some cases. Proper drainage implies sloping floors, which then requires that equipment have adjustable legs that can be used to level the equipment.

An industrial pilot plant should have sanitary design features appropriate to its use. A good principle is that dry processing areas should be kept dry, while liquid processing areas should be designed to drain well and to resist the strong cleaning agents often used in sanitation. Since food produced in an industrial pilot plant may be consumed by people in small market tests, the facility should comply with Good Manufacturing Practices. If products contain more than 2% meat or poultry, the facility must comply with US Department of Agriculture (USDA) regulations and probably needs to acquire its own establishment number, meaning that it has passed inspection by USDA. If the products made involve fruit juice, seafood, meat or poultry, the facility needs a hazard analysis critical control point (HACCP) plan, according to Food and Drug Administration (FDA) regulations.

Clearly, there are some design and operation consequences of manufacturing food for human consumption in a pilot plant. These inconveniences are offset by the ability to manufacture relatively small quantities, compared to the capability of a full-scale plant. Furthermore, it is well to realize that a pilot plant, in development mode, is intended to produce a lot of waste as the team learns how to make something new. It is better to do this on a small scale than on a large one.

Architectural finishes and details should be representative of those used in good practice on an industrial scale. This can be a challenge when the design professionals are experienced in laboratory, office and classroom design, but not industrial factory design. There are different practices in facility design for dairy, meat, baking, fruit and vegetable, candy and snack processing.

Good general choices include epoxy floor and wall finishes, stainless-steel drains, culinary steam supply, treated potable water and water resistant electrical outlets, as examples.

Finding the right equipment

Almost every pilot plant, academic or industrial, will have some or all of the following: jacketed kettles of several sizes (5–100 gal), positive-displacement and centrifugal pumps of several sizes (usually mounted on movable carts), several heat exchangers (plate, triple tube, shell and tube), plate dryer, freeze dryer, retort, clean-in-place (CIP) skid, ice cream freezer and/or a selection of valves, pipe fittings and sanitary hoses. Some may also have some packaging equipment, such as a can closer, aseptic bag filler or pouch filler and sealer. Support equipment includes bench scales, floor scales, bench instruments (pH meter, spectrophotometer, conductivity meter), computers and temperature recorders. Most of this equipment can be found as the smallest available offerings of typical vendors. One option for teaching and research is use of small-scale equipment offered by several firms. Because small-scale equipment embodies even more engineering effort than a larger-capacity unit, they may seem relatively expensive, but they are fully integrated, often are portable and are relatively easy to operate and maintain.

Third parties are another option

For industrial concerns embarking on a new venture, doing development work at a third party location can be an attractive option. Some universities have built centers that serve both their own teaching and research needs and are available for contract work. Examples include the University of Nebraska, which has a medium sized twin-screw extruder and Purdue University, which has particular strength in aseptic processing. The Guelph Food Technology Center, Guelph, Ontario, Canada, while near a university, is an independent center with a wide range of capabilities. The National Center for Food Safety and Technology (NCFST), Summit-Argo, Ill. is operated by the Illinois Institute of Technology with substantial support from FDA and has a large pilot plant (built originally by Corn Products) with a wide variety of aseptic, high-pressure and thermal processing equipment. The National Food Laboratory in Dublin, CA is operated by the National Food Processors Association and has special expertise in thermal processing.

In using a third party, firms need to balance the inconvenience and potential risk to confidentiality against the speed, cost savings and potential contribution of skills available at the center. With an outside center, there often are specialized skills and experience available to contract users. In the case of NCFST, there is the potential for direct collaboration with FDA scientists who may have a role in approving a novel preservation process.

Pilot plants are worth the investment

It may seem hard to justify the capital and operating costs of a proper pilot plant and, in fact, many food companies have closed the ones they had. But this may be a very short-sighted decision, driven by an inadequate understanding of costs and benefits.

Types of pilot plants

As discussed previously, academic institutions, food companies and equipment suppliers might have different types of pilot plants. The emphasis in a university is on education, research and service. Its pilot plant, if it has one – as many food science and agricultural engineering departments do – must be flexible, with plenty of plug-in utilities and roll-in/roll-out equipment. Often, depending on the institution's history, the pilot plant may focus on a specific industry such as dairy, baking or soy processing. Some universities have had a tradition of manufacturing food products, such as cheese, ice cream and sausage, which they sell to students and local residents.

Chemical engineering departments often have a unit operations laboratory, which is rarely much of a pilot plant in the sense that its equipment usually cannot be connected to form all or most of a process. Rather, the usual focus is on study and operation of an isolated single piece of equipment, such as a dryer, distillation column or chemical reactor. Equipment suppliers often have pilot plants intended to demonstrate the equipment they make. To do so well, they may have some supporting equipment, such as mixing tanks, conveyors, scales and pumps. Users of such facilities usually must provide their own raw materials, labor and packaging material (if used). The equipment manufacturers often provide technicians and commonly charge a fee for use of the facility. Such facilities may have some flexibility, but are often fairly spartan, as they may occupy a corner of a fabrication plant or shop and so may not provide a typical food processing environment. However, they are usually adequate for targeted testing, especially of equipment that is new to a potential customer.

Food companies can face daunting challenges in designing a good pilot plant, because of the wide variety of processes and products in which they are interested and the multiple and conflicting missions that may be assigned to the pilot plant. Usually, a food company pilot plant is the responsibility of a process development group (if there is one), the product development group or the engineering group. Ideally, each of these groups should exist and all should have an interest in the pilot plant.

Proper scale of a pilot plant

A perennial debate occurs over the desirable scale of an industrial pilot plant and how much it should resemble a production facility. On the one hand, small-scale equipment is easy to operate and clean, though it is not necessarily much less expensive than a larger unit. Some small-scale equipment can simulate multiple processes and thus may represent a cost saving over having multiple lines. However, for some operations, small-scale equipment may not exist. In other cases, such as cooking screw extrusion, scale-up from small to larger sizes may be unreliable.

One possible use of a pilot plant is manufacture of supplies of a new product for testing at various levels – central location, home use and controlled markets. Larger and longer tests may require substantial quantities of product, which can severely tax the capabilities of what otherwise is properly seen as a research facility. The culture and skills of research technicians are quite different from those of manufacturing staff.

Some food firms address this issue with a specialized type of pilot plant, often called a semi-works, which has more of a manufacturing atmosphere. It is usually intended to be the temporary home of a given process until the fate of a new product or line is determined. A good semi-works is basically a large room with utilities and drains into which a small, integrated line can be installed and then later removed, to be replaced with the next project. Often, a separate packaging area is provided, which may not change much if a company's products can use a common packaging approach.

Assuming that larger production runs are usually accomplished elsewhere – in a plant or semi-works – then the primary focus of a good industrial pilot plant is development. One consequence is that there will be a lot of waste, because it is normal in development to learn by trial and error and to experience frequent failure. This is one powerful reason to avoid doing development work at large scale in a manufacturing facility.

Challenges of using a production plant

In many companies where a good pilot plant does not exist, it is common to do formulation work on a lab bench top and then go directly to a plant trial. This produces a number of consequences. First, research personnel must get to the plant site, which for some reason seems often to be remote. Second, the plant must free up a line, provide staff and obtain any special materials, such as novel ingredients.

It is not uncommon that the line needs to be modified in some way. For example, the packaging machines to which a line normally delivers products may not be appropriate or an additional operation may need to be inserted. Third, the plant will charge back to research the material and labor costs of one or more shifts. It is common for commercial food lines to produce thousands of pounds of product per hour and to require 6–10 people. Even for foods based on flour or corn, thousands of pounds costs multiple hundreds of dollars. With more expensive ingredients, such as meat, the cost is obviously still higher.

Some plants are so tightly scheduled that the only times available for tests are weekends on which labor costs may carry a premium. Working and traveling on weekends can also be stressful for the research people involved. With all these costs and challenges, the costs for using plants for development are still understated because they ignore the lost opportunity costs of not using the plant for commercial production. This arises from the difference between an accounting perspective and an economic perspective. So long as the company could sell profitably any product it can make – and today that is likely to be true – the true cost of conducting development in a plant is the lost profit on the sale of the product it did not make.

Where the cost of materials for thousands of pounds may be multiple hundreds of dollars, the value of thousands of pounds of product is certainly thousands of dollars – an order of magnitude larger. Baking and snack lines can produce 3000–5000 lb of product/hour. These often have values of \$2–3/lb. A lost shift means lost income of \$48 000–120 000. If a company has six developers and each does about 15 plant trials/year, the lost income could be \$4.3–10.8 million/year.

Now, some plant trials always need to be performed and there are costs associated with running a pilot plant but, even when these costs are recognized, it is not hard to justify a substantial investment in a decent pilot plant.

A significant design issue besides scale is the degree of integration required. In many cases, sequential batch operation may be a reasonable approach. For example, most bread and cake products are still developed by batch mixing, rounding, proofing, forming (or depositing) and baking in deck or rotary ovens. At a commercial level, transfers are automatic and baking is in continuous conveyor ovens. Some fine-tuning may be required on translation from the lab or pilot plant to the full scale, but it usually goes smoothly. At another extreme, a near-full-scale aseptic processing and packaging unit might be needed because there is such integration among product treatment, package material sterilization and filling-space sterilization and protection. Some aspects of aseptic processing can be simulated with available small-scale equipment, primarily for product development, but some of the more important challenges are only seen on production equipment.

Worthwhile investment

It requires a good understanding of a company's core technologies to design a proper pilot plant, but the effort is almost always worth the investment because of the increased income, more efficient research and development (R&D) and reduced stress on both R&D and plant staff.

Scaling-up food processes

Scale-up is the task of producing an identical, if possible, process result at a larger production rate than previously accomplished (Valentas et al., 1991, p. 233).

Scale-up usually, but not always, requires experimentation at two scales, though not necessarily at the scale that is targeted. The key objective is to identify a criterion that remains constant regardless of scale. An example is the ratio

$$t/m^{2/3} \qquad \text{(A.1)}$$

where,

t is the time required, s, to reach a given internal temperature and
m is mass, kg.

This ratio remains constant in cooking objects of different mass but essentially the same geometric shape, such as a turkey or roast.

This result can be derived from fundamental principles of heat transfer and geometry, but often experimental data must be manipulated to derive the appropriate criterion. If the underlying physics and chemistry of a process are understood, the scale-up criteria may be known or a form suggested. In the fields of heat transfer, mass transfer and fluid flow, there are well-established criteria known as dimensionless numbers with such names as Prandtl, Nusselt, Sherwood and Reynolds. These typically combine important parameters in such a way that the units or dimensions cancel and thus are independent of scale.

One of the best-known dimensionless numbers is the Reynolds number for fluid flow, which is defined as:

$$N_{Re} = LV\rho/\mu \qquad (A.2)$$

where,
L is some characteristic dimension, such as pipe diameter, m
V is fluid velocity, m/s
ρ is fluid density, kg/m^3 and
μ is viscosity, Pa.s (which has units of kg/(m.s).

For flow through a pipe, if the Reynolds number is below about 4000, the flow is laminar and above that value the flow is turbulent. This has a significant effect on residence time distribution, as in hold tubes for pasteurizers or aseptic processes, previously discussed in Appendix II. The residence time of the fastest particle in laminar flow is about half that of the average particle, while in turbulent flow, all of the fluid particles have about the same residence time. One can imagine developing a process in small-diameter tubing and then wishing to scale up to a larger flow rate and larger tubing. It is important to maintain the same Reynolds number, if possible, to ensure the same process result.

Another instance where Reynolds number is important is in cleaning of process piping. For good cleaning-in-place (CIP), it is important that the flow be turbulent. In practice, in the USA, the minimum velocity in the cleaning cycle is specified to be 5 ft/s regardless of the pipe diameter. This means that the Reynolds number is not constant at different pipe sizes, but it is more convenient and easier to enforce a constant velocity. European practice is to adjust velocity to maintain a turbulent Reynolds number but not to expend pumping power needlessly by keeping velocity constant.

Often there are secondary criteria which prevent exact scale-up. For example, in fluid flow, there may be pressure drop considerations, which prevent exact duplication. In other cases, heat transfer may not scale up in the same way that the primary process criterion does. This situation often arises when scaling a kettle cooking or cooling process because the surface-to-volume ratio of a vessel goes down as the vessel gets larger while retaining geometrical similarity. This means that heating or cooling area will not remain in proportion to the mass of contents. One solution is to provide a supplemental heat-transfer surface either external to the kettle or by adding coils inside the vessel. Coils may change the mixing pattern in the vessel and can be hard to clean. An external heat exchanger requires additional investment, addition of a pump and extra piping.

The lesson is that scale-up can be complex in even the simplest-appearing situations. What about seemingly very complex processes, such as extrusion? Screw speed is one of the most important parameters in extrusion and, combined with the number of die openings (assuming constant die shape and constant mix formula), it should be a primary experimental variable. Often, specific mechanical energy input or total energy input (mechanical and thermal) correlates well with product properties. Experimentation is still required at several scales (e.g. screw diameters in extrusion) to permit confident extrapolation to larger machines.

Solids mixing is a common operation where experimentation can occur at one scale and then be scaled up reliably. It is known that the time to mix powders to some desired degree in a given mixer is a function of the Froude number Fr, defined as:

$$Fr = N^2D/g \tag{A.3}$$

where,
N is rate of rotation, s^{-1}
D is size of the mixer, m
g is acceleration of gravity, m/s^2.

The product Nt, the number of turnovers to reach a given degree of mixing, is a function of Fr and is determined by mixing at various values of Fr, usually by varying speed. (It is assumed that degree of fill is maintained constant, usually just above 50%.)

Once the appropriate Fr is determined and fixed, then the speed at a larger scale is inversely proportional to the square root of the size. That is, as a mixer gets larger, the speed to maintain the constant Fr decreases. As a result also, the time to mix to a desired degree increases because Nt is constant. It was long believed that mix times for a given mixture remained constant upon scale-up, but this analysis shows that this is not true. There are obvious consequences in process design.

Dimensionless analysis

When theory does not suggest the appropriate correlation or scale-up criteria, dimensionless analysis may help. 'Dimensionless analysis is the method of reducing the equations that describe a process into a form containing no reference to units of measurement, that is, a dimensionless form' (Valentas et al., 1991, p. 291). Unfortunately, dimensionless analysis cannot be applied to the effect of process variables on most product qualities. The problem with product qualities is that there is no absolute scale for subjective properties, such as taste or texture. However, the technique is very useful for such properties as temperature or degree of mixing.

It is not always necessary to develop new dimensionless numbers or groups – many have been found by researchers to be useful. Tables of common dimensionless numbers are in Valentas et al. (1991, p. 320) and similar lists can be found in other textbooks. For a given problem, one selects the appropriate dimensionless numbers, knowing the expected phenomena of interest (heat transfer, mass transfer, pressure drop, etc.) and conducts experiments in which the selected groups are the parameters.

If a correlation is found, then it can be used for scale-up.

An example of a useful result from such studies is the observation that power per unit volume should remain constant in fluid mixing scale-up, if possible. Secondary issues, as previously mentioned, may prevent exact application, perhaps because additional heat-transfer surface distorts the geometrical similarity or some other consideration applies. In fluid mixing, the shape of the agitator, shape of the vessel, degree of fill and the baffling must all be similar for small-scale experimentation to apply on a larger scale.

In dough mixing, which can be very complex, development time can be identical in a small and large mixer operated at the same speed if the two mixers are geometrically identical except for scale. However, that is rarely the case.

In another analysis, it is found that the dimensionless power number:

$$N_P = P/(\rho N^3 D^5) \tag{A.4}$$

is inversely proportional to Fr (at low values of Fr) for mixers of similar geometry but different scale and the same degree of fill.

This permits measurement of power consumption at one scale and confident extrapolation to a larger scale. The result applies to such devices as pan coaters as well as typical mixers. Energy per unit mass increases at constant Fr, which may mean more damage to products at larger scale.

It is important actually to operate processes at their design conditions and to resist the temptation to overfill mixers, for instance. Most people know that clothes dry faster when a clothes dryer is not too full. Operations such as packaging usually perform better when run at something less than their theoretical maximum, because there are fewer interruptions when running at a more 'comfortable' speed. These factors, while not expressed quantitatively, can be experienced and observed in most plants.

A challenging task not often taught

Scale-up is one of the more challenging tasks facing the food engineer or food technologist. Often, the underlying physics or chemistry is not well known, though when it is, great insight may be gained with careful experimentation.

The common technique of experimental design must be carefully applied using the correct combinations of variables. Scale-up criteria and dimensionless groups convert the basic variables of temperature, time, size, power, mass and pressure drop into parameters that have no dimensions and thus apply to any scale. If an experimental design is developed with the basic variables, such as power or time, it may become distorted and less useful when the variables are combined into dimensionless groups. Many experimental designs are orthogonal, meaning they are symmetrical in the experimental parameters. After variables are converted, this convenient relationship may be distorted. It is better to develop the orthogonal design with dimensionless parameters if possible. It takes some degree of intuition and physical insight to simplify seemingly intractable scale-up problems. Much of this wisdom comes with experience, but studying pertinent examples can help in acquiring these skills. Sadly, the topic is not often taught in engineering, let alone in food science, so must be acquired on the job.

Hazard analysis

Hazard analysis in a food plant is the first step in creating a hazard analysis and critical control point (HACCP) plan. As most people know, HACCP has become the industry standard approach to ensuring food safety. It is actually mandated by federal regulation in certain industries, such as seafood, juice and meat and poultry.

Several authorities on food safety and HACCP have pointed out that simply having a HACCP plan is not sufficient to guarantee safe food. In developing countries especially, HACCP plans can be misapplied. For example, a HACCP plan in the absence of Good Manufacturing Practices (GMPs) and Sanitation Standard Operating Procedures (SSOPs) will not be effective. (IFT has produced a CDROM entitled 'Prerequisite Programs for HACCP: You Can't Start HACCP without Them' that addresses this issue.)

Foreign matter

Foreign matter may be a physical hazard, depending on the product and the results of the hazard analysis. Possible sources may be the agricultural field, the processing plant, the distribution system or intentional contamination. The twelve most commonly identified foreign substances in food are:

- glass
- metal
- stones
- wood
- jewelry
- insects
- insulation
- bone
- plastic
- personal effects
- bullets
- needles.

Any of these could, in principle, cause injury, but there are sensible provisions and/or unit operations in the process that can be taken or installed to avoid or remove them.

For example, food processing systems almost always have a cleaning step to remove field debris, such as stones, dirt and small animals. Dry processes have several stages of screening to remove foreign matter. Wood, stones and insulation are so rarely found in foods that they do not represent a serious hazard. The unit operations alluded to above will almost always eliminate such materials. Assessing the relative risk is an important practice in establishing a HACCP plan so that attention is focused where it is needed.

Bullets and needles are found in meat as a result of careless or malicious hunters and of animals flinching as they are inoculated. Manufacturers of veterinarian supplies make their needles of easily detected metal so this hazard can be found and removed.

Plastic contamination, which can occur from drum liners and other packaging, is addressed by using colored plastic. Blue is suggested because few foods are blue, so visual inspection can find pieces of plastic.

Personal effects and jewelry are normally removed by workers and visitors to avoid loss into food. Many companies do not permit breast pockets on work gowns because of the potential for things to fall into product when the employee bends over. Employees carry pens, thermometers and watches in scabbards at their waist or in inside pockets. Bandages, if they must be worn, should be colored so they can be spotted. Some plants require wearing gloves over bandages on hands.

To address the issue of intentional contamination takes good management practices and employee education. The workers on a line generally know what is happening. If they understand that their livelihood depends on the production of safe food, they may deter the actions of a disgruntled colleague. Making the work environment safe and comfortable helps also to reduce the temptation to exact revenge on the company.

Mandated critical control points

There is concern about mandated critical control points (CCPs). The original HACCP concept relied on those closest to the process to identify the potential hazards and the relevant control points. As the approach has been adopted by regulatory agencies such as the Food and Drug Administration and the US Department of Agriculture, inspectors have been refusing to accept HACCP plans that do not conform to their preconceived ideas.

For example, FDA has required that there be a CCP at receipt of bulk shelf-stable juice or high-Brix concentrate, which is to be repackaged at a site different from where they were pasteurized or sterilized. A guidance document issued in April 2003 (www.cfsan.

fda.gov/~dms/juicgui8.html) gives very specific 'suggestions' about CCPs and procedures. Apparently, these arose from at least one instance of contamination that occurred when a sealed bulk load of juice was opened incorrectly during shipping.

The normal practice in the juice industry has been to pasteurize bulk juice even though it has been previously sterilized. Juice that has been heat treated does not pose a health hazard, though fresh juice has been implicated in some food-borne illnesses.

Those incidents led to the requirement of a five-log reduction in target pathogens. Heat treatment is the easiest way to conform, but other approaches are acceptable, such as vigorous surface cleaning (for citrus fruit), high pressure and pulsed electric fields.

The meat industry is concerned about the 'zero tolerance for visible fecal matter' requirement for meat. While obviously undesirable, fecal matter is not the real hazard in meat. Invisible microbes, such as *Salmonella*, *Listeria monocytogenes* and *Escherichia coli* O157:H7 are the hazards and are not found by visual inspection.

The meat industry does not produce a sterile final product in fresh meat. Meat is intended to be cooked before eating.

Consumer advocates worry that education of food preparers can never be so effective that all hazards are eliminated. Thus, there is a tension between the industry, which wants to produce as safe a product as possible, and those who want some absolute guarantee of safety.

There have come to exist three types of HACCP: scientific HACCP, government HACCP and customer HACCP.

Scientific HACCP is the original, which uses those close to the process to identify hazards, assess risk and identify critical control points. A CCP is not very useful unless something can be measured and steps taken to correct deviations.

Government HACCP, as previously mentioned, has become a regulatory tool in which some CCPs are mandated, whether they would have been identified under a scientific approach or not. In the case of the zero-tolerance rule, for example, it is permitted to steam-pasteurize or trim away visible contamination. This does not necessarily address the invisible contamination that may or may not exist. Some meat packers are routinely adopting carcass surface pasteurization, but then measures must be taken to ensure that recontamination does not occur.

Customer HACCP occurs when a buyer insists that a supplier have a HACCP plan in place and that it include certain CCPs.

A common one is metal detection, which is, in fact, quite common but may or may not actually represent a CCP under the scientific approach. The normal operation of the process may ensure that most foreign matter is removed, so further checking might not be required. However, to satisfy a customer, most manufacturers will comply.

The problem with proliferation of CCPs is that the resulting HACCP plan can become cumbersome to manage. There exists software to help prepare HACCP plans in a systematic way, which particularly emphasize assessing risk. For example, a small exposure to *Listeria* is not dangerous to healthy adults but can be fatal to unborn children, the elderly and those with compromised immune systems. Whether measures to prevent or remove *Listeria* contamination are critical may depend on who is the target consumer for a given product. However, there is in practice a zero tolerance for *Listeria* in most foods.

Proper design is key

Proper process design is the key to hazard prevention and removal. Prevention of contamination is the first priority. Good judgment is necessary in assessing risk and focusing on correct priorities. Controlling access to unprotected food while providing opportunities for visual inspection is a challenge. Finally, any HACCP plan is dynamic. One of the critical steps is verification that it is working. If the HACCP documents are dusty, that is a good sign that it has not been revisited and adapted to changing circumstance.

Preventing and detecting foreign matter in foods

In the previous piece discussing hazard analysis were listed the 12 most common foreign substances found in food as glass, metal, stones, wood, jewelry, insects, insulation, bone, plastic, personal effects, bullets and needles. Any of these could cause injury and thus pose a hazard, but most are routinely removed by standard operations in food processing. This piece discusses each of these materials in more detail and describes some of the instrumentation available for detection.

Types of contaminants

Preventing foreign matter contamination of foods depends on understanding the source of each potential material and taking appropriate steps to prevent contamination.

Even after installing such steps, most manufacturers rely on some final inspection to ensure safe and unadulterated food.

Glass

Glass chips may be created by breaking of glass containers or by accidental breaking of light fixtures or windows. Glass containers are routinely cleaned before filling and filling lines are designed to prevent jams and bottle-to-bottle contact. Nonetheless, glass containers do break. When they do, normal practice is to stop the line, clean thoroughly and put on hold products filled before and after the break. The number of such containers (or the time period involved) is a matter of company policy. Obviously, enough must be held and reinspected to ensure safety, but such reinspection incurs cost. Increasingly, glass containers are being replaced with plastic for use with soft drinks, baby food and mayonnaise, in part because such containers are unbreakable and also lighter.

Light fixtures should have shields, usually plastic sleeves on fluorescent tubes, to prevent contamination. Other sources of glass, such as laboratory vessels, should not be permitted in food-contact areas. Normal architectural practice is not to have windows in such areas, but many existing plants do have windows and some natural light is considered desirable. Windows can have plastic panes, often made of polycarbonate, or safety glass that will not shed pieces if broken. Glass is hard to detect because it is transparent and not electroconducting. More and more companies have established both glass breakage policies and programs to inventory all glass in plants. Many buyers also mandate these programs as part of their purchasing agreement.

Metal

Metal contamination may come from metal-to-metal wear, loose machine parts, staples, broken screens, wire snipped during maintenance, tools and broken structural members. Stainless steel is the most common metal encountered in food plants, since so much equipment is made of it, but iron, copper, aluminum and mild steel can all be encountered. Proper maintenance to ensure correct clearances in close-tolerance equipment, such as pumps, and careful attention in opening bags and performing repairs can prevent some metal contamination. Fortunately, metal is relatively easy to detect.

Stones

Field stones can be a common contaminant of many raw materials, especially cereal grains. Special equipment for cereals and other seeds rely on size and density differences to remove field stones, so they rarely are found in foods. Cherry pits and fruit seeds may also be found, despite efforts to remove them. Label warnings are common for cherry pits, since the best efforts to keep them out of pie fillings and jams are still not perfect.

Wood

A common source of wood contamination is from pallets, widely used in shipping raw materials and finished goods. Pallets should be kept in good condition and many plants have a special area for repairing pallets. A good practice is to use plastic or metal pallets in food-contact areas, keeping wood pallets in shipping and receiving areas. Sifting and screening easily remove wood pieces, so wood is rarely found in food.

Jewelry

Jewelry gets into food by falling from workers or visitors. The obvious and common practice is to forbid wearing of jewelry in food-contact areas. This includes wristwatches, rings with stones (wedding bands are usually allowed), earrings, body piercings and necklaces. Fortunately, most jewelry is relatively large and often is made of metal that can be detected, but small gemstones can be more difficult to find.

Insects

Many foods, such as grains, are almost always contaminated by insects. Some insects are routinely fumigated with chemicals, but the list of acceptable agents is reduced because most are toxic or may threaten the ozone layer. Some facilities can be heat treated to kill insects, but this may require that the plant, especially control systems, be designed for extreme conditions. Carbon dioxide can be used for fumigation, but can present a hazard to workers. Flours are routinely processed through a pin mill to break up and kill insect eggs that might hatch if left alone. Powdered foods are sifted and screened to remove insect parts and the normal processes for liquid foods kill and help remove insects. There are federally mandated action levels for insect parts in foods, meaning that a minimal level is permitted, on the reasoning that complete removal is impossible.

Insulation

Fiberglass and polystyrene foam are common insulation materials found in food plants and therefore potential sources of contamination. Spray-on fireproofing may also be found. Good practice is to sheath insulation in washable sleeves and to enclose fireproofed structural members. If pieces of insulation do break off, usually they are so large that they are removed by screening or other operations.

Bone

Bone can be found in any meat or meat-containing product and can be difficult to detect. Often meat is ground, so bone chips are also relatively small and more of a nuisance than a hazard. Meat grinders have bone-removal plates that do a good job, but efforts to increase yields may mean accepting more bone than is desirable. Use of meat recovered from mechanically deboned material may increase the probability of having bone chips. There are federal standards for calcium content of such recovered material to reduce bone content. USDA does not consider the presence of chicken bones in meats a hazard, as it is natural. Some buyers may have their own standards.

Plastic

The most common source of plastic contamination in foods is probably from packaging, such as polymer bag liners for drums of ingredients, shrink wrap or stretch wrap from pallets, plastic machine parts (such as gaskets) and food wrappers from snacks. The last can be prevented by forbidding eating in a food-contact area, which is common practice. The others are prevented by care in slitting bags, careful maintenance of equipment and isolating removal of pallet wraps from use points. Plastic is usually removed by screening but can be hard to detect. More and more processors package bulk powders in blue liners, as blue is easier to see and remove. Along these same lines, many buyers mandate the use of colored plastic liner bags.

Personal effects

These may include pens and pencils falling from shirt pockets, tools, notebooks, coins and other objects. Good practice is to forbid anything loose above the waist. Many uniforms and smocks do not have shirt pockets for just this reason. Most such objects are large enough to be easily detected and removed if they do get into the food stream. If they are found, there is a chance that it is because of a deliberate act.

Bullets

Sadly, it is not uncommon for meat animals to be shot accidentally or deliberately. While wounded, they often recover and the bullet or shot may remain in the meat. Typically, the bullet or shot can be detected in several ways.

Needles

Needles get into meat when an animal twitches while receiving an injection from a veterinarian and the needle breaks off. Such needles are deliberately made of carbon steel so they can be easily detected and removed.

Detection and removal methods

The three instrumental methods of detecting foreign matter are potentiometric (conventional metal detection, using the same principle used in airline passenger screening), X-ray and optical sorting. X-ray is quickly becoming almost an industry standard because it can detect contamination by non-metallic materials, such as bone and glass.

In addition to detecting non-metallic contaminants, X-ray is often used in place of a metal detector, where metallic packaging (e.g. foil or metallized film) prevents use of a conventional metal detector or seriously compromises its sensitivity. A common example would be pies on aluminum foil trays, or cookies in metallized film bags.

Also, some products are so conductive that the sensitivity of a metal detector (especially to stainless steel) is unacceptable. X-ray detects only density differences and is not influenced by product conductivity, so it is becoming more commonly used as a 'better metal detector'.

However, X-ray has its limitations. Detection relies on sufficient density and thickness of a contaminant so that it can be seen in contrast to the bulk food. Paper, plastic and many rubbers are hard to see by any instrumental means. Some food manufacturers have chosen gasket materials, such as Viton, that are visible by X-ray. Also, both X-ray and conventional metal detection lose sensitivity as the package size increases, so most X-ray inspection is of single packages rather than cases. X-ray inspection is more expensive than conventional metal detection, but prices have decreased over the past 20 years.

Conventional metal detectors are most sensitive to mild steel contamination but can detect stainless steel and other metals. Detection sensitivity is usually described in dimensions of millimeters, typified by small ball bearings. Thus, metal dust or shavings, pins and other small pieces may escape detection. Sensitivity varies with type of metal. Ferrous metals are most easily detected, followed by non-ferrous and stainless steel. As an example, a processor might establish sensitivities for the three metals as 2.5, 3.5 and 4.5 mm, respectively. Processors need to work with equipment suppliers to ensure that they do not strive to obtain a sensitivity that an instrument cannot achieve.

There are optical sorting technologies designed to identify and remove foreign matter as well as visually defective food. The devices use laser or other light sources and cameras to detect abnormalities and direct an air blast to remove them.

In the visible range of the spectrum, 'color' determines the amount of light reflected from the product. However, in the infrared (IR) range, reflectivity is determined by the physical characteristics of the product, such as water, oil, etc. Because of the composition of their molecules, products will absorb infrared energy at specific wavelengths. In the IR range, foreign material such as white rocks and clear glass absorb large amounts of IR energy, compared to dry white beans. This allows for a clear difference and separation, irrespective of surface color.

Finally, ferrous metal, especially small particles, can be removed by in-line magnets. Several firms make magnetic separators and all use rare-earth permanent magnets. A magnet is meant to complement metal detection by other means, since it can remove particles too small to be detected, including shavings of stainless steel that become ferromagnetic by work hardening from wear. It is important when using a magnet to observe what it is catching and investigate the source of the contamination.

Food plant security

The US Department of Homeland Security (DHS), the US Department of Agriculture (USDA) and the Food and Drug

Administration (FDA) are sufficiently concerned about potential terrorist threats to agriculture and food processing that they have devoted significant portions of their recent budgets to various aspects of the issue. It is well known that inadvertent contamination of food already causes significant numbers of cases of disease and death each year. What if someone maliciously sabotages our food? What can be done to prevent this?

Known instances of agro-terrorism have been documented and helped suggest good practices for food plant security. Disgruntled employees have instigated several instances of known sabotage involving food. These are especially insidious because the employees know the plant and processes and are not usually considered suspicious. Employees are one of the first lines of defense against contamination of foods, whether deliberate or accidental. They know that their jobs may be at stake if something goes wrong. Knowing who belongs where and challenging those out of place is fundamental to good security practices.

Plants are training their employees to look for identification badges and to challenge those without them, including visitors without escorts. Different-colored uniforms are issued for those working in different areas so people who are out of place are obvious. Plant-issued uniforms usually do not have pockets, primarily so that objects do not fall out and into food, but the same practice makes carrying and delivering a contaminant more difficult. Tools such as temperature indicators, stopwatches and samplers are typically carried in holsters hung from belts. In general, employees are trained to know who and what is normal and to be proactive and confident in reporting deviations.

The principles mentioned here, and many others, can be found in recommendations published by USDA (www.usda.gov/homeland-security) and FDA (www.cfsan.fda.gov/~dms/secguid6.html).

Physical security

A perimeter fence with strictly controlled entry can be a significant line of defense. Personal vehicles, trucks and pedestrian access should be limited and guarded. Many plants now have personal vehicle parking at a distance from the plant. Trucks should be sealed at the point of loading and seals must match bills of lading to ensure that ingredients and supplies have not been tampered with en route. Out-going products are likewise sealed after loading.

Remotely operated cameras on the periphery and in internal passages are another useful tool. Cameras not only discourage malicious acts but also assist criminal investigators in identifying likely suspects after the act. Access through closed doors should be by pass codes rather than magnetic badges, because badges are easy to steal. ID tags are useful and recommended but are notoriously easy to fake. Visitors should be escorted and truck drivers should be restricted to a lounge area with their own rest rooms.

Ingredients should be obtained from trusted suppliers who have an effective security plan and chain of custody of ingredients should be routinely documented. If letters of guarantee are not provided, ingredients should be held until their suitability is confirmed. Testing is typically for identity and conformance to specifications. Many agents of interest for food defense are difficult to detect, so improvement of rapid testing is a major area of research.

During processing, food should not be exposed to the environment unless necessary. This may require adding covers to conveyors and putting lids on totes.

Remediation

Research in several areas concerning food safety and security is being conducted. One area is the impact of ordinary food preservation processes on biological contaminants other than those usually targeted. These biological agents include common food-borne organisms, such as virulent *Escherichia coli*, but also potential biological weapons such as *Bacillus anthracis* (anthrax) spores and botulinum toxin. The behavior of some agents of interest is known from government agency research but is classified and so may be redetermined by academic researchers. It is suspected that certain select agents can survive the normal pasteurization process for milk, so the dairy industry has been advised to increase its thermal treatment of fluid milk. One result is that some processors observe a perceived reduction in quality, while others note beneficial shelf life impacts. Others have found that incremental changes in processes are more consumer-acceptable than sudden changes.

Researchers have developed a mathematical model of disease spread and agency response for various scenarios of deliberate contamination. One example is intentionally contaminated ice cream mix that is shipped around the country from the Midwest. Because of the wide dispersion of the product, it takes days before consumers begin to feel ill enough to seek a doctor or emergency room. Cases are scattered, so suspicion does not immediately fall on the contaminated product. By the time government agencies realize there has been an incident, a large portion of the product is out of distribution centers and in the hands of consumers. The only remedy is to alert medical personnel and recommend treatment.

Cleaning up a plant contaminated by various agents may be a challenge. As seen in the anthrax episodes of 2001, ordinary cleaning is not sufficient. Chlorine dioxide is evidently effective against spores, as is irradiation. But irradiation is impractical for equipment and facilities and some current food plants and processes are not usually designed for easy fumigation. Chlorine dioxide, for example, is highly corrosive and can damage electrical equipment. New plants and equipment should be designed with some consideration for how they would be decontaminated if necessary.

Disposing of large quantities of contaminated food or agricultural material is also a concern. Burying food with viable microorganisms may not prevent subsequent contamination of the water supply. Incineration could cause air pollution. During a simulation of response to an outbreak of foot-and-mouth disease, which is not a threat to humans but spreads rapidly among herds, one response suggested was to destroy about 50 million cattle – at which point, someone asked where to get 50 million bullets! The point of that exercise was to challenge the assumed reaction to such a threat, recognizing that the instinctive response might do more harm than good. In the case of foot-and-mouth disease, which has not occurred in the USA, eradication could be economically devastating. One suggestion is to learn to live with it, as South American countries have done.

The broader point is that our planned response to potential incidents may need some creative thinking. A major concern of researchers thinking about various possible threats is the loss of confidence in our otherwise enviably safe food system. Thus, remediation refers not only to treating sick people, recovering contaminated products and sanitizing contaminated plants, but also to restoring trust. As seen in some accidental events, the economic impact may be even greater than the health impact.

Additional benefits

Research to prevent and recover from deliberate food contamination will benefit food processors even if the feared event never occurs. The same policies necessary to ensure that ingredients are not contaminated will also ensure that they are safe and correct. The same policies and training that have employees watching for strangers also help prevent cross-contamination by careless workers wandering around. Closing up equipment to prevent easy access to food in process also prevents contamination from dripping condensate and dust.

Understanding thermal and non-thermal preservation processes and making them more severe in some cases, should extend shelf life while providing another line of defense against deliberate contamination. Of course, preservation processes directed at biological agents may have no effect against chemical contaminants, such as pesticides and other poisons. Fortunately, it takes significant quantities of such chemicals to cause widespread harm, so precautions against unauthorized access and other measures offer protection. For example, pesticides and cleaning chemicals needed in a plant should be stored in locked rooms or closets with restricted access. Quantities should be limited and users should be trained and carefully supervised.

Measures taken to confirm employee identity and suitability, such as background checks and eligibility for work, should be current policy anyway and help to avoid difficulties with government agencies, especially regarding undocumented workers. With rapid turnover among workers in many food plants, there is concern about infiltration by terrorists. Measures taken to reduce turnover may provide the dividend of improving security as well.

Food plants are required by the Bioterrorism Act of 2002 to register with the federal government and to comply with notification procedures for imported foods and ingredients. The normal concerns about food safety are reason enough to apply the practices and policies that also help to protect against deliberate acts of sabotage.

Sanitation

Sanitation is an important part of safe operation in a food plant. The term may refer to cleaning as well as sanitizing or disinfection.

Sanitizing

Microbes on food or food contact surfaces can be reduced by removal, killed by heat or killed by chemicals. Typical chemicals are oxidizers such as chlorine compounds, ozone and peroxyacids. Chemical sanitizers must meet specific criteria. They must be non-toxic at the levels likely to encounter indirect food contact. In concentrated form, they are potential hazards to those mixing or handling them.

Oxidizing chemicals can react with organic materials, such as soils, reducing their effectiveness against target microorganisms. Some chemicals may contribute undesirable flavors or odors to foods, if used improperly. Cleaning and sanitizing depends on having adequate time, temperature and complete contact. Crevices within which microbes and dirt can hide prevent complete cleaning of surfaces, such as those of cutting boards, unless special provisions are taken, such as scrubbing or immersion.

Cleaning chemicals are often compounded with detergents and foaming agents to enhance spreading on surfaces and encourage retention.

A challenge to sanitation is the development of resistance by some organisms to some sanitizers, especially the quaternary ammonia compounds. Those sanitizers that kill and then rapidly disappear (oxidizers) seem to create less opportunity for resistance to develop.

Sanitation Standard Operating Procedures (SSOP)

Written Sanitation Standard Operating Procedures (SSOP) are mandated by Federal regulation wherever Hazard Analysis Critical Control Point (HACCP) plans are required. Currently, seafood, juices and most meat and poultry plants must have HACCP plans and soon the entire food industry will have them as well. This means that all these plants need SSOPs as well.

An SSOP documents the chemicals, concentrations, application methods and timing for every part of the plant. Enclosed vessels and piping systems may be cleaned in place (CIP) under automatic control, while other types of equipment require cleaning out of place (COP), which typically means careful washing by hand. External surfaces are typically cleaned with portable spray equipment.

A cleaning and sanitizing regimen may involve several steps, such as rinsing, washing with alkali, rinsing, washing with acid, rinsing and sanitizing. Neutral detergents may be used in some applications. Because soils, equipment design and specific microbial flora vary from plant to plant and among industry segments, preparing a cleaning and sanitation plan, choosing chemicals and writing SSOPs may require outside expert assistance. This assistance is often provided by the suppliers of cleaning chemicals as part of their sales effort.

Some proprietary cleaning and sanitizing agents are based on peroxyacetic acid. The peroxyacetic acid compounds break down to acetic acid, octanoic acid and water and are used at such low concentrations that there is no residual vinegar flavor. There are computer-controlled formulation and dispensing systems, which keep track of amounts used, help prevent over or under use and can inform management that cleaning procedures are in fact being followed.

Ozone

Ozone (O_3) is a relatively unstable and very reactive compound formed by the action of electricity on oxygen. It is familiar as the source of the distinctive odor associated with thunderstorms, where it is formed by lightning strikes. It is also formed in the atmosphere by the action of chemical pollutants impacted by ultraviolet radiation from the sun. Because it is toxic, it is used as an indicator of air quality. Higher up in the atmosphere, it helps to shield life on earth from excessive ultraviolet radiation by absorbing much of the radiation before it can do damage to us.

Ozone can be used as a sanitizer for food contact surfaces and direct food rinsing. Ozone is approved as a sanitizer for contact with food and food equipment because it is effective against many microbes and leaves no residue after it reacts and decomposes. Unlike another strong oxidizer, chlorine, ozone does not react with organic materials to produce undesirable compounds and does not leave an unpleasant taste. Thus, ozone has begun to replace chlorine in treating drinking water, processing water for reuse and wastewater (after treatment) before discharge. Most bottled water is treated with ozone, again because it is effective while not affecting taste.

Ozone is a strong oxidizer but, since it is applied at much lower doses than chlorine, is not as aggressive as chlorine in causing corrosion. In testing, ozone has been found to be equivalent in antimicrobial kill rates to 200 times the concentration of chlorine. Extensive testing and installed plants for produce washing applications have had very favorable results (with one possible exception being mushroom washing).

Ozone is used in aquaculture to disinfect water and assist in filtration; in cooling-tower water to reduce fouling; in bottled water; and in many areas of food processing. In poultry processing, for example, ozone is used to purify the drinking water for chickens, to reduce airborne disease in chicken houses, to disinfect the chill water in a slaughter plant and to disinfect the slicing equipment. Often, it is necessary to combine other treatments, such as cleaning, with ozone to remove competing organic material.

Ozone has been used to deactivate pathogens on potatoes. Currently, potatoes are not usually treated before storage and so may suffer deterioration due to pink rot, soft rot and silver scurf. High concentrations of gaseous ozone applied as the potatoes are conveyed to storage can reduce the incidence of the pathogens. The ozone is applied in a covered conveyor.

Shell eggs can be pasteurized by a mild heat treatment (58°C for 40 min). The eggs are not cooked, but do show turbidity in the whites. When heated at a lower temperature for about half the time and then exposed to gaseous ozone under pressure, the eggs show more than 6 log reduction in inoculated *Salmonella* with less turbidity. It is believed that the heat treatment improves the permeability of the shell to ozone and that the ozone then reacts with the microbes. It may be that the lethal action of ozone is from free radicals made by interaction with other materials or with the microbes themselves, as well as the reactive oxygen radical released by ozone as it decomposes.

Not all applications of ozone work well. Oxidizing sanitizers such as ozone are indiscriminate in their attack on organic material and so can be consumed by extraneous organic material. Attempts to reduce the spread of pathogens among cattle by treating drinking water with ozone failed because of the high load of spilled feed in the water. Surface treatment of meat failed because the ozone bleached the color from the meat. Ozone reacts differently with various materials. For example, phenolics and flavor compounds in juice concentrates are very reactive, which means that ozone may not be very effective in pasteurizing such materials. On the other hand, egg albumin and high-fructose corn syrup (HFCS) are less reactive, which helps explain why the egg process works.

To generate ozone, there are units that concentrate oxygen from air using pressure swing absorption (PSA), some that use air directly and others that feed pure oxygen from another source. The most common is PSA, because the feed gas must be dried anyway (to prevent formation of undesirable by-products in the electrochemical reaction forming ozone) and the drying process is essentially the same as the concentration process. In aquaculture, where densities of fish or shrimp may be very high, pure oxygen may be available anyway, because it is used to keep the fish or shrimp alive and so can be used to generate ozone. Finally, in salt-water aquaria, it is desirable to preserve clarity by minimizing formation of small bubbles, so making ozone from air is preferred.

Any ozone system uses electricity to generate the feed gas, which may be air or oxygen concentrated from air, and the ozone. The ozone is used as a gas or is contacted with water for application. Care must be taken to ventilate the equipment properly as released ozone can be irritating to workers.

Another application is to release gaseous ozone in cold storage rooms to control molds and eliminate ethylene, which stored produce releases, and which can accelerate ripening in fruits and vegetables. Ozone is not a panacea or magic bullet, but it is a powerful and useful tool in the battle for food safety.

Antimicrobial coating for steel

A novel approach to sanitizing surfaces is to coat them with an antimicrobial substance. One coating contains an inorganic antimicrobial compound, a zeolite containing silver ions. The zeolite is suspended in an epoxy coating. The coating is applied to sheet steel on a coil coating line, which can coat miles of steel at a time. The coating is cured and then the coil is slit and cut to produce standard size steel blanks. These blanks or sheets are used to fabricate such products as insulated panels, food service equipment, air handling systems and ductwork.

The initial applications are in hospitals and clean rooms, but there is great potential in food plants. The compound does curb microbe growth. Ceilings are good candidates for application of the coating where condensation might occur, as in meat plants. Drip pans under cooling units have been notorious sources of potential microbial contamination.

The zeolite coating has the added benefit on stainless steel of reducing the impact of fingerprints. A humble but effective application for the coated thin sheet is push plates on rest room doors, spots that often become contaminated and may not be routinely included in cleaning and sanitation.

Methods are only as good as the human who uses them

Cleaning and sanitation may rely on some sophisticated chemistry, but they are only as good as the humans who execute the procedures. Specially coated steel takes some of the human element away, but food contact surfaces will still need to be cleaned, often by a person with a hose and a brush. Protection of the worker as well as the consumer is critical, especially from chemicals, which can be toxic. An additional complication is the sad fact that sanitation is often a low-paid position relegated to the late shift, with little supervision. Tools that document usage and control formulas help compensate for what may be low skill levels.

Waste treatment

Food and beverage plants can produce large quantities of relatively strong wastewater. Water is used in recipes and for washing raw materials, transporting materials in flumes, cleaning equipment, raising steam and cooling. Compared to sanitary wastewater generated by homes and apartments, industrial wastewater in general, and food wastewater in particular, is typically more concentrated in dissolved and suspended solids and more variable in flow and pH. Food wastewater may also be high in fats, oil and grease (FOG), which are of special concern because they can solidify and choke sewer lines.

Wastewater is traditionally characterized by biological oxygen demand (BOD), which is measured in the laboratory by culturing a sample with a population of microorganisms for five days. The reduction of oxygen in streams due to consumption of organic matter can lead to fish kills. Sanitary wastes often have BOD values of about 200 mg/l (same as parts per million), while food wastes can exceed 1000 mg/l. Chemical oxygen demand (COD) is an alternative measure that is faster to perform and usually gives a higher value because it includes some matter that may resist biological oxidation. Total suspended solids (TSS) is measured by filtration. Values of pH in food wastes can range widely because both acids and bases are often used in cleaning.

Wastewater cannot be discharged directly to a stream unless it has BOD, TSS, FOG and pH values essentially the same as those of the stream or even lower. Thus, something must be done to remove the organic matter and otherwise purify the water.

First reduce and segregate

Most food plants use more water than they must and could dramatically reduce their use if they tried. Doing so should be the first step in addressing a wastewater issue. Start by identifying all points of water use. It can be a surprise to discover, for instance, that there are small but steady streams of water flowing on filling machines to wash away spills. Perhaps these can be converted to intermittent sprays or mists or even turned off entirely. An ice cream plant saved about 12 000 gal/day by using a different filler with less water consumption.

Too often in food plants, hoses are left running because they do not have a shutoff valve on the end. These same hoses are used to chase spills to a drain. Hoses should have 'dead man' valves so that they only run when attended. Spills should be cleaned with scoops or shovels when possible. Most plants could probably use fewer hoses, but taking them out can be unpopular.

Water used for cooling is rarely contaminated but may be mixed with other wastes, adding to discharge volumes. It often is economical to install a cooling tower and recirculate cooling water. Finally, it may be effective to reuse water before finally discharging it. In one case, a clam processor used fresh water in several washing steps, including on freshly caught, muddy clams in the shell. By modifying the flow so fresh water was used on the final clam pieces and then the same water in counter-current flow, volume was reduced by a factor of three.

Municipal treatment

If the community in which a plant is located has sufficient treatment capacity, the most convenient approach is to discharge to that facility. There almost always is a fee for this service and there may be restrictions on waste volume and strength. Water conservation, as mentioned, should always be practiced, but may be essential where treatment capacity is limited. Some pretreatment may also be needed, especially for FOG.

Process wastewater and sanitary wastewater should flow through separate lines until outside the plant, where there should be an air break or catch basin, which can also function as a grease trap. This prevents contamination of the process area by backflow in the event of a blockage or flood. Floating grease is periodically removed and disposed of in landfill or by other means.

Land application

When a food plant is sufficiently isolated and has adequate land, it may safely dispose of wastewater by spraying it on land planted in grass or other cover crop. Wind, temperature and soil permeability all affect how much land is required and how well the system works. Seasonal canneries often used land application because they were frequently in rural areas and operated mostly during warm weather. As housing encroaches on once isolated plants, there can be complaints about odor and spray carryover.

Conventional treatment

Conventional wastewater treatment involves applying the natural processes of physical separation and oxidation in controlled circumstances to produce an effluent that is acceptable for discharge to the environment. There are many variations, but a common sequence is primary settling, in which heavy and light suspended matter is separated by gravity; followed by secondary aeration, in which BOD is consumed by microorganisms supplied with air, typically by strong agitation; followed by clarification, in which the microorganisms are separated by gravity to produce sludge and clear effluent. This process is called activated sludge because the sludge contains the microbes that are doing most of the oxidation.

Some processes use tertiary treatment, in which the effluent may be polished by powdered or activated carbon; filtered through sand or membranes; chlorinated or ozonated; or otherwise further treated. Disposal of sludge is a major issue because the microbes are highly hydrated and hard to concentrate – sludge can be only 1% solids. Some sludge is recycled to keep the process operating, but some must be wasted. It can be dried, spread on land, or digested using anaerobic treatment, in which air is excluded. Instead of oxidizing organic matter to carbon dioxide and water, as in aerobic treatment, anaerobic digestion produces methane and carbon dioxide. The mixture can be burned as an energy source to fuel a boiler or dryer.

Proprietary treatment processes

Conventional wastewater treatment, as briefly described here, is rarely a good choice for a food plant that must pretreat or fully treat its wastewater, because it requires a large amount of space, takes skill and training to operate and generates large volumes of bulky sludge. Some better choices are proprietary treatment processes that are more compact and often produce useful by-products. Here are a few representative examples.

Physical separation

Suspended solids also contribute to BOD and FOG, so physical removal can be an effective treatment option. However, conventional filtration may be difficult because the typical organic material is hydrated, has small particle size and may plug many filter media. One approach is to dissolve air in the waste under pressure or disperse fine bubbles. The bubbles of released dissolved air attract particles and float to the surface, where the scum is skimmed.

Aerobic treatment

A *membrane biological reactor* (MBR) retains the microorganisms at a much higher concentration than is possible in the typical aeration reactor/clarifier combination. This is expressed as the mixed liquor suspended solids value (MLSS) and is 15 000 mg/l in the MBR, compared to 2000–5000 in conventional activated sludge systems. The membranes are placed close together in a tank above an air diffuser. Bubbles provide the air and help keep the membrane surface clear. The membranes are porous enough that effluent moves through by gravity or is assisted by a suction pump.

About every 10 min, liquid flow is interrupted to allow the air bubbles to scour the membrane surface. About twice a year, the membranes are cleaned chemically with sodium hypochlorite. Membranes last 5–8 years if maintained well.

Anaerobic treatment

The anaerobic *mobilized film technology* (MFT) is an advancement of a technology, in which microbes are attached to small-diameter, inert media in an enclosed reactor. Within the system, the high density of microorganisms (20 000–80 000 mg/l) allows for ultra-high treatment rates and efficiencies. Biogas, mostly methane, is recovered from the top of the chamber. With rising fuel costs, the biogas can have significant value and is used in co-generation and to replace natural gas in boilers.

Co-manufacturing

Using third-party services – referred to as co-manufacturing or co-packing – for some or all parts of the food supply chain has been a significant element of food companies' strategy for many years. One example is renting warehouse space on a long- or short-term basis. Another is contracting for special packaging, such as promotional bundling (e.g., six-packs of soup) or addition of stickers. Many marketing-oriented firms had some or all of their products made by other companies. In recent years, as all parts of the supply chain are scrutinized for cost savings, both the use of third parties and the possibility of performing such services have become more common topics of conversation within food companies. Here are some of the issues and influences affecting such discussions.

Why does co-manufacturing make any sense?

One way to improve return on assets is to have fewer assets while maintaining income. Thus, if a third party has underutilized and appropriate assets and is willing to use them for a fee to manufacture someone else's product, both the customer and the asset owner are better off than they would be if the customer were forced to invest in new equipment and facility. This is the essential reason why co-manufacturing makes sense. However, each of the conditions mentioned can be significant, and additional factors can apply, as will be discussed later.

Several categories of products are good candidates for co-manufacturing:

- New products, with their risk of failure and the possibility that the developing company does not have appropriate manufacturing capacity (because the product is new)
- Well-established products that do not have a highly proprietary process
- Intermediate products, such as bakery premixes or products that can be made in bulk and packaged separately
- Specially packaged products, such as those for club stores or those carrying a promotional premium

- Products whose manufacture in a plant might interfere with other operations, such as those with strong odors or kosher products not acceptable for Passover use produced near Passover-certified products.

Co-manufacturing may also be driven by the ability to get to market faster, so long as the appropriate capacity is available. Almost always, especially for new products, there may need to be some investment, in packaging for instance. Who pays for that and how the costs are recovered are topics for negotiation. Co-manufacturers charge a fee for their services that covers labor, energy, overhead, amortization and profit. Raw materials and packaging materials may be provided by the customer or by the co-manufacturer. There is always tension concerning fees between the conflicting ambitions of the co-manufacturer and the customer. The customer wants the lowest cost possible. The co-manufacturer wants to earn a fair profit. Both need to earn a return on the assets employed. The co-manufacturer also bears some risk for the quality of the product and the working capital used to purchase supplies.

In a broad sense, the costs of self-manufacture and co-manufacture should be comparable, but there are some subtle factors. Some co-manufacturers have lower labor and overhead costs than large food companies. Existing assets probably have lower book value than new assets would have. Some co-manufacturers, often privately held, may accept a lower return than a large, public company. Owned assets generate depreciation, which is a positive cash flow, whereas, paying for another's assets, as a component of a fee, is a pure expense. Thus, the economic impact of having a product made by a third party may be positive, negative or neutral.

Co-manufacturing should be distinguished from private label manufacturing, though there are similarities. Private label often refers to food and grocery products that carry a store label or a label other than a national brand. The products are often made by relatively small food companies that offer a range of formulas within a family of products, e.g., soups, sauces, juices or cookies. Sometimes, large, branded manufacturers will offer their products for private label or 'generics'. One distinction is that most private label manufacturers prefer not to develop special products for each customer, but rather offer what they normally make. Co-manufacturers, on the other hand, usually are given formulas and processes by their customers.

Co-manufacturers usually have a specific skill set, such as dry blending, sifting and packaging of food and pharmaceutical ingredients. Customers of co-manufacturers have become more demanding through more-frequent and more-stringent customer audits, third-party inspections and certifications. Some co-manufacturers will buy or build facilities if they do not have existing capacity or space. Experienced co-manufacturers believe they can design, build and operate facilities at lower costs and more quickly than their customers can because of differences in culture and organization, among other reasons. Some facilities are dedicated to one customer, while others have multiple customers.

How to find a co-manufacturer

Many potential co-manufacturers advertise in professional and trade journals. They usually list their specializations – spray drying, dry mixing, pouch packing, extrusion, baking, etc. Many belong to various trade associations, but there does not appear to be one just for co-manufacturing. As mentioned earlier, large branded companies may agree to co-manufacture or may offer existing products under private label. Ordinarily, one's first interest, after finding a few candidates, is to establish that sufficient appropriate capacity is available. For instance, many firms make frozen or refrigerated dough and pastries, but most of them do not have ovens and so cannot co-manufacture a fully baked product. There are many small and medium sized bakeries, but few of them have freezing capacity, so they might not be suitable for a frozen, baked product. On the other hand, a firm making frozen pizzas might easily convert some assets to make frozen baked cake. One has to be creative. If time is less of a factor, then building or acquiring may be an option. A consultant may be useful in maintaining confidentiality while conducting a search for a co-manufacturer or in evaluating one's capability.

The overall concern of customers of co-manufacturers is quality. Price is significant, of course, and negotiations can be contentious, but once all parties understand the real costs and relative risks, it is usually possible to reach a fair arrangement. Customers agonize about losing control of products that carry their brand, so the best co-manufacturers have scrupulous quality and logistics systems. Some integrate their computer systems with customers so the co-manufacturer assumes responsibility for scheduling runs, ordering supplies and delivering product where it is needed.

In contrast, an older vision of a co-packer used to be an entrepreneur with a ribbon blender in his garage and the ability to fill drums or kraft bags.

Such a small operation would be hard-pressed to meet the requirements of inspections by the American Institute of Baking and the Food Processors Association today, let alone provide the range of services and the sophistication that the large co-manufacturers do.

Topics concerning unit operations and selected industries

Freezing

A number of interesting developments are occurring in the area of freezing research and applications.

Ice cream processing and formulation

A new process for ice cream, ultra-low-temperature ice cream (ULTICE), began with the observation that in conventional ice cream, about 40% of the water is frozen when the mixture exits a scraped-surface freezer at about 21°F (−6°C). The rest of the water is frozen in a hardening tunnel at about −40°F (−40°C), which leads to relatively large ice crystals, because it is frozen while static, and a rough texture. Fully frozen ice cream is still plastic, meaning it can be pumped and frozen at much lower temperatures, with agitation, giving smaller ice crystals and better texture.

A twin-screw extruder cooled with liquid nitrogen is used as a freezer. The mix is fed by pump and kept under pressure so that entrained air is retained. Exit temperatures are close to 0°F (−18°C) and no further hardening is needed, but the ice crystals formed are small because of the agitation provided by the extruder. Traditional hardening tunnels have significant capital costs and consume energy. Not only does ULTICE, as the process is called, give an improved product, but it also uses less energy.

Natural ice modifying proteins can be used as food ingredients in frozen products. These are the compounds that enable fish to survive in Arctic waters and plants to tolerate cold. They can be nucleating or anti-nucleating in their effects. At low concentrations in ice cream, they can prevent recrystallization of ice, but at higher concentrations they may negatively affect texture by promoting non-spherical crystals.

Versatile freezing equipment

Equipment developed originally for ice cream hardening has found important new applications. The automated tray freezer system has found applications in the poultry and bakery industries. The system has several decks or paths through a large freezer box. An automated loader can read bar codes and deliver packages to any of the decks. Each deck can have a different residence time, hence the name VRT, for variable residence time. Most applications are for cases or other relatively large packages, which might otherwise be frozen in static blast freezers.

Static freezers require considerable labor to load and unload. To get high density, they are closely packed, which can inhibit air flow and may require that all packages receive the longest residence time required by any size. Residence time is related to size by about the square of the characteristic dimension.

Thus the advantage of the VRT system is that each package size gets the residence time it requires. The same system can handle various size packages, which are sorted as they are discharged. The system also reduces freezing time by providing high air velocities and good exposure to the cooling air. Compared to a static blast freezer, the VRT machine is more expensive to build, but it offers savings in labor and energy costs and helps with order tracking.

Research in freezing

Air impingement heat transfer, which has been applied in baking and other ovens, is being applied to freezing. Air impingement uses nozzles to direct cold air at 30–40 m/s at the surface of pieces to be frozen. The concept is to reduce the insulating boundary layer at the surface, which controls the external removal of heat. It does not affect the internal heat transfer, which is by conduction and which depends on the thermal conductivity of the material. By reducing the external heat transfer resistance, the approach ensures that the rate is governed solely by the internal properties, which should then give the fastest freezing rate.

Fast freezing normally gives the highest quality by reducing moisture loss and by forming small ice crystals, which do less damage to texture. Tests on hamburger patties have shown positive effects on quality. Optimizing air-impingement freezing can be complex, as it is sensitive to the distance from nozzle to food, to velocity and to the pattern of nozzles.

Cryogenic freezing involves the use of liquid nitrogen and liquid carbon dioxide to remove heat from foods. Industrial gas companies provide both equipment and cryogenic gases. Cryogenic freezing equipment is normally less expensive than mechanical refrigeration equipment because it does not require the compressors, evaporators and condensers of a mechanical system. However, the operating cost of cryogenic freezers is usually higher because one must continuously buy the gas. The cost is sensitive to the cost of electricity, since operating the liquefaction compressors is the major cost. Relative supply and demand of the cryogenic gases and of oxygen, which is separated from air when liquid nitrogen is produced, also affect prices.

Which gas to use depends on the application and, usually, local costs. Sometimes nitrogen is plentiful and inexpensive because it is produced as a by-product of purifying oxygen for steel making or other industrial processes. Sometimes carbon dioxide is available from fermentation or from ammonia plants.

Cryogenic freezing equipment is tailored to the gas. Most of the cooling with nitrogen comes from sensible heat, so the liquid is injected counter-currently to the product flow and warmed vapor is exhausted near the entrance of the typical tunnel. With carbon dioxide, the heat removal is by sublimation of the dry ice snow, so the liquid is injected concurrently with the food and vapor is exhausted near the exit. Both gases can displace oxygen, causing an asphyxiation hazard if they are not properly exhausted.

Cryogenic freezing is especially appealing when products are frozen before packaging and when weight loss is important. The very low temperatures reduce moisture loss and so increase yield. They also form small ice crystals, which usually helps quality. However, freezing too fast can have a negative impact on quality by causing stress cracking in some foods.

An interesting variation on cryogenics is an experimental system in which air is liquefied on site and used as a cryogen without separation. This makes some sense when local electricity costs are low. The benefits of low temperature are achieved without a third party or any delivery costs. On the other hand, a small liquefaction plant is probably less efficient than a larger one because of economies of scale and the greater integration of heat recovery in a large plant. In addition, this technology might be a little sophisticated for some food plants.

Drying

Drying or dehydration of foods may be one of the oldest preservation methods known. Research has been performed on it for many years and, surprisingly, it is still an active topic. Reams of paper have been used to present equations for describing drying or dehydration of foods, but still it seems that many approaching the subject struggle with understanding what occurs and how best to develop a drying process. Here is a brief tutorial.

Why dry?

One of the more obvious motivations for drying foods is to preserve perishables by reducing the water activity (a_W) below that needed by pathogens or spoilage microorganisms to grow. This level varies with the food and the microorganism but is generally below about 0.6. Water activity is related to but not equal to moisture content. It is measured experimentally and is equal to the relative humidity of the atmosphere at a given temperature with which a food material with a given moisture content is in equilibrium; i.e. neither the food nor the atmosphere changes in weight after being in contact, in a closed container, for some time.

Drying also reduces weight, may reduce volume and may cause other changes that are more or less desirable, such as color changes. For example, baking is a drying process in which color and flavor changes are desirable. For dried onions, on the other hand, the objective is to maintain a light color if possible.

Some drying processes convert a liquid into a powder that is not only more stable but also more convenient to use, such as soluble coffee or dried milk.

Drying basics

Water, or occasionally another liquid such as a solvent, is removed from a solid matrix by converting it into a vapor and removing the vapor from the chamber in which the wet material is placed. The conversion of liquid to vapor requires energy, the heat of vaporization, which for water is about 1000 BTU/lb. Delivery of this energy to the liquid requires heat transfer, which may be by convection, radiation, conduction or a combination of several mechanisms.

The heat source may be burning natural gas (or, rarely, another fuel) in air, indirect heating with steam or electricity or solar energy. Heat transfer is governed by the temperature difference between the heat source and the surface of the wet material. In the cases of conduction and convection, the rate is proportional to the temperature difference. In the case of radiation, the rate is proportional to the difference between the absolute temperatures each raised to the fourth power.

So long as there is free moisture at the surface of the material, the surface temperature is equal to the wet bulb temperature – the temperature of a water-saturated wick that is in equilibrium with the humidity of the surrounding air. This can be found from psychometric charts, which give the properties of water in air at various temperatures and humidities.

In the early stages of most drying processes, there is enough free moisture and it migrates easily enough to the surface, that the surface is 'wet' and the removal of moisture occurs from the surface. As drying proceeds and moisture is removed, the interface at which liquid is converted into vapor retreats within the wet material.

So long as the surface is wet and other conditions remain constant, the rate of removal of moisture – the drying rate – is constant. For most materials, there is a moisture content, called the critical moisture content, at which the drying rate begins to decline because of the previously mentioned retreat of the liquid–vapor interface. While not quite correct, it is useful to picture a retreating interface leaving behind, from the surface inward, a dry layer that is both a thermal insulator and a barrier to vapor diffusion.

It is the growth of this layer that causes the drying rate to decline.

The critical concept here is that there are four rate processes that can control overall drying:

- external heat transfer (from source to surface)
- internal heat transfer (from surface to liquid interface)
- external mass transfer (from surface to bulk environment, usually air)
- internal mass transfer (from interface to surface).

The exact mechanism of mass transfer inside the dried layer varies with materials and conditions and probably involves vapor diffusion, capillary diffusion of liquid and adsorption and desorption of water on the dried surface. In practice, it is usually modeled as vapor diffusion with a diffusion coefficient that is smaller than that for free diffusion in air, because of the additional resistance of the porous dried layer.

How to affect drying rates

Given this admittedly brief description of the governing rates, what can be done to affect drying rates? First, it is necessary to understand potential constraints. For economic reasons, it is common to want to achieve the highest possible drying rates, but other considerations may apply. For example, the most obvious way to increase heat transfer is to increase the temperature of the heat source. However, as previously mentioned, there may be concern about color development in certain foods, while others may scorch or burn if heated too much.

Lowering the humidity of the environment lowers the surface temperature as long as there is free water at the surface, so this can increase the temperature driving force and also increases the mass transfer driving force. However, there is a cost associated with this approach. Incoming air can be dehumidified by cooling or by using adsorbents, but then it takes additional energy to heat the cold air or regenerate the adsorbents. Air that has picked up moisture can be discharged, but that means throwing away the energy it contains. In practice, hot air is normally recirculated to save energy, but this allows humidity to build up somewhat. Enough air is discharged to exhaust the moisture that is removed, typically by adjusting dampers.

Increasing air velocity would appear to be another way to improve heat and mass transfer because heat and mass transfer coefficients typically increase with velocity. However, experimentally, air velocity usually has only a small effect on drying rate. There are also constraints on it, including the cost of operating blowers and the risk of blowing dried product off the trays or belts.

It is important to realize that temperature, humidity and velocity can only affect the external rates, while during much of a drying process the internal rates are controlling. Sadly, there is not much that can be done to affect the internal rates.

One option is to reduce the critical dimensions of the material. Thus, vegetables are sliced thinly or made into relatively small cubes. A drum dryer spreads a thin layer of liquid or paste over a heated metal drum and scrapes a dried flake off after one revolution. A spray dryer creates small droplets from liquid or concentrate, which fall through heated air and are collected as a fine powder.

Lowering the pressure by drawing a vacuum lowers the temperature at which water vaporizes and also reduces the resistance to vapor flow in the dried layer, thus increasing the drying rate. Maintaining a vacuum adds the cost of running a vacuum pump or steam ejector and, usually, of removing water from the exhausted air to reduce the load on the pump.

Drying equipment

The most common industrial dryers are conveyor or belt tunnels, which may be multipass and which often have several temperature zones, cooling zones and controls on air recirculation. Other dryer types include batch tray dryers, which may also use vacuum; drum dryers; spray dryers; fluidized bed dryers, in which air velocity is sufficient to entrain wet particles; tunnel dryers, in which trucks loaded with trays of food are pushed successively through a chamber; air impingement dryers, in which jets of heated air are directed perpendicular to the belt carrying product to be dried, to increase heat transfer; and rotating tray dryers, in which wet powders are transferred, through holes in the trays, from one tray to another with plows.

Drying equipment requirements include sanitary design, so they can be cleaned; gentle material handling, as many dried foods are fragile; energy efficiency; flexibility of control; durability; and cost effectiveness.

In spite of the extensive research on modeling, when one considers a new dryer, it is helpful to have a practical guide to design. Such a guide has been provided by Guillermo H. Crapiste and Enrique Rotstein in their chapter, Design and Performance Evaluation of Dryers in Valentas et al. (1997). Some experimental data are almost always needed, but this chapter gives adequate mathematical equations with which to correlate data and calculate drying times.

In practical terms, dryers differ in their quality of construction, uniformity of airflow, ease of cleaning, ease of control, flexibility and ease of changing loading, temperatures, airflow and cost. For food use, they are normally made of stainless steel, but some may be welded, while others are bolted together. Large dryers may be built in modules or as one unit. Even the amount and quality of insulation may vary. It is common to recycle large volumes of air to save energy and to adjust humidity, and the precision with which this is done can vary from one design to another.

As Crapiste and Rotstein point out, drying rates may depend on internal or external heat or mass transfer. It is usually relatively easy to maximize external heat transfer by raising temperature and air velocity. The limit is that temperature at which scorching of the surface occurs. Internal resistances are functions of the physical properties and size of the raw material. More porous materials offer low resistance to moisture removal but are also good thermal insulators. Reducing pressure lowers the temperature at which water vaporizes and may reduce mass transfer resistance while increasing heat transfer resistance. Raising pressure can have the opposite effect. In fact, raising the pressure in freeze drying, which usually occurs under very high vacuum, especially with either helium or air, can improve drying rates for some materials.

Freeze drying

Freeze drying is the process of maintaining conditions such that water is frozen and sublimes directly from ice to vapor. This avoids the collapse that occurs in many foods when they are normally dried, as moisture is removed and the remaining matrix sags to fill the voids. Freeze drying also prevents case hardening, which occurs as solubles migrate to the surface and are left behind. The more open porous structure and the lack of surface case hardening means that freeze-dried materials rehydrate well. Because the process occurs below the triple point of water, about 0°C (usually lower because of freezing point depression by dissolved solids), there is less volatile flavor loss and usually less undesirable color development.

To maintain freeze drying, the vapor pressure of water in the environment must be below 4.59 mm Hg, which is usually achieved by maintaining a high vacuum. However, freeze drying can occur at higher total pressures and, for some materials, there may be benefits from using a slightly higher absolute pressure. The reason is that internal heat transfer often governs during freeze drying and a slightly higher pressure increases apparent thermal conductivity of the dried layer.

Manipulating texture by drying

Sometimes during drying it is desirable to have shrinkage, as in pasta, where a dense texture is sought. In other foods, expansion to give a porous structure is the objective, as with crisp rice and crackers. Under identical conditions of temperature, airflow and humidity, different rheological properties will lead to different results, as illustrated by pasta made from durum wheat flour or bread flour, which have different protein contents. Given an understanding of the raw material properties, process conditions can be modified to adjust the end properties. Likewise, raw materials might be modified, by enzymes, for instance, to tailor the physical properties to achieve the desired final product.

Osmotic drying is a popular topic of academic study but is only used in a minor way commercially. Probably the best-known product is dried cranberries in which the infused sugar from osmotic drying is a valued ingredient. For commercial success, osmotic drying depends on reuse of a strong syrup, which draws water from the raw material. Sucrose syrup, for instance, has been reused up to 20 times in dehydration of apple cubes. The syrup was reconcentrated by evaporation and, while it picked up some reducing sugars and a little color, it appeared to stabilize, suggesting that further reuse is probably justified. Other fruits, such as cherries and blueberries, are osmotically dried. Since osmotic drying only removes some water, such products are normally finish dried with air. The added sugar not only reduces water activity, but also adds to the taste and texture.

Drying remains an important preservation method for many foods, especially in developing areas of the world, where stability at ambient conditions is particularly valuable. Seasonal crops like potatoes and onions can be kept in a convenient and lightweight form for use in a variety of foods.

Thermal processing of solids

Solid foods such as spices, herbs and teas can be contaminated with bacteria, molds and insects because they are agricultural products and are often grown and harvested under dusty conditions in developing parts of the world. To avoid transmission of plant pests and potential contamination of foods and mixtures in which the materials are used, they are often treated by various means, including heat, irradiation and fumigation, to reduce the microbial load and to kill insects, eggs and larvae.

Another instance in which solids may require treatment is fresh and ready-to-eat meats, which may have surface contamination by salmonellae or *Listeria*. Ready-to-eat meats, such as frankfurters or lunchmeat, are fully cooked but are subject to post-processing contamination before packaging. Fresh meat, especially chicken, is likely to have *Salmonella* because that microoorganism is common among chickens. It is desirable to reduce the microbial load to extend shelf life and to reduce the risk of cross-contamination from people handling raw meat and then contacting other foods.

Many imported spices and herbs are treated by irradiation or by exposure to chemical sterilants, such as ethylene oxide. While these treatments are well accepted in the USA, there can be objections to them in Europe and elsewhere. Also, foods treated by irradiation or chemicals may not be considered 'organic'. Ethylene oxide is toxic and flammable, so care is required in its application. Irradiation requires special facilities for applying gamma radiation from isotopes or an electron beam, which has limited penetration capability and so requires that the material to be treated be presented in a relatively thin layer.

Thus, there is an opportunity for an alternative treatment that leaves no residue but is effective in reducing microbial and insect contamination. For treating meat, it is desirable to deliver a microbial kill without cooking fresh meat or overcooking ready-to-eat meat. For spices, herbs and teas, it is important to retain the delicate flavors, color and essential oils. Microbes are more vulnerable to wet heat than to dry heat, so live steam is a promising treatment agent. However, many of the foods needing treatment are dry and could be vulnerable to caking or deterioration caused by excess moisture. Some clever techniques have been developed to apply steam to dry materials without causing damage from excessive heating or moisture.

The Safesteril process

The *Safesteril* process was developed by a French company, ETIA, Compiegne Cedex, France, which is represented in the USA by BNW Industries, Tippecanoe, Ind. BNW primarily manufactures the *Belt-O-Matic* conveyor dryer.

The heart of the process is an electrically heated screw turning in a Teflon-lined trough. The screw heats the powder being treated and prevents condensation of the live, atmospheric steam to which it is exposed. Residence time is controlled by screw speed and ranges up to 20 min. The trough is 6–8 m long and 600 mm in diameter. Volumetric capacity is 1.6–4.8 m^3/h.

After heating, the powder passes to a cooling unit, where chilled water is passed through a hollow screw while cool, dry air is passed through the product. In both the heating and cooling steps, the heat transfer is between the screw and the material being processed. It is not entirely clear what the steam does, because the major thermal contribution from steam is usually from condensation, giving up the latent heat. In this process, there should be no condensation. The steam does help exclude air which could cause oxidation and helps keep the equipment hot. After cooling, the material is packaged, which requires a clean environment to avoid recontamination.

In this process, as in the others described below, the specific conditions required to achieve a desired reduction in microbial load depend on the initial load and the properties of the specific material. The rate of reduction is generally a first-order process in which the rate constant increases exponentially with temperature. However, for a mixed load of microbes, there can be a wide diversity in thermal sensitivity. It is common to design a process for the most thermally resistant microbe, but it is not always clear what that may be.

When present, spores are generally the most resistant form of microorganism and spores of *Clostridium botulinum* are a special concern for low-acid foods that may encounter an anaerobic environment. Molds, yeasts and insects are generally fairly sensitive to heat and may be the targets of concern in many dry foods. A constraint on permissible conditions is the retention of flavor, color, texture and volatile essential oils.

The SteamLab approach

Another approach to steam sterilization of solids was developed by SteamLab Systems GmbH, Hamburg, Germany. The system uses specially constructed chambers ranging in volume from 400 to 12 000 l, producing 200–6000 kg of powder/h. Products are loaded in special equipment, which guarantees treatment of every particle and prevents cross-contamination in the machine. Loading equipment could be trays, porous packages such as cloth bags, or specially designed bins.

A vacuum is applied, which helps to remove some surface contamination and, more important, removes air from the chamber. Then saturated steam is introduced which, at the reduced pressure, is at 150–270°F (65–132°C), depending on the goal of the treatment. Sensitive herbs are treated very gently at 165–210°F (74–99°C) and powders with heat-resistant spores at >250°F (121°C). For disinfestation of insects and eggs, 160°F (71°C) is sufficient, because the effect of the very deep vacuum helps destroy the eggs.

The saturated steam becomes superheated at lower pressures because its temperature is above the boiling point of water at a lower pressure and so can deliver some sensible heat before reaching its saturation condition at a given pressure. By removing air, the system removes a potential insulating layer around the material, permitting rapid access of the steam to the spores. The product is held for a predetermined time, then vacuum is again applied, rapidly cooling the product and exhausting the steam. Atmospheric pressure is then restored and the product is moved through a second door to a clean room where it is conditioned if necessary and packaged. The system is able to treat almost all powders, although some may cake or lump from picking up moisture in the treatment and therefore require milling or screening before packaging.

The process has been applied to more than 300 kinds of ingredients, including herbs, spices, dried mushrooms, cereal, nuts and dried fruits. Cycle times are about 30 minutes and the chambers can be filled about 50%.

Flash pasteurization

A system using principles similar to those applied in SteamLab's system was conceived by and is still being studied at the Eastern Regional Research Center of the US Department of Agriculture's Agricultural Research Service, Wyndmoor, Pa. The process evolved so that vacuum is not used until after steam exposure, where it accelerates cooling.

The original focus of the work was reduction of surface contamination on chickens, a particularly challenging target because of the odd shape and roughness of the skin. A prototype was constructed that automatically cycled between vacuum and steam application, with a goal of 1.5 s/treatment. The technology was transferred to Alkar-RapidPak, Inc., Lodi, Wis, for commercialization.

Given the difficulties posed by treating chickens, the research turned to smooth surface products such as frankfurters and sausages, where 2- to 3-log reductions in *Listeria* were achieved. Alkar-RapidPak was able to eliminate the vacuum step, using a blast of steam alone, followed by vacuum cooling. The commercial unit treats eight packages of franks at a time just before the packages are sealed. Other smooth-skinned products, such as fruits, can also be treated successfully.

This treatment, combined with use of growth inhibitors, may meet USDA's Food Safety and Inspection Service requirements for Alternative 1 *Listeria* testing and certification and relieves the manufacturer of some testing requirements. The usual antimicrobial growth inhibitors are sodium diacetate and potassium lactate, which are said not to affect the flavor of sausages.

Process development paradigm

The general idea of using direct steam contact for surface sterilization and pasteurization of solids has been implemented in several distinct ways that have been commercialized. The challenge has been to avoid damage from moisture and overheating while achieving the required time and temperature regimen. Vacuum and a chilled screw have been used to achieve rapid cooling after steam exposure. In a way, the story is a paradigm of food process development, in that solutions are found for specific problems and then generalized to other applications.

Mixing of liquids and of liquids with solids

Mixing two liquids together seems deceptively simple at first glance. Even mixing solids into liquids appears easy, until one tries to do it on a scale of hundreds or thousands of gallons. Mixing plays a major role in food processing. Fruit juice concentrates are routinely diluted with water and added sweetener to make beverages. Milk and sweeteners have emulsifiers and flavors added to make ice cream. Soft drinks are made by mixing sweetener, flavor and water with carbon dioxide. Salad dressings are made by mixing oil, vinegar and flavors. Sauces and soups are made by mixing tomato paste, vegetables, spices and water. The list of examples could go on at great length. What are some of the operating principles and equipment choices?

Operating principles

All mixing involving liquids uses some form of energy to promote convection, the bulk movement of fluid and to reduce droplet size in the cases involving otherwise immiscible fluids such as oil and water. The natural process of diffusion uses differences in concentration to drive a non-uniform mixture toward a more uniform composition, but diffusion is very slow. Most people have witnessed the example of pouring cream into coffee or tea. If done carefully, it is possible to float cream on top of the beverage. Just a few stirs with a spoon produce a uniform tan-colored drink. This is convection in action on a very small scale with thin liquids.

As fluids used become more viscous, as two immiscible fluids are dispersed, as the scale becomes larger and as solids are dispersed, much more energy is required and the issue becomes how best to deliver it. Mixing can be in batches or continuous. For many purposes, batches are preferred so that the composition can be checked before the next operation. On the other hand, batch operation may require multiple units so that supply of a mixture to subsequent operations is continuous. Batch operations also can be labor intensive and, if tests are indeed made on each batch, productivity can be low. Nonetheless, batches are common in the food industry, where formulas change often and multiple flavors may be processed and packaged on the same line.

Liquids and solids are mixed and blended for many reasons in food processing. Some common examples include dispersing gums and stabilizers in ice cream mix; dissolving salt and sugar in water to make brines; suspending vegetables and meat pieces in broth for soups and sauces; mixing oil, eggs and vinegar to make mayonnaise; and dispersing water in flour to make bread dough.

Some of the parameters that distinguish different regimes of mixing include the proportion of solid to liquid, the viscosity of the final mix, the solubility of the solids and the presence of other materials, such as a second liquid phase.

Many equipment choices

Batch tanks are usually cylindrical vessels with dished bottoms, but they may also have flat or conical bottoms. One simple approach to mixing is to circulate the contents with a pump. This can take a long time if the batch is large and it may degrade fragile particles, such as meat or vegetables in soups. A more common approach is to circulate the contents within the tank with an agitator.

Agitators may be shaped like propellers, paddles or turbines. Propellers, which have smooth blades twisted to move at an angle through the fluid, are relatively energy efficient and appropriate for low-viscosity fluids. The shaft should be mounted at an angle to the centerline of the tank to promote good circulation. Propellers can generate a vortex, which may incorporate air into the fluid. This is not always desirable.

Propellers can also be mounted through the side of a tank or through the bottom. The advantage in these cases is a shorter shaft, which may have less tendency to deflect. Deflection puts additional strain on the bearings supporting the agitator. However, passing a moving shaft through a tank wall or bottom requires a mechanical seal to prevent leakage. Such seals then require maintenance and may be difficult to clean.

Paddle agitators typically have two, four or more vertical blades, often mounted on a horizontal disk rotated by a vertical shaft. Several paddles can be mounted on the same shaft in large tanks. Paddles do not promote vertical circulation in a tank unless there also are baffles along the sides. Turbine agitators have a rotating impeller inside a stationary cage. The clearance between the impeller and the cage can be quite small, leading to very high shear rates. High shear means imposition of considerable energy in a relatively small volume, which is good for breaking up droplets and aggregates of solids, such as starches and gums.

High-shear mixers

The Breddo Likwifier is familiar to many food processors. It looks much like a bar blender or kitchen food processor, except that it is much larger. The machine was developed to help disperse dairy stabilizers, which have a tendency to form 'fish eyes' lumps of powder that are wet on the outside, which prevents the inside from being wetted. It takes high local shear to break down such particles and completely hydrate the powder. The Likwifier uses a bottom-entering agitator shaft with slanted blades to create high circulation rates and high local shear rates.

A bottom-entering shaft has the advantage that it can be shorter and thinner than a top-entering shaft to deliver the same power because the impeller is close to the bottom and thus immersed in the liquid. By being submerged deeper, the agitator also incorporates less air than would an impeller located higher in the vessel. On the other hand, a bottom-entering shaft requires a good mechanical seal to prevent leaking of the liquid or contamination from the outside. Mechanical seals are subject to abrasion and wear from the solids being mixed and often require disassembly for cleaning. This can create damage from misalignment during reassembly. Breddo has developed a water-flushed seal in which most of the parts are outside the vessel. The water flushing also cools the seal, reducing wear. Many of the company's vessels are square, making them self-baffling while still easy to clean. They also make round vessels, and both round and square vessels may be jacketed for heating or cooling. Some mixers have scraped-surface agitators to promote heat transfer and to help circulate viscous mixes.

Microfluidics, Newton, Mass offers Sanitary Laboratory Homogenizers. Lightweight, versatile, portable and easy to use, these patented homogenizers are suited for a range of applications, including emulsions, dispersions, cosmetics, pharmaceuticals, liposomes and food and beverage products. Microfluidizer processors impart controllable shear rates on the product stream by producing process pressures from 2500 psi to more than 40 000 psi. This is accomplished with a combination of constant-pressure intensifier pumps and fixed-geometry interaction chambers, resulting in nanoparticles with extremely narrow distribution, translating into highly stable products with long shelf life.

A special category of high-shear mixers is rotor/stator mixers, in which a specially designed impeller rotates, usually at high speed, inside a stationary ring containing slots. Fluid is drawn into the rotating part and expelled through the slots, creating very high shear in a small volume. Some companies making high-shear rotor/stator mixers, and often other types as well, include Charles Ross and Son Co., Hauppauge, NY; Quadro Engineering, Millburn, NJ; Lancaster Products, Lebanon, Pa; Silverson Machines, Inc., East Longmeadow, Mass; and IKA Works, Inc., Wilmington, NC.

Ross makes a full line of mixing equipment and may be best known for 'can' mixers, in which the vessel can be removed and used to transport its contents to packaging or further processing. Quadro makes a family of devices in which fluid is pumped through a high intensity zone, where it is combined with solids then transferred to another vessel. The company also offers in-vessel dispersers, where the solids are introduced directly to the high-shear zone rather than being added to the surface of the fluid.

Lancaster builds a unique family of machines in which the vessel or pan rotates in one direction while various tools, including side and bottom scrapers and rotating impellers rotate in the opposite direction. The application seems best suited for viscous pastes in which, without the extra tools, the fluid would not move naturally into the high-shear zone.

Silverson makes equipment comparable in function to that of Quadro, in which a low-pressure zone is created by the rotation of an impeller in a chamber so that fluid and solids can be combined and pumped to the next step in the process. Sometimes, in circulating systems, the fluid is recycled back to the feed tank until a batch is uniform.

IKA makes a line of high intensity mixers, often as complete systems, some with rotor stator agitators and others with helical or spiral agitators.

Mechanical design important

In considering a mixer type and specific vendor, it is well to understand the various design issues involved. When power is applied through a shaft to a body of fluid, various mechanical forces are created, especially if the fluid is viscous and there is a high concentration of solids. One force tends to push back on the shaft. A thrust bearing resists this force. There can be forces tending to bend the shaft, which are resisted by the thickness and material strength of the shaft. The shaft and impeller also impose their own weight on the drive system. The longer the shaft and higher the speed, the more tendency there is for misalignment, with the risk of bearing failure. As previously mentioned, if the shaft enters through the liquid, there must be a mechanical seal. If the vessel is under pressure, even a top-entering shaft must have a seal to prevent leakage of gas.

Every vessel has a working volume which is less than its actual volume, usually about 70%. There is also a minimum volume below which the agitator is not submerged. Without the resistance of fluid, a running agitator can damage itself if not properly designed.

For food processing, it is important that mixers be easily cleaned, which means that they are usually built of stainless steel, with polished surfaces and rounded joints. If designed for cleaning in place, it is important that cleaning spray balls or nozzles cover all surfaces. Connections should be made as close to the vessel wall as possible to make cleaning easier. In food applications, it is common to use several mixing devices, such as a slow scraper along the sides and bottom of a shallow tank with a higher-speed agitator elsewhere in the tank to disperse solids. Food mixing tanks may be jacketed for heating and cooling and the agitation may be primarily intended to promote heat transfer rather than intense mixing.

Drives are usually electric motors but, for light applications, drives can be pneumatic motors, driven by compressed air. These are especially convenient if flammable liquids are present, as is often true for flavors and essential oils.

Homogenizers and colloid mills are special cases of mixers designed to make stable emulsions and dispersions. These usually involve pumping fluids at very high pressures through small openings or passing the fluid through very small clearances between a moving and a stationary plate.

Most vendors offer lab- or pilot-scale versions of their designs that can be used for scale-up. Remember that the correlations for power and mixing effectiveness are highly dependent on the specific impeller and vessel design. With some experience, an appropriate choice among the many possibilities can be made.

Scaling up

Practical batch sizes for liquid mixing depend on viscosity. An old rule of thumb is 5000 gal for viscosity of 200 000 cP and 20 000 gal for 100 cP. Emulsification and dispersion occur at a finite rate, which may need to be determined experimentally. Mix time is best expressed as blend number N_B:

$$N_B = Nt \tag{A.5}$$

where,
N is speed of the agitator, s^{-1} and
t is time, s.

Thus, if speed is in revolutions/s, time is in seconds and the result is dimensionless. This value, the number of revolutions until a satisfactory mix is achieved, often correlates with the Reynolds number, Eq. (A.2). Experiments in mixing must preserve geometric similarity between scales for correlations to be useful. Often, the size of an agitator has a relation to vessel diameter, such as 50%. For good mixing, vessels should be about the same height as their diameter, though other proportions are used.

As in other mass transfer and fluid flow situations, it matters whether the flow is turbulent or laminar. For mixing using an impeller, typically a multibladed rotor on a shaft, the flow pattern is characterized by the Reynolds number, N_{Re}, Eq. (A.2) adapted for an impeller by using the diameter of the impeller and its tip speed. High values of Re indicate turbulent flow, while low values indicate laminar flow. Mixing is more effective with turbulence, but this may be difficult to achieve with high-viscosity mixtures.

The power consumed by an agitator is a function of N_{Re} and typically depends on the impeller and vessel design. The dimensionless power number N_P, Eq. (A.4), can be correlated with the dimensionless N_{Re} for use in scale-up. For miscible liquids, time to reach a satisfactory degree of homogeneity is often estimated as requiring about 4 or 5 turnovers of vessel contents.

Many foods are non-Newtonian, meaning that their viscosity changes with shear rate. Often, foods are pseudoplastic, which means that their viscosity decreases as shear rate increases. Shear rate roughly correlates with agitator speed. Blending tends to improve with increasing Reynolds number, which also increases with speed.

A particularly useful scale-up parameter is power per unit volume, often expressed as horsepower per gallon (or per 100 gal, to avoid using fractions). Representative values are 2–5 hp/100 gal to disperse solids or make emulsions. Lower values are adequate for dispersing light fluids or dissolving solids. Higher values, up to 7.5–10 hp/100 gal, are encountered with more-complex mixtures, even up to 100 hp/100 gal for thick pastes and doughs. In continuous mixing systems, the corresponding parameter is horsepower per unit flow, such as gallons per minute.

The critical issue in continuous mixing is not usually the mixing but accurate feeding of all the components. This is one reason some units are often used in a batch mode – feeding is then less critical and the quality of the batch can be confirmed. In continuous blending of fluids, especially for beverages, an in-line refractometer may be used to control one or more flows as the mix goes through an in-line agitator or static mixer. (Static mixers have no moving parts. Rather, they contain precise flow diversion elements within a pipe.) Refractometers, however, are notorious for occasional drift in their accuracy as the optical windows get dirty. One of the great needs for continuous fluid blending is reliable instrumentation.

Mixing of fluids may be one of the most common unit operations in food processing. Constraints and challenges abound – sanitation, scale-up, consistency, efficiency, productivity and maintaining quality, whether that be related to particle identity, flavor, or mouth feel. There are many useful technologies – low cost or expensive, low-shear or high-shear, simple or complex. In the end, a process developer needs a good selection of options in the lab and pilot plant and enough understanding to apply them properly.

Size reduction

Size reduction can be a critical operation in food processing. For example, cereal milling relies on size reduction by crushing or fracture to yield a variety of particles, which can be sorted by screening to give fractions that are higher in fiber, protein or starch. Milling works because cereal grains are relatively hard and break under stress. Proper control of moisture is important to control the physical properties and thus give the desired particles without excessive dust on the one hand and without flaking on the other hand. (Of course, under different circumstances, specifically higher moisture content, flaking is the desired result, using very similar equipment.)

Grinding of meat is a size-reduction operation which is essential to the production of sausage, hamburger, lunchmeats and other processed meats. Rather than with moisture, the physical properties are controlled by temperature. Meats are typically ground at near-freezing temperatures, where the meat is firm and can still be cut. If the temperature is too low, the meat fractures into undesirable fine fragments and if the temperature is too warm, the meat smears and does not produce the distinct pieces that are generally desired. For some processed meats, a fine emulsion is sought, so warmer temperatures may be accepted, even preferred.

Random or uniform particles

Size-reduction processes may be divided into those that produce random particles or pieces and those that produce pieces that are more uniform. A random process produces a size distribution. In some cases, the extremes – the smallest or the largest – may be undesirable, while in others the mix can be used completely. If only one portion of the size distribution is sought, there must be a separation or fractionation process. If smaller particles are desired, the larger ones may be screened out and recycled. Very fine particles are often discarded as waste but, in some cases, may be treated to create larger particles by agglomeration. An example of this situation is sugar grinding followed by granulation to create a size distribution suitable for tableting or compacting. Many familiar confections are made from crystalline sugar and liquid sweeteners this way.

A versatile machine for creating particle size distributions is a hammer mill, such as those made by Prater, Inc., Cicero, Ill. This firm offers hammer mills, fine grinders and classifier mills. Hammer mills have a rotor inside a perforated cage or screen. The rotor has blades attached in any of several patterns. The blades swivel at the attachment point and can be reversed as they wear to extend their life before being replaced. A fine grinder has fixed blades and closer clearances between the blade tip and the screen. The classifier mill incorporates a separation step to retain oversize particles for continued grinding and is commonly used for sugar.

Mills are routinely used on cereals, though roller mills give a more narrow size distribution. They are also used to make breadcrumbs, recycle breakfast cereals and finish dry mixes, especially those in which fat may be incorporated.

One way to avoid excessive fines is to stage milling with intermediate screening. The desired size range of particles is removed after each step and the overs are ground again. This creates a more complex process but may result in higher yield.

Dust is frequently an issue in hammer milling, so hammer mills are often enclosed in blast-proof rooms and must have explosion-proof electrical controls. Because typical applications are for dry materials, they may be constructed of carbon steel, but they can also be built of stainless steel if required.

Another variation on random milling is attrition milling, in which particle-to-particle contact in a high-velocity air stream causes particle disintegration. The air stream may carry off lighter and smaller particles or the entire stream may be separated by screens or sifting. Sugar is often ground this way. Particles must be hard and brittle to perform properly.

Uniform cutting

Where a mill might be compared to using a hammer, coffee grinder or mortar and pestle, cutting is more like using a knife. If one wants a slice, strip or dice, one can use a knife to make one, two or three cuts of a food. Chefs know how to do this very fast and accurately without losing a digit.

Urschel Laboratories Inc., Valparaiso, Ind, specializes in making machines that slice, cut and dice many different foods. Physical properties, size and capacity dictate which machine is appropriate. The most complex machines make three cuts to give dice, cubes or other shaped pieces with quite regular dimensions. Urschel makes all of its own parts, including fasteners. The plant in Valparaiso has three foundries, for stainless steel and bronze. Each of the many varieties of machines is built to order, one at a time, by a team. Every part is kept in stock and shipped all over the world as needed.

Replacement parts are a significant portion of Urschel's sales because the knives and cutters eventually wear out. Some can be resharpened using another machine made by Urschel, but most are replaced. Familiar foods probably cut on Urschel machines include potato chips, pickles, mushrooms and celery. There are few foods they cannot cut, but they are most dominant in fruits and vegetables.

Deville Technologies Inc., Montreal, Quebec, Canada, has focused its cutting and shredding machines on cheese and related products and also makes machines to cut and shred meats, fruits and vegetables. Deville was originally part of a firm that built cheese plants and developed shredding technology that was spun off to form Deville.

The machines can accept larger blocks of cheese, up to 40 lb (18 kg) and shred at rates of 10–20 000 lb/h (4500–9072 kg/h). The same machine can dice meat at similar rates. One Deville machine replaces three or four competing devices. An important part of its sanitary design is a drive separate from the cutting area. This reduces the opportunity for contamination by lubricants.

A unique form of uniform cutting is offered by Grote Co., Columbus, Ohio. Originally, the Grote slicer was devised to cut and place pepperoni on pizzas. It still is in wide use on commercial lines, but that market is no longer Grote's primary target.

The slicer has a series of tubes sized to take the specific product, such as pepperoni, bacon or fruit. The tubes rock back and forth over a moving band-saw blade, cutting a slice with each pass and dropping it precisely under the tube. Thus, as originally conceived, a bundle of tubes could cover a pizza crust with meat all at once. As the feed piece is depleted, the operator replaces it with another.

A current high volume application is slicing and placing bacon for pre-cooking. One machine can place pieces across a wide belt feeding an oven, whereas several conventional slicers would otherwise be needed.

Another interesting application is prepared sandwiches, where meat and cheese can be sliced and placed on pieces of bread directly, without the labor of hand placement. Pre-sliced vegetables for salads and slices of fruit for drying are two other applications.

In general, Grote focuses on the 'slice and place' market. Like Urschel and Deville, Grote builds its own machines. Grote has also cooperated with Urschel to integrate machines for special situations.

Often requires other steps

Size reduction is a common unit operation in food processing. Unlike in other industries, there often is a requirement for precise shapes made from irregular raw materials. There is the usual concern for sanitation and the hazard of metal contamination.

Cutting agricultural raw materials introduces the risk of stones or other objects that could damage equipment, so pre-screening, inspection and cleaning are important. Metal detection almost always follows cutting or slicing.

Random size distributions are often produced by chopping, hammer milling and roller milling, depending on the physical properties. Additional separation steps can improve yield at the cost of greater process complexity. Finding a use for fines, including agglomeration to make larger particles, is often necessary.

Concentrating proteins

Proteins are recovered and purified from a variety of sources for their nutritional and functional properties. In particular, proteins from oilseeds such as soy are valued components of human foods and animal feeds. Oilseed meals, after vegetable oil has been pressed and solvent extracted, may be extracted with acids and bases to dissolve proteins and separate them from carbohydrates. After neutralization, protein concentrates and isolates are produced, which may be formed by extrusion or spinning into fibers to simulate meats.

Proteins from other sources may be soluble, film-forming or emulsifying in addition to providing vital nutrition. For example, whey protein fractions recovered by membrane processes from cheese whey can be used to form edible films and coatings. Whey films can replace shellac in polishing chocolate confections and form moisture barriers between sauce and crust in frozen pizzas and other foods.

Concentrating milk protein

Several factors have combined to make ultrafiltration of raw milk on the farm attractive. Dairy herds have gotten larger and more remote as dairy farms consolidate and seek less expensive land. Many dairy farms are members of large cooperatives, which also process milk into cheese and other products. The relatively weak dollar has made milk proteins attractive on the world market.

The process involves concentrating milk fat and protein while allowing water, lactose and salts to permeate a membrane under pressure. The relatively porous membrane permits a higher flow at lower pressure than that required by a reverse osmosis membrane, which might retain more of the soluble and low-molecular-weight material. Since the concentrate is intended for cheese making, in which the sugars and salts are normally lost anyway, it is economical and efficient to remove them on the farm and save the cost of transporting the water. The farmer is first paid for his raw milk as normal, according to weight and fat content. The equipment may be owned by the farmer or by the processor.

Concentrating meat protein

When meat animals are butchered, considerable quantities of trim are produced. These are sorted according to their lean meat content and sold to sausage makers or ground for hamburger. The higher the lean content, the more valuable the trimmings. Surplus fatty trimmings are rendered to recover the fat from beef as tallow and lard from pork.

Rendering involves cooking in large vessels, usually by direct steam injection, followed by centrifugation and drying of the fat and the protein fraction. The protein from edible rendering may be used in animal feeds, while that from inedible rendering is used as fertilizer. If the trimmings have been handled in a sanitary fashion, the rendering is done under relatively mild conditions and the fat is considered edible. Tallow and lard are valued in baking and frying, though nutritional concerns about saturated fats are affecting their use. The aqueous phase from the centrifuge is called stick water and may be concentrated as a source of beef flavor. If the stick water is not concentrated, it represents a significant waste disposal challenge. If the raw material is not considered edible, the rendering conditions are typically more severe and the fat is used for chemicals, such as soap and fatty acids.

A special form of rendering is used for bones, which after the fat and protein are cooked away are then extracted for gelatin. The strongest and most valuable grade of gelatin is used for photographic film. The next strongest is used for pharmaceutical capsules (and paint balls) and the weakest form is used in foods. Gelatin is highly purified in the recovery process and is a uniquely functional protein.

In South America, especially Argentina and Brazil, range-fed beef is quite lean and relatively inexpensive. More than 100 years ago, the South American industry sought ways to export its beef without the benefit and cost of refrigeration. One innovation was to produce beef extract by cooking beef cuts in water and then concentrating the broth. Fat in the broth is separated, dried and sold as edible tallow before the aqueous phase is concentrated by evaporation.

At first, the fully cooked beef was discarded, but then the concept of canning the beef with curing agents to make corned beef was developed. The unique trapezohedron metal can still characteristic of canned corn beef was developed so that nested empty cans could be shipped economically. Later, uncured cooked ground beef from the extraction process was canned and sold as a protein ingredient for chili, taco filling and other cooked products, where the relative absence of beef flavor can be compensated for by spices and flavorings.

An additional product line is a frozen cooked beef roll, made from larger cuts of meat, which are also cooked for extract, then stuffed into a cellulose casing and frozen. These rolls may be sliced for frozen dinners or sandwiches or diced for use in soups and stews. The canned ground beef is sold as a high-protein ingredient, permitting the use of less-expensive fatty cuts or trim in a given formula while still achieving a target protein content for nutritional or functional reasons.

To prevent the introduction of foot-and-mouth disease to the USA, all meat from South America must be cooked before being imported, so the processes in which extract is manufactured and an inexpensive food ingredient is also created make a virtue from a necessity.

Retaining functionality in lean beef

Beef Products, Inc., Dakota Dunes, SD, has developed a unique process to concentrate lean meat from fatty trim in a sanitary and cost-effective way. The company has four plants, all located close to large Midwestern meat-packing plants, from which they can obtain a reliable supply of fatty trim with low transportation costs. The overall concept is to concentrate the lean meat without losing its functionality. Unlike the South American process, there is no cooking step, so the company operates under extremely sanitary conditions.

The first step in the process is to remove any sinews by grinding and separating hard or tough pieces. Then the mass is tempered to near-post-mortem temperatures, about 105°F (41°C), at which point the fat is liquid but the meat does not cook. A centrifuge separates the lean phase from the liquid fat. The lean slurry is exposed to ammonia to increase the pH in a microbial reduction step. The fat phase is vacuum dried to produce edible tallow.

The slurry is then frozen in sheets on a roller freezer, a 14-ft × 12-ft (4 × 3.6 m) stainless-steel drum. In 90 seconds, the sheet is frozen and scraped from the drum, broken into flakes and packaged in 60-lb (27 kg) cartons. The entire process takes 7–9 minutes, which is a very short residence time for any food process. All make-up air for the plant is washed and cooled with chilled sanitizing solution. The plant is designed for cleaning in place, including the drains, which are known potentially to be harbors for microorganisms such as *Listeria*. In some rooms, the walls and ceiling are stainless-steel panels, which facilitates washing and sanitation.

Processes provide ingredients and inspiration

Cooked ground beef, boneless lean beef and milk protein concentrate are complex mixtures obtained by sophisticated processes, providing valuable ingredients to the processed food industry. They also provide inspiration for other creative process developments, such as applying the same operations to other raw materials.

Extraction

Extraction describes a wide variety of unit operations found in the food industry, including the manufacture of soluble coffee and tea, vegetable oils, fruit juices and flavors and the removal of undesirable substances such as caffeine. Strictly speaking, some of these operations should be called leaching, washing or expression, but it is common to call them extraction.

Operations may seem relatively simple, as when fruits are crushed and their juices removed by pressure. However, to enhance recovery, the remaining pulp may be washed with water and sometimes the pulp is treated with enzymes to convert some of the insoluble material into juice solids. Thus, the apparently simple operation adds a biochemical reaction and a washing step. The recovered juice is more dilute than straight-run juice and is usually concentrated by evaporation.

Common features of extraction

This dilution illustrates a universal feature of extraction with solvents (which washing with water is): there is an inverse relationship between recovery and concentration – using more solvent removes more of the solute, but the resulting solution has a lower concentration. Usually, the solute is the desired component, so the excess solvent must be removed and that usually involves some cost. This means that, in extraction processes, there is almost always an optimum way to operate, determined by the costs of concentration and the value of the recovered material.

Water is an inexpensive solvent but, in other operations, the solvent may be an organic fluid, such as hexane, alcohol or ether. There are both economic and safety motivations to recover as much solvent as possible. Another universal feature of extraction processes is that the solvent saturates the residue as well as appears in the extract solution. Thus, the residue usually is 'dried' to drive off the retained solvent and the extract solution may be evaporated for the same purpose.

Vegetable oil manufacture illustrates this practice. Olives and oilseeds such as soy, cotton, peanut, canola and sunflower are usually crushed to express first-run oil. Some seeds may be cooked first or after crushing. Since pressing alone leaves some residual oil, the crushed meal is usually extracted with solvents, often hexane, which is flammable. Solvent-extracted oil may be considered inferior for some purposes but, after refining, may be difficult to distinguish from first-run oil. Olive is a case where the first-run ('virgin') oil is considered superior in flavor. Because of the heat generated in pressing and cooking, extracted oil may contain free fatty acids, which are removed in refining. Gums and other impurities are often found as well; some, such as lecithin from soy, are recovered as valuable products in their own right.

The solvent-extracted meal is heated to remove solvent, which must be recovered by condensation to reduce cost and to prevent discharge to the atmosphere, where it is a contributor to air pollution as volatile organic compound (VOC). Obviously, there is some risk in heating a flammable material. Since the meal is often valued as animal feed, minimal heating is desired to maintain nutritive value.

Meanwhile, the solvent and oil solution is evaporated to remove solvent and concentrate the oil. Since there is usually a large difference in boiling point between the oil and solvent, the separation is relatively easy and mostly complete, but there can be some residual solvent in the oil. Few separations are 100% efficient, so there usually is some solvent loss, which contributes to cost.

Coffee and tea extraction

Coffee and tea solubles are removed industrially much as they are in the home, by contact with hot water. Again, there is an inverse relationship between recovery and concentration. At home, the second pot of tea using the same tea bag is noticeably weaker. Recovery is increased, but at a lower concentration. Avid coffee brewers know that over extraction does not result in better coffee; in fact, it is usually worse, because the more flavorful compounds are also most easily extracted and the later extracted compounds are bitter or acidic.

In commercial operations to produce soluble coffee and tea, yield is important, so extraction is very thorough and complete. The joke in the industry is that there should be only air left in the vessels when the process is finished. It is not unusual to use high temperatures and pressures to increase yield by breaking down the otherwise insoluble material. One should not be surprised that commercial soluble coffee and tea do not taste like their freshly brewed counterparts.

Coffee and tea can also be decaffeinated using extraction. This illustrates a case of selective dissolution. Caffeine is soluble in some solvents, such as methylene chloride, while the carbohydrates, acids and phenolics are not. An early process directly contacted coffee beans or tea leaves with solvent to remove caffeine. However, some solvents are carcinogenic and left residues in the beans, so an improvement was to contact a water extract with the solvent, which was mostly immiscible with water. This improvement comes at the cost of complexity: first, the beans are contacted with hot water, then the water is contacted with solvent, the solvent is removed from the water, the water is removed from the beans, the solvent is removed from the caffeine and the coffee solubles are removed from the water stream and returned to the beans somehow.

The modern decaffeination process uses supercritical carbon dioxide, which leaves no residue and is selective for caffeine.

Supercritical fluid extraction

Gases can be compressed at high pressure to form a phase that has both liquid and gas-like properties. The compressed gas, called a supercritical fluid because it is above the substance's critical pressure, can have high solvent power but low viscosity. Release of pressure dramatically reduces the solvency, precipitating the solute quickly. Carbon dioxide is popular for such use because it is inexpensive, non-explosive and non-toxic.

Supercritical extraction is not a panacea. In addition to decaffeination of coffee and tea, it is in use to remove nicotine from tobacco, to impregnate wood, to replace harmful solvents in dry cleaning and to prepare fine particles of drugs for pharmaceuticals. One hundred and forty million pounds (63 504 000 kg) of coffee is treated with supercritical fluids to remove caffeine each year.

Thar Technologies, Pittsburgh, Pa., has applied supercritical fluid extraction to a wide variety of products and uses, including spices, flavors, foods, nutraceuticals, solvent removal, coatings, impregnation, vegetable oil refining and others. Supercritical fluid technology offers advantages such as the absence of any organic solvent residue and selective extraction and fractionation of different compounds. Another major application of supercritical fluids is extraction of hops to yield an easy-to-use flavor concentrate for beer.

Research on supercritical fluid extraction is also conducted at the US Department of Agriculture's National Center for Agricultural Utilization Research in Peoria, Ill. A major focus is on extraction of oil from various seeds and on subsequent refining of the oils. The Center has also applied supercritical fluid extraction to analysis of toxicants in meats, grains and commercial food products. The supercritical fluids replace organic solvents in the laboratory.

Other extraction equipment

Crown Iron Works Co., Minneapolis, Minn. makes specialized extraction equipment primarily applied in the oilseed industry. The company's extractor uses a chain to drag oilseed flakes through solvent-filled chambers in a counter-current path. This equipment illustrates two more common features of extraction: the importance of solid size and shape and the concept of counter-current flow.

Solids containing a solute of value or interest typically are composed of inert material, such as carbohydrate or protein, that entraps the solute. To remove the solute, solvent must penetrate the inert matrix and then diffuse out. This diffusion process is often the rate-limiting step. To reduce the time required, it is common to grind the particles to a fine powder or to make thin flakes, if possible. Powders may be difficult to handle and may plug equipment. Flakes are often easier to move. Sometimes, of course, one cannot change the shape of the substrate.

Counter-current flow refers to the practice of contacting exhausted substrate with fresh solvent while fresh substrate sees the exiting solvent. This is easy to arrange when contacting one liquid with another. One typically relies on density differences to separate the fluids. With solids, it may be more complex to simulate counter-current flow. One way is with complex piping and valves in which the relative position of vessels containing the solids is changed periodically. Another is by physically moving the solids, as is done in the Crown contactor.

Littleford Day, Florence, Ky applies its *Ploughshare®* technology to special batch extractions, using choppers and plows in a vessel to promote agitation and contact. Material is contacted in the vessel with solvent, the solution is removed through filters, heating the vessel evaporates the residual solvent, then the extracted solids are discharged.

Designing and operating an extraction process is a challenging task, even for experienced engineers. However, it is useful for anyone in the food industry to know a little of the potential applications and to understand some of the basic principles.

Physical separations

In food processing, some separations are good and some may be bad. For example, milling of flour relies on separating wheat bran from white flour by screening to produce an important food. On the other hand, settling of pulp from fruit juice is usually undesirable. Physical separations rely on some difference in size or in properties, such as density. Other separations, such as distillation, absorption, chromatography and extraction may rely on differences in chemical or physicochemical properties, such as vapor pressure, chemical affinity or even shape.

Separation by size: screening

Screening is used to remove foreign matter, to sort raw materials by size and to separate components that are mixed together. Screens are made of wire mesh, perforated metal sheets and woven cloths. Openings may be square, round or other shapes. Material to be treated is spread on the surface and usually is agitated by moving the screen, sometimes in a circle and sometimes back and forth. The movement is intended to expose each particle to the openings in the screen and eventually to move the 'overs', those too large to pass through the openings, off the screen. Because most food particles are irregular in shape, screening is a statistical process – some fraction of 'throughs' or 'unders', those which should pass through the screen, are actually retained and some particles with a relatively large dimension may pass through by presenting a small aspect to the opening. Retention of undersized particles is increased when the load on the screen is high, because there can be a reduced chance that all particles will see an opening and the undersized particles are swept along with the overs. This means that screens should be carefully sized for the anticipated feed rate.

Screens with large openings have higher capacity than those with smaller openings, in part because there is less open area for a given screen surface with smaller openings. Often, several screens are used in series to create a number of fractions. These may each have a use, or some may be recycled for size reduction or, more rarely, agglomeration. Screening commonly follows a size-reduction step such as hammer milling, crushing, roller milling or grinding. Most size-reduction processes produce a range of particle sizes, only some of which are desirable. Sometimes the fines are the desired product and other times an intermediate size is the target. If too great a step is taken in size reduction, as by using a fine screen in a hammer mill, many fines are created. Roller mills can produce a narrower particle size range but will still produce fines, depending on the hardness of the material. It is good practice to use several steps of size reduction with intermediate screening to maximize the yield of desired particle sizes.

Screens may inadvertently contribute to particle size reduction if the feed particles are fragile and the agitation is vigorous. Thus, selection of the screen size, material and agitation speed are all critical to a screening process. Agglomerates or granules formed by attaching small particles together in a fluidized bed dryer can be shaken apart on a screen if the speed is not controlled carefully.

Separation by gravity: settling and centrifugation

Particles suspended in a liquid may rise or fall, depending on their density relative to the liquid. As the particles move through a liquid, their velocity is affected by the drag or frictional force exerted by the liquid. The rate of settling (or rising, when the particle is less dense than the liquid) is directly proportional to the square of the diameter of the particle and inversely proportional to the viscosity of the liquid. This relationship says that large particles settle much faster than small ones and that thick or viscous fluids suspend particles better than thin or less-viscous liquids.

Naturally occurring gums, called pectin, in fruit and vegetable juices help keep pulp particles suspended. For most juices, this is desirable, though there are cases where clear juices are preferred. When juices are released by crushing or reaming fruits or vegetables, enzymes that can attack pectin are also released. If not inactivated by heat, the enzymes reduce the juice viscosity and accelerate settling of pulp. This phenomenon is one reason that most fruit and vegetable juices are pasteurized. (Another reason is that fruit and vegetable juices can be contaminated with pathogens, such as *Escherichia coli*.) The amount of pulp can be controlled either by allowing it to settle or by centrifugation.

In centrifugation, a suspension is rotated very rapidly in a cylinder or chamber so that the force exerted on the particles is greatly increased, up to several thousand times the force of gravity. In one type of centrifuge, a disk-stack, many thin conical plates are rotated in a chamber. The fluid flows in the spaces between the plates. A particle only needs to travel a short distance before encountering a plate and being diverted to the edge of the chamber. The clear fluid exits from the center of the machine and the concentrated pulp exits from the perimeter. Pulp removed from some citrus juices may be added to other juices, permitting the marketing of juices with 'less pulp', 'some pulp' and 'more pulp'.

Centrifuges may also be used to remove oil from water, fine particles from water and protein from fat in rendering. Even with pasteurization, suspended pulp in fruit and vegetable juices may settle on standing. One solution is simply to advise the consumer to shake well before using. Another is to reduce the particle size of the pulp, often by homogenization, high-pressure shearing. Where permitted, gums and hydrocolloids might be added to increase viscosity. Good sanitation can help, especially in climates where there is dust in the air. It is possible that dust can act as a clarifying agent, by helping pulp particles collect together and form larger particles that then settle more quickly. Filtering the air that comes in contact with juices is good practice.

When clarity of liquids is desired, fining agents, such as clay, egg white or gelatin might be added to help particles that form haze agglomerate and then settle. Beer, wine, drinking water and clear juices are made this way.

Separation by filtering

Filtering can accelerate removal of suspended particles from liquids. In clarifying fluids, precoat filters may be used, in which an inert solid such as diatomaceous earth, cellulose fiber or rice hulls might be added to create a filter cake. In other filter applications, especially where the solid is the desired product, plate-and-frame or pressure filters are used. Many leaf filters rely on the pressure of the feed fluid or mechanical pressure to compress the solids in the filter cake. Some use compressed air to displace liquid from the filter cake and to help dry the cake. Each chamber of the press has a filter cloth that can be conveyed into place automatically. When the press is opened after a cycle in which the chambers are filled with slurry and then the cake collected, the cloth conveys the cake to a collection point. The cloth is simultaneously cleaned as it is replaced in the chamber. This press is not thought suitable for juice expression because the air could cause oxidation, but it is widely used in starch production from corn and potatoes, where efficiency of cake washing is valued. Simple plate-and-frame filter presses can be labor intensive by comparison.

Other types of filters include rotary vacuum filters, membrane filters and cartridge filters, often using disposable elements. Rotary vacuum filters use a perforated drum covered with a porous cloth on which a filter aid might or might not be deposited. One food application is recovery of sugar from candy waste, where various candies are dissolved in hot water, mixed with activated carbon to remove color and flavors and then filtered. The carbon is discarded and the sugar solution is concentrated and reused.

A plate-and-frame filter press is used in chocolate processing. Ground cocoa nibs are pumped into the press, a collection of chambers covered with a heavy cloth (like canvas) on a sturdy frame, and liquid cocoa butter passes through the cloth while cocoa is retained in the chamber. In a labor-intensive sequence, the press is opened by releasing the hydraulic cylinders holding it closed and the cocoa cake is dropped into a screw conveyor. The cocoa is ground and may be further treated with alkali to modify color and flavor.

Opportunity remains

Many filters have high maintenance costs because they have multiple moving parts, are subject to high pressures, often are subject to abrasive and corrosive materials and are frequently assembled and disassembled because they are used in batch operations. Thus, even though filtration is a relatively mature technology, there continues to be opportunity for improved designs.

Ultrasonics

Ultrasonics refers to sounds, really pressure waves, generally above the frequency that humans can hear, starting at 20 kiloHertz (20 000 cycles/s). The energy of ultrasound is inversely proportional to the square of frequency so 'power' ultrasound used for processing is 15–40 kHz, while frequencies greater than 100 kHz are used for imaging, medical diagnostics and other applications. Humans can hear 1 kHz and some can detect 20 kHz, so hearing protection and sound-absorbent enclosures may be necessary in these ranges. An electrical device, called a generator that can be tuned to create vibrations at the desired frequency, generates ultrasound. These vibrations, of relatively low amplitude, are transmitted and the amplitude magnified through a second device, called a *coupler*. Finally, the vibrations are delivered to a third device, called a *horn* or *tool*, which actually comes in contact with the material to be treated. Sound waves are attenuated rapidly in air, i.e. they quickly lose their energy and so the horn must be in physical contact with the material, which may be solid or fluid.

Those applications that involve liquids require immersing a tool in the liquid. For small volumes, the liquid may be enclosed in a test tube or small vessel, as for cell disruption in the lab. For larger volumes, the liquid may be pumped through a chamber where it is exposed to ultrasonic energy. As an ultrasonic tool vibrates in a liquid, it generates very high localized shear. This may also generate localized heating by viscous friction. The shear contributes to mixing and emulsification. The heating can accelerate chemical or biochemical reactions. Under some conditions, very small bubbles of vaporized liquid may form and quickly collapse, creating cavitation and very intense, though short-lived, heating. The combination of heating and enhanced mass transfer helps to promote reactions, as well as dispersion and homogenization.

Food applications and equipment

One of the first applications for ultrasound was in welding plastic packaging, such as polystyrene clamshells. This works because the horn, which has a blunt face, very rapidly rubs the two sides of a plastic package against each other, generating heat by friction, which melts the thermoplastic and forms a seam. This is an alternative to hot bar or impulse sealing, where the heat is transmitted through the packaging material by contact. For thick materials, a hot bar may be in contact for so long that it damages the outside surface of the seal area, whereas ultrasonic sealing generates the heat just where it is needed.

Ultrasonic sealing also can push aside potential seal contaminants, such as meat fibers or sauces, which might occur in filling pouches, particularly retort pouches. For that application, the sealing tool might have more of an edge and form a narrower seal than when sealing thicker materials.

Another common application is cutting of sticky or multitextured foods, such as cakes, pies and pizzas. The rapid vibration of a properly designed ultrasonic tool 'saws' its way through the food with less pressure applied than a conventional knife would need.

Blades can be fabricated up to 10 inches (254 cm) wide. Typically, ultrasonic cutting tools are made of titanium because it is light, very strong and does not corrode. The weight is important, because the mass of the tool, or more properly its inertia, consumes the ultrasonic energy. Titanium is expensive and in demand for aerospace and defense applications, so ultrasonic cutting can be an expensive option but, for some materials, it may be the only choice.

Depending on the arrangement of the tools, different shapes can be produced. For example, a row of relatively narrow ultrasonic knives can slit a ribbon of food. Cutting a sheet of candy, for instance, into long ribbons and then cutting crosswise can yield bars or cubes. Likewise, a sheet of cake can be cut into portions. Kraft has a patent on a hand-held cheese snack that reveals the use of ultrasonic cutting. The tops of pies or wraps can be scored easily with an ultrasonic knife without crushing the pastry shell.

Among the foods commonly cut by ultrasonics are frozen cakes and pies, frozen fish, snack and nutrition bars, fresh/frozen prepared meats, dough or baked cookies, soft and hard cheeses, fresh/frozen vegetables, candy and confections and ice cream bars.

Some other interesting food applications for ultrasonics are:

- peeling
- disintegration of cells
- extracting (extract intracellular components or obtain cell-free bacterial enzyme)
- activation (acceleration) of an enzyme reaction in liquid foods
- acceleration of a microbial fermentation
- mixing
- homogenizing
- dispersion of a dry powder in a liquid
- emulsifying of oil/fat in a liquid stream
- spraying
- degassing
- inspection
- deactivation of enzymes
- microbial inactivation (preservation)
- crystallization

- meat processing
- stimulation of living cells
- defoaming
- enhanced oxidation.

Among original equipment manufacturers (OEM) offering ultrasonic processing equipment are Matiss, Saint-Georges, Quebec, Canada, Marchant Schmidt, Inc., Fond du Lac, Wis. and FoodTools, Inc., Santa Barbara, Calif. and South Haven, Mich.

Other applications

Ultrasonics has many other applications besides those mentioned above.

Ultrasonic imaging

Ultrasonic imaging uses vibrations of significantly lower power and higher frequency (>1 MHz) transmitted to a target by contact to detect differences in density by differences in the ability to transmit the sonic energy. Many are familiar with the technology from pre-natal imaging of unborn babies or diagnosis of cardiac conditions. The same concept can be applied to seals in food packages to detect potential leaks. Because of the time it takes to form a useful image, ultrasonic seal testing is typically done off-line, but it does have the advantage of being non-destructive, so that tested-satisfactory packages are not wasted.

Ultrasonic imaging is used to test welds and to detect buried flaws in solids such as metal structures, pipes and vessels. The response to ultrasound can be correlated with some useful physical properties of food solids, such as texture and strength.

Material handling

Conveying of sticky and fragile foods, such as candy bars and snack cakes can be challenging, especially when changing direction or when aligning for packaging. A typical approach uses a deflector plate or rod, which may accumulate soil from products or accumulate products that stick. An ultrasonic tool can be used instead, as very little will stick to it because of the rapid vibration.

Likewise, another traditional trouble spot in conveying is the transition from one belt to another. Usually, there is a 'dead plate' on which product slides to prevent pieces from dropping through the unavoidable gap between conveyor rollers. If this plate is vibrated ultrasonically there is less sticking.

Cleaning

Ultrasonic energy can accelerate cleaning of soils from solids and surfaces. This is typically a batch operation applied to relatively small pieces such as jewelry, but one can imagine using it on tools and even ultrasonic horns after they have been used for a while.

Offers opportunities

Ultrasonics can be a specialized and versatile technology with numerous applications in food processing. It has not realized its full potential, in part because the equipment is fairly expensive and is almost always custom fabricated. The full benefits of ultrasonic energy for extracting valuable materials, accelerating reactions and homogenizing emulsions have not been achieved and offer opportunities to creative engineers.

Fermentation

Fermentation of foods can be considered spoilage that does some good. It has been said that if cheese were invented today, it might not be approved. As it is, some of our favorite and nutritious foods are created by fermentation.

Fermented foods

A wide variety of foods and beverages are produced through fermentation.

Beverages

Wine and beer are ancient products, but mead was probably the first fermented beverage. It is made by diluting honey with water or fruit juice and allowing yeast to convert sugars (fructose and glucose) to alcohol and carbon dioxide. Since honey can be found naturally and could easily be diluted with water and since wild yeasts abound, it is likely that this combination occurred and the resulting intoxicant beverage became popular. Mead is notorious for giving memorable hangovers when used in excess, so the benefits and consequences of fermentation were probably discovered at the same time.

Fermentation of fruits and grains is a more complex process, requiring extraction of juice from grapes, apples or other fruits and malting of grains. While barley is favored for fermentation because it has high concentrations of diastase enzymes that convert starch to sugar, wheat, rye, corn and rice are also used. The beverages that result from fermenting each of these grains include beer, sake and whiskies. Whiskies are made by distilling mashes from grains to concentrate the alcohol and flavors. Brandies are distilled from fruit wines.

Alcohol fermentation uses yeast under anaerobic conditions, that is excluding most air. When yeasts ferment in the presence of air – aerobic fermentation – little alcohol is produced. There are many useful strains of yeast and pure cultures are normally used in controlled fermentations, with many breweries and wineries maintaining proprietary strains. A special mold, *Botrytis cinerea*, sometimes grows on grapes and contributes a unique flavor to certain wines. The mold helps moisture to evaporate, concentrating the sugars and leading to a sweet wine.

The residue from fermentation of fruits is called lees and it may be distilled to produce alcohol for fortification of wines such as port and sherry. After distillation, the material is difficult to dispose of because it has had most of its readily biodegradable content removed. Often, it is spread on fields as a soil amendment.

Spent grains from beer, fuel ethanol and whiskey production are high in protein and are used for animal feed. If necessary, they are dried, but that expense can be avoided if a farmer will take them wet.

Vegetables

Sauerkraut and pickles are examples of foods preserved by fermentation. Sauerkraut undergoes three to five stages of bacterial conversion in which sugars are converted to organic acids. Salt, which is required to inhibit the growth of spoilage and pathogenic microorganisms, is added to shredded cabbage and the mixture is stored in large vats, with air excluded by flexible covers.

Normally, the desired organisms are inoculated, though the natural flora may also be used. Some gas may be produced. Natural juice extracted by the added salt creates a brine. Cooler temperatures are preferred to help control the rate of conversion, which can take weeks, but very low temperatures can prevent bacterial growth altogether.

Special cucumbers, bred to respond well to the conversion process, are converted to pickles in much the same way – storage in large vats with added salt and other flavors, such as garlic. Elucidating the exact mechanisms of conversion and improving process control are still subjects of research, even for such familiar old products.

Bread

Early breads were probably simple grilled wafers like tortillas and chapattis made from ground seed grains and water. It was observed that if dough were left alone, it grew and changed texture when baked. Before the malting process was understood, the ancient Egyptians actually used a baking process with barley to make their beer.

Yeast-raised cereal products, such as bread and doughnuts, rely on the unique ability of wheat to hold a foam structure. Wheat contains gluten, a protein hydrocolloid, which forms a strong network when hydrated by water. As yeast converts sugar and starch to carbon dioxide and some alcohol, the gas is trapped in the gluten-and-starch matrix. Heating helps to further expand the dough and the removal of water solidifies the foam into the familiar bread structure.

Heating in a steam atmosphere leads to a chewier and tougher crust, characteristic of many artisanal breads. San Francisco sourdough bread, made by returning a portion of the previous fermentation to the next, relies on a symbiotic combination of unique bacteria and an unusual yeast to create its distinct flavor. The bacteria have an absolute requirement for maltose, which was a previously unknown feature of any known strain of bacteria. Thus it had not previously been isolated because no isolation medium was routinely used with only maltose as an energy source. The yeast does not metabolize maltose. This meant that the yeast and bacterium were uniquely suited to live together. The bacteria produce organic acids which inhibit other strains of yeast from growing, which meant there was little competition for the special yeast.

Once this combination was identified and isolated at the US Department of Agriculture's Western Regional Research Center in Berkeley, Calif., in the late 1960s, it became possible to make authentic San Francisco sourdough bread anywhere, whereas previously all such efforts had failed.

Meats

To make a good sandwich on sourdough bread, one needs tasty Italian salami. The best salami is made by an extended fermentation and drying process, in which salt and starter culture are added to ground pork before it is stuffed into a slightly porous cellulose casing. The green salamis are hung in a temperature- and humidity-controlled room for about 30 days. They can lose about 30% of their weight by drying but, before that occurs, lactic acid bacteria convert sugars to organic acids. Often a white mold grows on the outside of the casing, but it does not contribute significantly to the flavor and is perfectly safe to eat.

The low water activity achieved by drying and addition of salt in combination with the acid produced by the bacteria makes the product safe and almost shelf stable. Most such products are sold and kept refrigerated, but probably do not need to be.

Dairy products

Legend has it that yogurt and cheese may have been discovered by Mongol horsemen carrying mare's milk in animal skins. Milk, of course, is nutritious but very perishable. Some forms of naturally occurring spoilage were found to give more stable and good-tasting products. The variety of cheeses available is astounding – there are hundreds of types of cheeses found in most European countries. The varieties are distinguished by the milk source (cattle, sheep and goats are most common), the way in which milk solids are concentrated (usually by precipitation with rennet or acid) and how the concentrated milk solids are fermented. Blue cheese, for example, involves both bacterial and mold fermentations.

Aging, salting and packaging also help distinguish cheese varieties. Reactions include acid formation, gas formation, hydrolysis of fat and hydrolysis of protein. Preservation is by a combination of low water activity, high acidity and the antimicrobial action of chemicals synthesized by the bacteria and molds.

New directions for food fermentations

The newer uses of fermentation for food additives such as enzymes, amino acids, vitamins, gums and acids often involve specially developed microorganisms. Genetically modified organisms (GMOs) in the form of modified bacteria can be used to produce food ingredients such as lysine. A food or feed containing added lysine produced this way would not contain any GMO, but one wonders if people anxious about GMOs would then be concerned.

Yeasts have been modified to reduce diacetyl in beer (a flavor defect) and to make better use of sugars in bread fermentation, but these developments have not been commercialized, possibly because of concerns about GMO labeling and regulation.

Producing enzymes is a developing trend for fermentation. Some examples are: pectinase (used to clarify fruit juices), phytase (used in animal feed to make available the phosphorus in phytate found in corn and otherwise not digestible) and glucose oxidase and beta-gluconase (used in baking to retard staling).

There is increasing interest in omega-3 fatty acids for use in baby foods. The oils containing omega-3 fatty acids can be extracted from some fish oils, but they are also produced by fermentation of algae and fungi. In baby foods, the fatty acids help mimic the composition of mother's milk. There is also some assertion of benefits to adults, though whether the specific fatty acids are any more helpful than other unsaturated fatty acids is not clear.

Fermentation is used to increase the value of food by-products. One example is conversion of lactose found in cheese whey, the dilute liquid left after precipitation of milk solids, to alcohol, acetone, butanol and lactic acid. Lactic acid, in turn, can be polymerized into a 'green' plastic, i.e. one made from renewable resources. A joint venture of Dow and Cargill, called Cargill Dow LLC, Blair, Neb., is commercializing that process using lactic acid fermented from glucose.

A continuing challenge

Understanding some of the complex but empirical processes described above is a continuing challenge to food scientists and engineers. It is common for several microbes to operate symbiotically or sequentially, modifying their environment to favor some organisms and exclude others. Complex flavors are created by conversion of sugars, proteins and fats. Textures are modified by gas generation, liquefaction of solids and creation of chemicals.

Encapsulation

Encapsulation and microencapsulation are fascinating and versatile technologies that offer many opportunities for food processors and formulators. In general, encapsulation means the enclosing or capturing of one substance by another. The core or base may be a liquid or solid and the coating or matrix may be a polymer, carbohydrate or other material.

The purpose may be to protect the core from the environment (moisture or oxygen), protect it from other ingredients, mask flavor or odor, make a liquid into a flowable powder, control release of the core or create unique effects.

Microencapsulation was originally developed by Barrett K. Green of the National Cash Register Corp. (NCR). Green invented a process called coacervation, in which a soluble polymer, such as gelatin, is induced to come out of solution and form a shell around dispersed droplets of an oil in a water medium. The gelatin shell is hardened by the addition of glutaraldehyde and the microscopic beads are collected and dried.

In the original application, the oil contained a colorless reactive dye and the beads were coated on one side of paper sheets. The facing side of a second sheet was coated with acidic clay. When the beads were burst by the pressure of writing, the dye reacted with the clay to form an image. This is the principle of carbonless copy paper. Today, the beads usually use urea-formaldehyde polymers rather than gelatin.

Some encapsulation technologies include:

- coacervation
- in situ polymerization
- vapor phase deposition
- Wurster coating (named for its inventor, otherwise known as bottom-spray fluidized-bed coating)
- interfacial polymerization
- pan coating (like jellybeans)
- matrix/entrapment.

Combining so many techniques with a wide variety of materials gives literally thousands of possible microcapsules.

Core materials have included acids, antioxidants, adhesives, bases, bleaches, catalysts, cosmetic ingredients, cosmetic oils, dietary supplements, dyes, dye solutions, highly reactive materials, flame retardants, flavor oils, fragrance oils, herbicides, lubricating oils, metal powders, moisturizing oils, oxidizers, peroxides, pesticides, pigments, preservatives, salts, solvents and vitamins.

Sometimes the microcapsules are dispersed in an ink so they can be applied to paper, as in scratch-and-sniff strips for advertising inserts.

Pharmaceutical ingredients are enclosed in coatings that may have a distribution in thickness so that the ingredients are released over a range in time. Sometimes the coating is designed to survive the stomach environment and let the core be released in the lower gut.

The acidic component of baking powder can be protected so that it is only activated after the dough or batter reaches a certain temperature, preventing premature release of the leavening agent.

In matrix encapsulation, the core material is dispersed within another material, which may dissolve or erode to release the active ingredient. One special example of this approach is Fuisz technology. The Fuisz approach uses a molten matrix, which is sprayed from a spinning nozzle, somewhat like cotton candy, but instead of long threads, very small beads are produced. Various carbohydrates may be used. Several years ago, Sunkist developed a similar technique for encapsulating citrus oils and flavors.

One interesting food application is to encapsulate gums used for thickening, which can be hard to hydrate and form 'fish eyes' when dispersed in water. The microcapsules disperse quickly in water and may permit smaller quantities of gum to be effective. Microcapsules can contain 10–50% of active material.

Southwest Research Institute (SwRI) has a long history of research into microencapsulation. The institute has a unique process using co-extruded jets which naturally break up because of hydrodynamic instabilities. To control particle size, the jets can be vibrated. One typical application is encapsulation of sodium bicarbonate in fat for delayed release in baking.

An interesting specific application of encapsulation is the double fortification of salt with iron and iodine, using dextrin encapsulated potassium iodate to prevent chemical reaction between the iron and the iodine. It has been routine to fortify salt with iodine to combat goiter. Salt might be a good vehicle with which to combat anemia by adding iron to the diet. However, the iron and iodine, if unprotected, react and discolor the salt. Microencapsulation by spray drying with dextrin, once the correct particle size was established, protects the iodine from reaction.

There are many industrial applications of microcapsules beyond foods. In fact, foods are a relatively minor application. The typical applications are pesticides, insect pheromones and fragrances, using inedible polymer coatings.

Much of the technology for microcapsules is now in the public domain, older patents having expired. There is still much art in achieving the desired result. Most of the processes produce a range of particle sizes and coating thicknesses. Sometimes this is positive, as when a range of release times is sought. In other cases, release over a narrower period is the target, so a more narrow size range is preferred. Dispersing in an ink or carrier may be easier if the size range is narrow.

Obviously, for food applications, both the core and matrix must be safe and approved for food use. This is why many such coatings are based on dextrin, fat, gelatin or sugar.

The cost of microcapsules has relatively little to do with the materials. It costs about the same to encapsulate mineral oil as it does some rare fragrance. This is because production rates are relatively small, there are many delicate operations (dispersing, coating, recovery and drying) and there is much skilled labor involved. Thus, it is not a solution to every formulation problem. However, in many cases, it may be the only way to incorporate reactive ingredients, such as minerals and vitamins, or highly volatile but critical flavors and aromas.

The technologies that have evolved may also inspire other creative thoughts. An old example might be *Pop Rocks*, which could be considered encapsulated carbon dioxide in sugar, resulting in both a novel confection and an ingredient. Pan-coated candies are larger scale versions of one technology; microcapsules are small-scale versions of that familiar art.

Coating

Coating is a critical operation widely found in food processing. Examples are batters and breading on chicken, fish, potatoes and snacks. Icings and frostings on baked goods are coatings. Chocolate is used to coat various centers, such as nuts, raisins, cherries, mint patties, cookies, crackers and cakes. Hard and soft sugar shells are coated onto nuts, gums, gels, chocolate lentils and tablets.

The critical issues in coating include adhesion, uniformity, texture of the coating and surface appearance, in many cases. Replenishment of the coating material, pot life and proper formulation are also important.

Battering and breading

Many fried foods, or foods that are finished by frying, are coated first with a relatively thin liquid, such as egg, milk or water with some flour and seasoning, called batter, and then with a dry powder or thick liquid paste. The dry powder may be breadcrumbs, seasoning, flour, starch or a mix of such ingredients.

Equipment to apply batter usually involves a flexible conveyor chain, often of parallel rods, running through a chamber or bath containing the batter. Pieces to be coated are laid on the chain and immersed in the bath. Usually, there is a portion of conveyor above the bath to allow draining of excess coating back into the bath. A second, thicker coat can be applied in the same way in a second bath, or dry powders can be dusted onto the wet pieces. Some pieces may need to be turned over to get full coverage.

After coating, pieces may be partially or fully fried and then most are frozen and packaged. Flavored French fries have a thin batter with seasoning applied. Chicken nuggets, fish sticks, poppers (fried peppers) and mushrooms are made in a similar way.

To achieve consistent organoleptic properties of the coated food, it is important to control the viscosity of the batter. The viscosity of the batter is dependent on the temperature and the temperature has a tendency to rise as a run proceeds, so good control of batter temperature is important.

A critical issue in this type of coating is the pot life of the batter. Because of its high moisture content and the fact that other foods are constantly being immersed, the batter can become contaminated with bacteria and begin to spoil. It also can contribute to contamination of the food to which it is applied. Frying helps to reduce the bacteria count in many cases, but battered and breaded frozen foods are rarely sterile. If they are allowed to thaw and warm up, then are frozen again, they can be a source of food poisoning.

Because batter is continuously removed on the coated food, a given batch of batter is eventually consumed. It is good practice to keep the bath relatively small and to dump and replace the batter after a controlled period of time, usually just a few hours. Leftover batter should not be reused.

Coating with solids is challenging because it involves handling powders, which can bridge, flood and form clumps. Usually, powders for coating are fed from a hopper by a specially designed screw or vibratory feeder. The powders are spread over the target pieces by a slot or vibrating table to form a curtain through which the pieces pass. Excess powder falls through the open-chain conveyor and is recycled to the hopper, often manually.

Fried snacks, such as potato and corn chips, are coated with dry seasoning in a rotating drum with several baffles. The process relies on the hot surface frying fat to help the seasoning adhere. Control of particle size of salt and seasoning is important to obtain consistent coating.

Dry flavors and seasonings such as salt, powdered cheese and dry onion or garlic may not adhere well to some snacks, while other snacks, with a residual layer of frying fat, may pick up and retain plenty of applied powder. Shiny snack pieces such as pretzels are especially challenging because the sodium carbonate or bicarbonate bath in which they are dipped before baking seals the surface and creates the characteristic surface finish. For these and other baked pieces, it is customary to spray a light coat of oil first and then apply the powder.

There are many ways to apply oil and powders, but one common method is to use a rotating metal drum with internal lifters. One supplier is Spray Dynamics Ltd., St. Clare, Mo. Drums come in diameters of 28–60 inches (71–152 cm) and lengths of 3–18 ft (0.9–5.5 m).

Typically, the drums rotate at about 10 rpm and are filled so that there is a bed from about 6 o'clock to 9 o'clock as one looks into the end of the drum. Pieces are introduced at one end and exit from the other. Flow is controlled by the rate of feed, the rotation speed and the elevation of the feed end of the drum.

It can be a challenge to measure the residence time of pieces, but one way is to spray paint some pieces, drop them into the feed and retrieve them from the exit, measuring the time when they appear. Depending on the piece shape, weight and flow through the drum, there is some back mixing, so there is a residence time distribution. Typically, the target is about 30 seconds average when just applying oil or other liquid and 60 seconds when applying both oil and solids.

Oil is applied through a spray bar with up to six piston nozzles whose stroke and frequency of pulsing can be adjusted. Oil or other liquid flow is tested by capturing the liquid in a cup for a short length of time. A calibration curve can be prepared for a given system and given liquid. Sometimes the oil is heated, while other times it is not. It is usually desired that the oil be relatively viscous so that it adheres to the piece. Typical oil applications are 2–20% by weight; the higher values are used for crackers.

Dry seasoning is applied with a screw feeder inserted at the exit end of the drum. It is adjusted by varying the screw speed and by blocking some of the holes in the feeder tube. Seasoning is caught on a tray for a short time period and weighed. Target dry application is 5–12% by weight. Seasonings vary widely in bulk density, so feeder tube diameter and even drive motor power must be adapted to the material. Straight salt is much more dense than dry cheese. Cheese and other seasonings may be cohesive, meaning they stick together well, which can inhibit flow from the feed hopper. It is not unusual for seasoning feed to be interrupted and some product to escape unseasoned.

It is one thing to set the flows in the anticipated ratios; it may be quite another to confirm that the desired final composition is achieved. Some pieces are so uniform that the difference in weight between uncoated and coated pieces can be measured by weighing the same number of pieces from the feed and exit streams. For other, more variable, pieces, it may be necessary to measure a tracer like salt or oil by chemical analysis.

An alternative to oil to achieve adherence is an aqueous starch solution, which acts like a glue for the dry seasoning. However, this approach then requires removing the water using heated air. This could be done in a separate dryer or in a special drum with perforated walls and a plenum or second shell so that hot air can be passed through the bed. The equipment to dry the pieces adds an extra cost and additional handling if using a separate dryer would increase breakage.

There are other ways to apply oil and dry seasoning, including simply spraying the products on a flat belt as they exit an oven and sprinkling salt or seasoning from a feeder over a belt, but these only treat one side of the product. However, that is adequate in some cases.

Coating with liquids

Breakfast cereals, pet foods and some snacks are often coated with liquids by spraying in rotating drums. Breakfast cereals often have vitamin mixtures and sweeteners applied to dry flakes or extruded pieces. Pet foods have fat, liquid flavors and dry powders such as yeast and egg applied. Raisins may be lightly coated with oil to prevent clumping and inhibit drying.

One of the more interesting applications is a dough-coated peanut, said to be popular in Japan. That operation uses a centrifugal batch coater in which the bottom spins to expose centers, in this case peanuts, to the liquid. The coating layer is built up by drying and then repeated spraying.

A continuous coater uses a rotating drum with perforated sides through which air is pulled after contacting the pieces. Such equipment can help control allergens in a plant by removing dust and powders.

Continental Products Corp., Milwaukee, Wis, promotes use of its proprietary Rollo-Mixer for coating, agglomerating and impregnating solids with liquids. The Rollo-Mixer is offered in sizes ranging from 3.5 cu ft to 1500 cu ft (0.1–42 m^3) of effective mixing volume. The principle is to expose all the surface area of all the solids to a spray of liquid by rotating a drum at a low speed (3 rpm). On each rotation, there are 25 divisions of the solid mass, achieved by a special design of the internals.

As with other solids mixers and contactors, the working volume of the machine is less (about 50%) than its total volume, to allow the solids to be moved and exposed.

Chocolate coating

Chocolate coating is a special case in which solidification rather than absorption or drying converts the liquid to a solid shell. Chocolate and other fat-based coatings, such as compound coatings and yogurt coatings, melt at about 100°F (38°C). Chocolate, in particular, has a relatively sharp melting point near body temperature, which accounts for its popular sensory impact. Fat-based coatings are applied warm to a piece that is cooler. It is important that the piece be neither too cool nor too warm. The molten coating is applied by dipping; with a waterfall, in an enrober; or by spraying successive layers in a batch or continuous pan coater. After the coating is applied, it is cooled to convert it into a solid. In an enrober, the cooling occurs in a refrigerated tunnel. Chocolate-coated candy bars and cookies are made this way. Cakes are usually iced, meaning they are not completely covered and the icing is not usually all chocolate. Some snack cakes are covered with compound coating using an enrober. Compound coatings are a mixture of cocoa with a vegetable oil instead of cocoa butter, which perform like chocolate but are less expensive.

Pan coating

In pan coating, pieces or centers are loaded into a spherical vessel mounted on a rotating shaft. The speed of rotation and the angle of the shaft are varied. Vessel diameters range from 12 to 18 inches (30–46 cm) holding a few pounds to 36–48 inches (91–122 cm) holding 150–300 pounds (68–136 kg) per batch. The motion of pieces against each other distributes the coating and polishes the product. Depending on the center, it may be necessary to apply a gum or starch layer before and after the chocolate, to improve adherence and to help protect the chocolate. A glossy appearance is achieved by applying an alcohol solution of shellac and then carnauba wax.

A substitute for shellac for glazing chocolate can be made from whey proteins. The whey is applied in an aqueous solution and therefore takes longer to dry than the alcohol solutions. It may also be necessary to apply a gum or starch solution to promote adherence.

A very wide range of products is made by coating centers with sugar or chocolate in panning. Centers may include nuts, fruits such as raisins or cranberries, soft gels as in jelly beans, hard candy, chocolate lentil-shaped pellets and, in the case of pharmaceuticals, tablets of drugs. The common feature is that the centers acquire a coating from successive applications of syrups or melted chocolate which are transformed into a solid shell by various means. There is a great deal of art in the specific operations, which are often done in batches and still involve manual labor and close attention.

The conversion of a liquid to a solid shell is a phase transformation that may be assisted by temperature and humidity control. In the case of chocolate, the transition is from a melt to a crystallized solid fat using cold air. In the case of shells over soft centers, a sugar syrup that also contains color and flavor is dried with dehumidified air and the addition of dry solid sugar. In the case of a sugar shell over harder centers, a sugar syrup is dried using warm air. Normally, the centers are loaded by hand, syrups and solid sugar are spread by hand and finished pieces are unloaded by hand. One person can tend about four pans at a time in many cases.

Polishing pans have ribs on the inside surface to help mixing. The flow patterns of pieces and syrup in the different sizes and shapes vary. The pans are about 30% full by volume after coating is finished. This is as full as they can be without pieces falling out. Some operators may attempt to increase the angle of the pan to increase the weight per batch, but there is an optimum angle that ensures constant movement and constant coating in the pan. The product can also limit pan loads. Lower loads are used for soft centers, which could deform under their own weight.

The various flavors of jelly bean coatings behaved sufficiently differently that a given operator tends to specialize in one or two colors, illustrating the artisinal character of the operation.

Reducing the labor involved while achieving greater consistency is one objective of automated pans. Automated panning systems load, coat and unload pieces using conveyors and a programmed controller. Sugar coating is often about 30% of the piece final weight, while chocolate is often 50%. Batch times for chocolate are 2–3 h. The automated equipment permits coating and polishing in the same unit, while batch systems require transfer to another pan. A big advantage is its use of a very shallow bed depth, which protects soft centers, reduces batch times and enhances uniform coating. The equipment is more expensive than a comparable set of conventional pans and is best suited to relatively large batches of 500–3000 kg, compared to about 200 kg in a typical single pan. Automation can also be flexible, in contrast to intuition, which might suggest it to be best to run the same product a long time.

The ability to reproduce the steps of a process exactly is one advantage of automation. An example of one extreme is the manufacture of jawbreakers, which are 100% sugar, starting with literally a grain of sugar and building layer upon layer over a period of perhaps a week.

Some panning operations can take several days, while most take about 5 hours. It is common to remove pieces for overnight drying before final waxing and polishing.

Hard sugar shells use relatively simple syrups of sucrose and water, while soft shells use sucrose, corn syrup and water. Colors and flavors are often added in the last few stages.

From fried chicken to jelly beans, coating operations have certain principles in common but use dramatically different types of equipment. The results are some of our favorite foods. The possibilities for creative new products from coating processes seem endless: hard or soft candy centers; fruits and nuts; hard or soft sugar coatings; sugar-free coatings; chocolate centers; chocolate coatings; and sugar coatings over chocolate coatings over a choice of centers.

Confectionery and chocolate processes

Controlling crystallization is one of the most critical objectives of most confectionery processes. It is an interesting and baffling phenomenon, influenced by many factors, which are not well understood. Confections, of course, are immensely varied and popular foods, usually based on one or more sweeteners and often incorporating chocolate or cocoa as well. The processes and equipment used have evolved over the years, mostly in an empirical fashion.

Some research in confections has focused on prediction of whether crystallization will occur in a specific system and, if so, at what rate. To understand these issues, it is helpful to review briefly how some familiar candies are made.

Candy making in brief

Sugar-based candies are classified as high boiled or low boiled, depending on the amount of residual moisture. Hard candies are glasses – amorphous, non-crystalline – while softer candies may have fine crystals. It should be noted that while sucrose is the most common sweetener, other carbohydrates such as sugar alcohols and various oligosaccharides may be substituted to reduce certain properties of sucrose. Substitute sweeteners may have fewer calories, be less cariogenic (cavity inducing in teeth) or be less glycemic (harmful to diabetics) than sucrose. These substitutes often are more expensive than sucrose, may require modifications to processes to achieve the same or similar final results and do not always taste the same as sucrose. For example, some sugar alcohols have a cooling effect in the mouth, while other substitutes have a warming sensation. The combination of two sweeteners may more closely approximate the taste of sucrose than either alone.

When sucrose is used, it generally is combined with glucose or dextrose from corn syrup. The glucose helps inhibit crystallization of sucrose. In addition, flavors and acids are often added to candies. The acids may catalyze inversion of sucrose to its constituents, glucose and fructose. Invert sugar can be stickier than sucrose and glucose in the glasses that are hard candies.

After the desired amounts of sucrose, glucose and water are measured, the mixture is cooked to dissolve the solids and evaporate some of the water. At low moisture contents, it is challenging to measure solids concentration accurately, so boiling point is used as an indication of concentration. Thus, many processes require that a mixture be cooked to a given temperature. High temperatures accelerate inversion and color formation, so some candies are cooked under vacuum or quickly discharged from atmospheric cookers into a vacuum chamber for rapid cooling.

For some products, such as toffee and caramel, color formation is desired, so milk proteins are often added to react with reducing sugars, such as glucose, to form new flavors and dark colors. Fats may be added to help make a cooled candy soft and to contribute to flavor and mouth feel.

Because some added flavors are volatile, they may be added after a molten candy mass has cooled somewhat. This can become a challenging mixing problem, because the candy mass is very viscous. If the mass has the correct moisture content and is deliberately agitated and aerated by pulling, many very small crystals of sugar can form, resulting in an opaque and chewy taffy. With lower moisture content and very rapid cooling, the result is a clear glass. While it is warm, the glass can be folded to incorporate flavors, acids and colors and then formed into pieces by stamping in molds or cutting from a correctly sized rope.

Crystallization

Research has been directed at understanding the complex phase behavior of these systems. The ratio of sugar to water and the ratio of sucrose to inhibitor (glucose) help to define three regions of crystallization: one where there is never any crystallization; one where crystallization is immediate; and one where crystallization may be slow or fast. It is not clear what is the best way to portray this complex behavior, but the insights already have helped in troubleshooting by candy manufacturers. A state-diagram approach is used where possible (in hard candy and fondant), but it is not yet possible to define adequately the phase boundaries for the more complex candies such as jellies and caramels.

Among the defects in candies is crystallization when it is not desired. For example, if all the sucrose crystals are not dissolved in a candy glass, they can serve to nucleate crystal formation, weakening the candy piece structure. If the surface of a glass gets wet, the lower viscosity may make surface crystallization possible.

Chocolate processing

Chocolate is an old food, discovered first by the Aztecs of Mexico and brought to Europe by the Spaniards. Now cocoa beans are grown in many tropical places, including Africa and South

America. Cost and quality can vary widely. Traditionally, cocoa beans from several sources have been blended to achieve a consistent flavor and to control costs. Cocoa farmers tend to be small and poor and have not always received a fair price for their crop. Fair-trade cocoa refers to an effort to help producers receive a higher return, responding to consumers' appreciation of the issue and their willingness to pay a higher price for the final products.

Single-origin cocoa recognizes that consumers can appreciate the subtle flavor differences among beans grown in various areas, even among different estates. An origin might be a region of the world, a country, or a single farm. One lesson, then, from chocolate is the potential for market segmentation, as contrasted with the more common objective of consistency in flavor.

There is increasing recognition of the potential health benefits of chocolate resulting from its high concentration of phytochemicals and antioxidants. Manufacturers are introducing new products with dark chocolate, single-origin cocoa, fair-trade cocoa and higher concentrations of cocoa. Furthermore, cocoa processing to make chocolate is one of the few examples where there are multiple paths or potential flow sheets, most of which are in use.

In processing generally and specifically in food processing, there usually is one best way to accomplish some desired end. This is usually discovered incrementally over time and all manufacturers eventually arrive at the same conclusion. With regard to chocolate, this is not the case.

Steps in processing cocoa

Chocolate flavor development begins shortly after harvest. Cocoa beans are found in a fleshy fruit that is collected from trees about twice a year. The fruits are cut open and the seeds spread in a thin layer on the ground to ferment and dry in the sun. As the fruit flesh disappears and the seeds dry, their color changes and their characteristic aroma develops. The seeds are typically packaged in 60-kg jute bags and sold through cooperatives, government agencies or directly to manufacturers, depending on the country and local practice.

Depending on whether a single-origin or certified product is being made or not, beans from one or several sources are blended according to a company's recipe before roasting. The cocoa beans consist of a hard shell and a softer nib on the inside. Beans can be roasted before or after removing the shell. There are advantages and disadvantages of each approach, giving rise to one of the steps for which there are process alternatives.

If the shell is removed before roasting, there is less loss of valuable cocoa butter soaked into the discarded shells after roasting. The roaster is also used more efficiently, as only nibs are handled. On the other hand, the shell is easier to remove after roasting. A compromise process heats the whole beans to dry the shell and make it easier to remove, then the nibs are roasted. This introduces an additional piece of equipment.

After roasting, the nibs are ground to a fine slurry such that the suspended particles are too small to be detected by the tongue. Grinding may be on a multiple roll refiner, in which up to five polished steel rolls are mounted in a stack very close together and the slurry passes from one to another until the desired particle size is achieved. Grinding is very important to the mouth feel of the eventual chocolate. The suspended particles are cocoa and the liquid is cocoa butter, a unique vegetable oil. Cocoa butter gives chocolate one of its special sensory properties, its ability to melt just at body temperature, because it has a sharp melting point of about 37°C. However, it also has a complex polymorphism, meaning that its solid form can take several crystal forms, only one of which is stable. To ensure that products containing cocoa butter maintain a stable state after cooling, the molten mass must be kept within a precise temperature range, neither too warm nor too cool.

The slurry is known as chocolate liquor and is one component of chocolate. Additional cocoa butter, sugar, milk powder (for milk chocolate), lecithin as an emulsifier, and other flavors can be added to make a final product. To get additional cocoa butter, some chocolate liquor is filtered under high pressure (because of the fineness of the particles), yielding cocoa powder as press cake and cocoa butter as filtrate. It is important to reduce the cocoa butter content of the cocoa powder as much as possible, because it is the more valuable product, so the press cake may be extracted with solvent or it can be ground up to yield a cocoa powder with a residual fat level (say 10–24%) that is appropriate for a final application.

The cocoa powder is an important product for making chocolate drinks, compound coatings, confections and other foods. The solubility and color of cocoa powder can be modified by the addition of a particular alkali to the cocoa liquor or to the press cake, leading to another set of alternative process options, namely, use alkali (and which one) or not, and add it at various points if used.

The chocolate mass then undergoes a process unique to chocolate, conching. This typically occurs in a special mixer, a large vessel with rotating mixing arms that have heavy, rolling disks attached. During conching, heat is generated, which helps to drive off some residual moisture and volatile flavors. Almost certainly, some chemical reactions occur among the various compounds present, including caramelization of sugars, Maillard or browning reactions between proteins and sugars and probably others. There may be further size reduction.

Efforts have been made to shorten significantly the time of conching or to separate some of its functions, such as evaporation, because conching of high-quality chocolate can take many hours and requires some skill. Most such efforts have not succeeded. Another lesson, one also seen in the aging of cheese, wine and whiskey, is that some processes just cannot be accelerated successfully. In the case of chocolate, the high viscosity, relatively low temperature and mild agitation means that the reactions will occur slowly because diffusion of reactant molecules is so slow under these conditions. At the end of conching, additional cocoa butter is added to control the final viscosity of the chocolate, depending on its intended use.

Chocolate confections are made by combining cocoa butter, cocoa powder, sweeteners, milk powder and inclusions such as nuts. To meet chocolate standards of identity (set by government regulation) takes more cocoa butter and less cocoa powder than the natural proportions of the cocoa bean, so cocoa powder is a major by-product of chocolate manufacture. Cocoa powder comes in a wide variety of colors, particle sizes and flavors and is widely used in baking and the manufacture of compound coatings.

Chocolate is used in candy bars, as an enrobing for ice cream, as a coating for baked goods, as a sauce and as an ingredient. Chocolate is supplied as liquid in bulk, as slabs or blocks, as drops or small pieces, and in other solid forms.

For most uses, chocolate must be tempered, which means heating carefully to a high-enough temperature to melt all forms of cocoa butter, which can crystallize in two forms, one of which is unstable and can cause visual defects in candy. Chocolate is then maintained at the proper temperature in use by circulating through double-walled tubing heated by hot water. Storage tanks are also double walled, agitated slowly and heated.

Uses for chocolate

A major use of chocolate is in confections. The largest companies tend to make their own chocolate from beans, while smaller companies buy from specialized firms. There has been a growing trend for larger companies to outsource their chocolate supplies, allowing them to focus resources and assets on their consumer brands and their marketing. Some of the processes used by candy companies include shell molding, enrobing, panning and molding.

For less expensive uses, such as enrobing baked snack cakes or cookies, compound coatings are made by mixing cocoa powder, sugar, emulsifiers and a compatible vegetable fat that has melting properties similar to those of cocoa butter. Such fats are made by partial hydrogenation or fractional crystallization. In Europe, it is permitted to add up to 5% of such fats to chocolate, primarily as a cost reduction and still call the product chocolate. There is a movement to allow this practice in the USA, which is controversial. Because the properties of the substitute fat can be manipulated, the resulting mixture may be easier to handle in manufacturing and also less expensive than chocolate.

Enrobed coatings for many baked goods are compound coatings rather than chocolate. The substitute fats may be other relatively hard fats, such as palm oil or coconut, may be fractionated from animal or vegetable fats or may be hydrogenated vegetable oils. Hydrogenated oils can have high *trans*-fatty acid contents, which are now considered potentially harmful to people, so their use is likely to be reduced in the future.

Confectionery defects

One of the defects of chocolate and compound coatings is bloom, a discoloration of the surface. There may be sugar bloom or fat bloom. Sugar bloom occurs when moisture on the surface of chocolate extracts some sugar and then evaporates, leaving a white deposit. Having the temperature too low on the outlet of a cooling tunnel can cause condensation on the exiting candy, leading to this effect.

Fat bloom was thought to be caused by a polymorphic transition in cocoa butter. It is now believed that such a transition is a result, not the cause. Fat bloom can occur in well-tempered chocolate that has been stored too long. Some research groups use a color meter to quantify bloom under different circumstances. Other research groups have used an atomic force microscope (AFM) to quantify the roughening of the surface caused by bloom.

A third form of bloom has recently been identified. When chocolate is solidified without tempering, as might happen when a chocolate bar melts in the car and then resolidifies, the bloom that appears is different from either sugar bloom or fat bloom. The bloom scraped from the surface of one of these bars is highly concentrated in cocoa solids and sugar crystals and is almost devoid of fat, as shown by the use of a differential scanning calorimeter (DSC).

Most people have considered this type of bloom to be identical to fat bloom caused by temperature cycling during storage and nut oil migration, but it is clearly a different mechanism (and composition). Storage bloom is all fat, but this bloom on untempered chocolate has essentially no fat. It may be related to the polymorphic transition of cocoa butter, but in this case the transition leads to a separation of the particulate matter as the cocoa butter contracts during polymorphic transition.

Trends in confectionery processing

One trend is the effort to maximize health benefits from chocolate by increasing desirable flavonoids using lower-temperature roasting. Another is to use aerated chocolate to lower density without affecting appearance or texture. Technologies originally developed for pharmaceutical delivery are being applied to confections, such as oral strips – rapidly dissolving pieces of polymeric gums that carry intense flavors – and breath fresheners.

There is a general trend toward greater automation in confectionery manufacturing. Where many processes were traditionally batch, such as cooking and pan coating, now they are more likely to be continuous, primarily to reduce labor. For example, a belt coater can handle 1000 lb (454 kg), whereas it would take five conventional pans to process the same amount. Moguls, starch-depositing machines on which are made such products as jellybeans and candy corn, are now 40 inches (102 cm) wide instead of 30 (76 cm). The drying rooms in which starch-deposited candies are cured now have better control of temperature and humidity, increasing uniformity and reducing the time before the candy can be further processed by coating or packaged.

Culinary techniques in food manufacturing

What culinary techniques are used in the food industry and how are they used? Several industrial chefs say that many culinary techniques and skills are applied in food manufacture and some are more difficult to translate to large scale than others.

Scaling-up cooking techniques

Here are some important culinary techniques and how they are applied on a larger scale.

Stewing is one of the easiest techniques to scale-up, since it is simply cooking in liquid, which can be done in steam-jacketed kettles or simulated by retort cooking in containers, such as cans or jars. Many foods that are later frozen are prepared in kettles.

Braising involves long, slow cooking in moist heat. It might be simulated by retort cooking, but would probably need a browning step.

Frying, cooking in hot oil, is relatively easy to scale-up by using larger oil baths with conveyors to move products in and out. Manufactured foods are typically par-fried (partially fried) rather than completely fried so that they can be finished in the home or restaurant.

Roasting is dry heating and can be accomplished in an oven, but at commercial scale, where times may be shortened and temperatures higher, color and flavor may need enhancement.

Grilling is cooking by direct contact, conduction and usually is characterized by char marks on the meat or vegetable. On a commercial scale, the marks can be simulated by printing with color, or using rollers or branding bars but, again, because time of exposure to heat is reduced, flavor and color may need to be added.

Sautéing is dry heating in small quantities of fat. A chef normally moves foods around in a pan to cook evenly and avoid burning. This is more difficult with a fixed piece of equipment, such as a jacketed kettle. Vessels with agitators or heated screws can simulate the process.

Research chefs are contributing to the trend of incorporating more sophisticated ingredients and tastes into manufactured foods. One of the building blocks a chef uses that is becoming commercially available is *mirepoix*, a combination of minced onion, carrot and celery that is often the basis for sauces and soups. Frozen and dehydrated vegetables are available as substitutes for fresh, though many manufacturers do use fresh vegetables if they can get them reliably.

Brown butter is simply butter that has been heated to promote Maillard reactions between sugars and amino acids. It is a natural source of sweetness and flavor in making sauces. Brown butter can be made onsite in a separate step or purchased from another source as an ingredient. Olive oil or olive oil flavor is a more common ingredient and gives a more sophisticated character than a less expensive oil. However, it is also more vulnerable to oxidation and so must be stored properly and not overheated.

New ingredients such as aseptic, seedless tamarind paste can contribute a unique sour and sweet flavor to foods while still being relatively convenient to use.

Fabricating a practical cut of meat

One culinary technique is shaping, as when a chef debones a leg or shoulder of a meat animal and then ties the muscle back together for faster and more uniform roasting.

One example was to replace pork loin. Pork loin is normally too expensive to use in quick serve restaurants. Instead, it is used to make Canadian style bacon, pork roasts and chops. Ham muscles were tumbled and massaged to improve binding and then filled into a tubular casing. A unique step was freezing the meat at this point to help it hold its shape. The casing was then removed and the meat wrapped with a layer of ham fat before being put into a cooking net. Wrapping meat with fat is called barding, in contrast to larding, in which slivers of fat are threaded through a cut of meat. Larding is uncommon, as natural marbling is achieved by animal breeding. The cylindrical piece of meat was then cooked by infrared heating to melt most of the fat and develop a brown, caramelized surface.

The product was not commercialized, but it does illustrate the application of some culinary skills and the way a chef approaches a product development task.

Another meat application uses braising. Braising is long, slow cooking with moist heat to tenderize tough meat cuts. In a kitchen, it normally begins with browning of the meat before a liquid such as stock, wine or water is added. In commercial bag cooking, there is no browning.

Instead of browning in a pan, a conveyor grill was used to brown beef short ribs before braising them in polymer bags. The bags were emptied of purged liquid and fat before freezing the meat for later use. In a kitchen, the braising liquid is normally the base for a sauce, but that may be impractical on a commercial scale, so sauces must use other sources of flavor, such as meat extracts.

Chefs on the plant floor

Fresh, chilled foods for food service and retail sale, such as sauces, gravies, entrees, soups and desserts are prepared in small batches in steam-heated kettles, filled hot into containers such as bags for foodservice and tubs and small bowls for retail, then very rapidly cooled in an ice water tank. Refrigerated shelf life is about 60 days.

The unique characteristic of one manufacturer is that the products are cooked much as they would be in a restaurant kitchen, by chefs with culinary training. Wherever possible, fresh ingredients are used, such as garlic and potatoes. Oil is heated, garlic is sautéed, minced onion, carrot and celery are added and, in general, the product is built step by step.

Concessions to scale include mechanical peeling where possible, mechanical slicing and dicing and automatic depositing into containers after transferring from the cook kettles. Many materials, such as eggplant, are prepared by skilled hands.

The step-wise process and the use of well-trained labor obviously adds to cost but pays off in high quality. The components of a scaled-up process include availability of fresh ingredients, careful choice of scale of operation and careful material handling to avoid damage to particulates such as pasta and meat pieces.

Reproducing the chef's touch

Components of airline meals and other foodservice items have been prepared for many years. An interesting example is omelets, which are normally cooked by a chef in a special pan one at a time. One plant has a carousel of about 30 typical omelet pans carried by a chain over a series of gas flames. Oil is automatically deposited, followed by a precise dose of liquid egg and, after a few seconds, a filling such as cheese (if needed). Then one of the few operators loosens the egg with a spatula, another folds the omelet in half and, finally, the omelet is tipped into a cavity in a plastic tray which is conveyed to freezing. The hot empty pan is quickly wiped clean, and the cycle repeats.

A similar continuous system is used to make stir-fried dishes. These processes illustrate another approach to scale-up: replicate and automate, rather than make larger batches – slices from a large loaf of cooked egg would not be mistaken for individual omelets.

Chefs struggle with the 'machine-made' look of much manufactured food and seek ways to preserve the human touch. Size reduction – slicing, cutting and dicing – is a troublesome area. Automation is necessary to reduce hand labor and also to help with portion control, but too much uniformity is a sure sign of 'factory food'. One solution is to have cutting machines set to different sizes. Another is to use some hand cutting – selectively and just enough to make a visual difference.

The diverse range of culinary techniques enriches the variety and enhances the quality of manufactured food, but the engineer is often challenged to reproduce the techniques accurately and efficiently on a large scale.

Refrigerants

One does not usually associate refrigeration with the baking industry, but it turns out that the industry is possibly breaking new ground for all food processors as it deals with the need to replace conventional refrigerants and cooling equipment.

The class of chemical compounds known as chlorofluorocarbons (CFCs) have many useful purposes because of their chemical inertness, thermodynamic properties and low toxicity. However, it has been found that these chemicals can decompose in the atmosphere and release chlorine, which then participates in the destruction of stratospheric ozone. This makes them ozone-depleting substances (ODS), according to the Environmental Protection Agency (EPA). Ozone helps protect us from exposure to excessive ultraviolet radiation.

Many useful and common refrigerants were CFCs, such as R-12 and R-502 (which contains a CFC in a mixture). Under an international treaty, the Montreal Protocol, these refrigerants are no longer manufactured and special provisions are required for their recovery from systems. As anyone needing to repair an automobile air conditioner has probably discovered, the consequence is a high cost because of scarcity of R-12 and the costs of recovery and purification.

Another class of compounds, hydrochlorofluorocarbons (HCFCs), are being manufactured for refrigeration and air-conditioning applications for a limited time, until 2020, as substitute refrigerants. R-22 is an example and is widely used. After 2010, it will not be used in original refrigeration equipment but will still be available for ten more years (or until supplies run out) for maintenance of existing systems. R-22 is also used in polymer manufacture and so will be manufactured for many years, but about 50% of its use now is in refrigeration. This poses a dilemma for manufacturers of the chemical that has not yet been resolved.

Chemical companies have developed substitute refrigerants with various properties. Some refrigerants are mixtures of other compounds. All must be of the class of chemical compounds known as hydrofluorocarbons (HFCs), which contain no chlorine and thus pose no threat to ozone. Examples include 134a, 404A, 507A, 410A, 407C and 417A. Different materials are appropriate for different refrigeration services.

For example, 404A and 507 are used for low temperatures, as in freezing; 134a is used for medium temperatures, as in coolers; and 410A and 407C are used for higher temperatures, as in air conditioning. All the refrigerant suppliers provide essentially the same chemical entities, competing primarily on price and service. Atofina Chemicals, Inc., Philadelphia, Pa is a major supplier of HFCs (*Forane* refrigerants) and is the result of a merger between the French companies Elf Aquitaine and TotalFina. The other major suppliers are DuPont, with its *Suva* line, and Honeywell, through its acquisition of Allied Signal, with its *Genetron*.

ICOR International, Indianapolis, Ind., imports a mixture of HFCs called NU-22 or 417A, which is offered as a direct replacement for R-22 and R-502 and is compatible with the mineral oil lubricants now used in refrigeration compressors. ICOR claims that its material can be used in all refrigeration ranges. Other HFCs require a different, synthetic lubricant called polyolester (POE). These lubricants can be hygroscopic and decompose if moisture contaminates them. Furthermore, when converting machinery to the new lubricants, several exchanges of oil must occur, creating a potentially large quantity of waste-contaminated lube oil onsite. With any change in refrigerant, there usually needs to be some adjustment to controls, perhaps including replacement of expansion valves and other parts. Capacity may also be affected. ICOR claims that its product reduces capacity slightly but also reduces energy consumption.

According to the US Department of Justice, all this became important to the baking industry after a baking company experienced very high rates of R-22 leakage from mixers that were cooled by direct expansion. The connecting piping was subject to vibration. Even though allowable leak rates were quite high (35% of refrigerant content per year), rates exceeding these were experienced, probably because of poor maintenance. EPA concluded that bakeries posed a high hazard of releasing ODS to the atmosphere and began scrutinizing them more closely. Potential fines and penalties are high – thousands of dollars per day per unit (or appliance, as EPA calls them).

There was a rush of demand for HFC refrigerants, especially those which can be used directly, such as 417A. Replacement refrigerants must be accepted under EPA's Significant New Alternative Policy (SNAP), in which proposed chemicals and mixtures are reviewed for safety in their proposed use. No single refrigerant is SNAP approved for all applications, but some, such as 134a, 404A and 507, have fairly wide approval and have been accepted by most equipment manufacturers for use in their equipment.

One obvious modification that many bakeries are pursuing is to convert from direct-expansion cooling to indirect cooling using a fluid such as propylene glycol to cool equipment and cooling the glycol with refrigerant. This reduces refrigerant piping and ensures that if connections are exposed to vibration leak, they will leak a non-toxic and non-ODS material. In many food plants, refrigeration is provided by a central ammonia system. Ammonia poses its own hazards, but such systems are efficient and are usually large enough that they have their own trained operators and maintenance people.

The experience of the baking industry is likely to be extended to other segments of the food industry where CFC and HCFC refrigerants are now used in processing equipment. They will face the issues of whether to replace existing compressors, what refrigerant to use, what to do with waste oil and recovered refrigerant and whether their systems can tolerate reduced capacity.

References

Altomare, R.E. (1994) Heat transfer in bakery ovens. In *Developments in Food Engineering, Proceedings of the 6th International Congress on Engineering in Food*, edited by Yano, T., Matsuno, R. and Nakamura, K. Blackie Academic & Professional, London.

American Meat Institute (2004) *Final FDTF Principles & Expanded Definitions, 2 page summary*. American Meat Institute, Washington, DC.

Barbosa-Canovas, G.V. (2005) *Food Engineering. Encyclopedia of Life Support Systems*. UNESCO Publishing, Paris.

Bartholomai, A. (ed.) (1987) *Food Factories Process, Equipment Costs*. VCH Verlagsgesellschaft mbH, Weinheim.

Boulton, R.B., Singleton, V.L., Bisson, L.F. and Kunkee, R.E. (1998) *Principles and Practices of Winemaking*. Aspen Publishers, Inc., Gaithersburg.

Burstein, D. and Stasiowski, F. (1982) *Project Management for the Design Professional*. Whitney Library of Design, New York.

Clark, J.P. (1993a) Plant design – basic principles. In *Encyclopaedia of Food Science, Food Technology and Nutrition*. Academic Press Ltd, London, pp. 3605–3608.

Clark, J.P. (1993b) Plant design – designing for hygienic operation. In *Encyclopaedia of Food Science, Food Technology and Nutrition*. Academic Press Ltd, London, pp. 3608–3613.

Clark, J.P. (1993c) Plant design – process control and automation. In *Encyclopaedia of Food Science, Food Technology and Nutrition*. Academic Press Ltd, London, pp. 3613–3617.

Clark, J.P. (1997a) Cost and profitability estimation. In *Handbook of Food Engineering Practice*, edited by Rotstein, E., Singh, R.P. and Valentas, K. CRC Press, Boca Raton, Chapter 13, pp. 537–557.

Clark, J.P. (1999) Food plant design and construction. In *Wiley Encyclopedia of Food Science and Technology*, 2nd edn. John Wiley & Sons, New York, pp. 946–953.

Practical Design, Construction and Operation of Food Facilities
ISBN: 978-0-12-374204-9

Clark, J.P. (2005a) Food plant design. In *Food Engineering, Encyclopedia of Life Support Systems*, edited by Barbosa-Canovas, G.V. EOLSS Publishers/UNESCO, Paris, pp. 683–696.

Clark, J.P. (2005b) Food process design. In *Food Engineering, Encyclopedia of Life Support Systems*, edited by Barbosa-Canovas, G.V. EOLSS Publishers/UNESCO, Paris, pp. 697–706.

Clark, J.P. (2007) Food processing plant design. In *Encyclopedia of Agricultural, Food and Biological Engineering (EAFE)*. Taylor & Francis, New York.

Clark, J.P. and Balsman, W.F. (1989) Computer integrated manufacturing in the food industry. In *Proceedings of 5th International Conference on Engineering and Food* (ICEF 5), edited by Spiess, W.E. Elsevier, London, and *Engineering and Food*, Vol.1, Elsevier, London 1990, pp. 781–789.

Connor, J.M. (1988) *Food Processing An Industrial Powerhouse in Transition*. Lexington Books, Lexington.

David, J.R.D., Graves, R.H. and Carlson, V.R. (1996) *Aseptic Processing and Packaging of Food*. CRC Press, Boca Raton.

Fast, R.B. and Caldwell, E.F. (eds) (2000) *Breakfast Cereals and How They Are Made*. American Association of Cereal Chemists, St Paul.

Geankoplis, C.J. (1993) *Transport Processes and Unit Operations*, 3rd edn. Prentice-Hall, Inc., Englewood Cliffs.

Goldratt, E.M. (1990) *The Haystack Syndrome*. North River Press, Croton-on-Hudson.

Goldratt, E.M. (1994) *It's Not Luck*. North River Press, Great Barrington.

Goldratt, E.M. and Cox, J. (1986) *The Goal A Process of Ongoing Improvement (rev.)*. North River Press, Croton-on-Hudson.

Harmon, R.L. and Peterson, L.D. (1990) *Reinventing the Factory*. Macmillan, New York.

Holdsworth, D. and Simpson, R. (2008) *Thermal Processing of Packaged Foods*. Springer, New York.

Imholte, T.J. (1984) *Engineering for Food Safety and Sanitation*. Technical Institute of Food Safety, Crystal.

Jowitt, R. (1980) *Hygienic Design and Operation of Food Plants*. Ellis Horwood Ltd., Chichester.

Kotter, J.P. (1988) *The Leadership Factor*. Macmillan, New York.

Lewis, M.J. and Young, T.W. (2002) *Brewing*, 2nd edn. Kluwer Academic/Plenum Publishers, New York.

Lopez, A. (1975) *A Complete Course in Canning*. The Canning Trade, Baltimore.

Lopez-Gomez, A. and Barbosa-Canovas, G.V. (2005) *Food Plant Design*. CRC Press, Boca Raton.

Maroulis, Z.B. and Saravacos, G.D. (2003) *Food Process Design*. Marcel Dekker, New York.

Maroulis, Z.B. and Saravacos, G.D. (2007) *Food Plant Economics*. Taylor & Francis Group LLC., Boca Raton.

Martin, C.C. (1976) *Project Management: How to Make It Work*. AMACOM, New York.

Matz, S.A. (1988) *Equipment for Bakers*. Pan-Tech International, McAllen.

McCabe, W.L. and Smith, J.C. (1976) *Unit Operations of Chemical Engineering*. McGraw-Hill, Inc., New York.

McCorkle, C.O. (1988) *Economics of Food Processing in the United States*. Academic Press, San Diego.

McGee, H. (1984) *On Food and Cooking*. Scribner, New York.

Merrow, E.W. (1989) *An Analysis of Cost Improvement in Chemical Process Technologies, R-3357-DOE*. The Rand Corporation, Santa Monica.

Merrow, E.W., Chapel, S.W. and Worthing, C. (1979) *A Review of Cost Estimation in New Technologies, R-2481-DOE*. The Rand Corporation, Santa Monica.

Merrow, E.W., Phillips, K.E. and Myers, C.W. (1981) *Understanding Cost Growth and Performance Shortfalls in Pioneer Process Plants, R-2569-DOE*. The Rand Corporation, Santa Monica.

Myers, C.W., Shangraw, R.F., Devey, M.R. and Hayashi, T. (1986) *Understanding Process Plant Schedule Slippage and Startup Costs, R-3215-PSSP/RC*. The Rand Corporation, Santa Monica.

Ramaswamy, H.S. and Singh, R.P. (1997) Sterilization process engineering. In *Handbook of Food Engineering Practice*, edited by Valentas, K.J., Rotstein, E. and Singh, R.P. CRC Press, Boca Raton.

Schonberger, R.J. (1986) *World Class Manufacturing*. Macmillan, Inc., New York.

Schultz, G.A. (2000) *Conveyor Safety*. American Society of Safety Engineers, Des Plaines.

Seiberling, D.A. (1997) CIP sanitary process design. In *Handbook of Food Engineering Practice*, edited by Valentas, K.J., Rotstein, E. and Singh, R.P. CRC Press, Boca Raton.

Singh, R.P. and Heldman, D.R. (2001) *Introduction to Food Engineering*, 3rd edn. Academic Press, London.

Steffe, J.F. and Singh, R.P. (1997) Pipeline Design for Newtonian and Non-Newtonian Fluids. In *Handbook of Food Engineering*

Practice, edited by Valentas, K.J., Rotstein, E. and Singh, R.P. CRC Press, Boca Raton.

Tetra Pak (1998) *The Orange Book*. Tetra Pak Processing systems AB, Lund.

Troller, J.H. (1983) *Sanitation in Food Processing*. Academic Press, London.

Valentas, K.J., Levine, L. and Clark, J.P. (1991) *Food Processing Operations and Scale-Up*. Marcel Dekker, Inc., New York.

Valentas, K.J., Rotstein, E. and Singh, R.P. (eds) (1997) *Handbook of Food Engineering Practice*. CRC Press, Boca Raton.

Valle-Riestra, J.F. (1983) *Project Evaluation in the Chemical Process Industries*. McGraw-Hill Book Company, New York.

Van Arsdel, W.B., Copley, M.J. and Morgan, A.I. (1973) *Food Dehydration*. AVI Publishing Company, Westport.

Walters, J.D. (1987) *The Art of Supportive Leadership*. Crystal Clarity, Nevada City.

Wheatley, M.J. (1992) *Leadership and the New Science*. Berrett-Koehler, San Francisco.

Index

Food Science and Technology
International Series

Maynard A. Amerine, Rose Marie Pangborn, and Edward B. Roessler, *Principles of Sensory Evaluation of Food*. 1965.
Martin Glicksman, *Gum Technology in the Food Industry*. 1970.
Maynard A. Joslyn, *Methods in Food Analysis*, second edition. 1970.
C. R. Stumbo, *Thermobacteriology in Food Processing*, second edition. 1973.
Aaron M. Altschul (ed.), *New Protein Foods*: Volume 1, *Technology, Part A*—1974. Volume 2, *Technology, Part B*—1976. Volume 3, *Animal Protein Supplies, Part A*—1978. Volume 4, *Animal Protein Supplies, Part B*—1981. Volume 5, *Seed Storage Proteins*—1985.
S. A. Goldblith, L. Rey, and W. W. Rothmayr, *Freeze Drying and Advanced Food Technology*. 1975.
R. B. Duckworth (ed.), *Water Relations of Food*. 1975.
John A. Troller and J. H. B. Christian, *Water Activity and Food*. 1978.
A. E. Bender, *Food Processing and Nutrition*. 1978.
D. R. Osborne and P. Voogt, *The Analysis of Nutrients in Foods*. 1978.
Marcel Loncin and R. L. Merson, *Food Engineering: Principles and Selected Applications*. 1979.
J. G. Vaughan (ed.), *Food Microscopy*. 1979.
J. R. A. Pollock (ed.), *Brewing Science*, Volume 1—1979. Volume 2—1980. Volume 3—1987.
J. Christopher Bauernfeind (ed.), *Carotenoids as Colorants and Vitamin A Precursors: Technological and Nutritional Applications*. 1981.
Pericles Markakis (ed.), *Anthocyanins as Food Colors*. 1982.
George F. Stewart and Maynard A. Amerine (eds), *Introduction to Food Science and Technology*, second edition. 1982.
Hector A. Iglesias and Jorge Chirife, *Handbook of Food Isotherms: Water Sorption Parameters for Food and Food Components*. 1982.
Colin Dennis (ed.), *Post-Harvest Pathology of Fruits and Vegetables*. 1983.
P. J. Barnes (ed.), *Lipids in Cereal Technology*. 1983.
David Pimentel and Carl W. Hall (eds), *Food and Energy Resources*. 1984.
Joe M. Regenstein and Carrie E. Regenstein, *Food Protein Chemistry: An Introduction for Food Scientists*. 1984.

Maximo C. Gacula, Jr. and Jagbir Singh, *Statistical Methods in Food and Consumer Research*. 1984.
Fergus M. Clydesdale and Kathryn L. Wiemer (eds), *Iron Fortification of Foods*. 1985.
Robert V. Decareau, *Microwaves in the Food Processing Industry*. 1985.
S. M. Herschdoerfer (ed.), *Quality Control in the Food Industry*, second edition. Volume 1—1985. Volume 2—1985. Volume 3—1986. Volume 4—1987.
F. E. Cunningham and N. A. Cox (eds), *Microbiology of Poultry Meat Products*. 1987.
Walter M. Urbain, *Food Irradiation*. 1986.
Peter J. Bechtel, *Muscle as Food*. 1986. H. W.-S. Chan, *Autoxidation of Unsaturated Lipids*. 1986.
Chester O. McCorkle, Jr., *Economics of Food Processing in the United States*. 1987.
Jethro Japtiani, Harvey T. Chan, Jr., and William S. Sakai, *Tropical Fruit Processing*. 1987.
J. Solms, D. A. Booth, R. M. Dangborn, and O. Raunhardt, *Food Acceptance and Nutrition*. 1987.
R. Macrae, *HPLC in Food Analysis*, second edition. 1988.
A. M. Pearson and R. B. Young, *Muscle and Meat Biochemistry*. 1989.
Marjorie P. Penfield and Ada Marie Campbell, *Experimental Food Science*, third edition. 1990.
Leroy C. Blankenship, *Colonization Control of Human Bacterial Enteropathogens in Poultry*. 1991.
Yeshajahu Pomeranz, *Functional Properties of Food Components*, second edition. 1991.
Reginald H. Walter, *The Chemistry and Technology of Pectin*. 1991.
Herbert Stone and Joel L. Sidel, *Sensory Evaluation Practices*, second edition. 1993.
Robert L. Shewfelt and Stanley E. Prussia, *Postharvest Handling: A Systems Approach*. 1993.
Tilak Nagodawithana and Gerald Reed, *Enzymes in Food Processing*, third edition. 1993.
Dallas G. Hoover and Larry R. Steenson, *Bacteriocins*. 1993.
Takayaki Shibamoto and Leonard Bjeldanes, *Introduction to Food Toxicology*. 1993.
John A. Troller, *Sanitation in Food Processing*, second edition. 1993.
Harold D. Hafs and Robert G. Zimbelman, *Low-fat Meats*. 1994.
Lance G. Phillips, Dana M. Whitehead, and John Kinsella, *Structure-Function Properties of Food Proteins*. 1994.
Robert G. Jensen, *Handbook of Milk Composition*. 1995.
Yrjö H. Roos, *Phase Transitions in Foods*. 1995.
Reginald H. Walter, *Polysaccharide Dispersions*. 1997.

Gustavo V. Barbosa-Cánovas, M. Marcela Góngora-Nieto, Usha R. Pothakamury, and Barry G. Swanson, *Preservation of Foods with Pulsed Electric Fields*. 1999.
Ronald S. Jackson, *Wine Tasting: A Professional Handbook*. 2002.
Malcolm C. Bourne, *Food Texture and Viscosity: Concept and Measurement*, second edition. 2002.
Benjamin Caballero and Barry M. Popkin (eds), *The Nutrition Transition: Diet and Disease in the Developing World*. 2002.
Dean O. Cliver and Hans P. Riemann (eds), *Foodborne Diseases*, second edition. 2002. Martin
Kohlmeier, *Nutrient Metabolism*, 2003.
Herbert Stone and Joel L. Sidel, *Sensory Evaluation Practices*, third edition. 2004.
Jung H. Han, *Innovations in Food Packaging*. 2005.
Da-Wen Sun, *Emerging Technologies for Food Processing*. 2005.
Hans Riemann and Dean Cliver (eds) *Foodborne Infections and Intoxications*, third edition. 2006.
Ioannis S. Arvanitoyannis, *Waste Management for the Food Industries*. 2008.
Ronald S. Jackson, *Wine Science: Principles and Applications*, third edition. 2008.
Da-Wen Sun, *Computer Vision Technology for Food Quality Evaluation*. 2008.
Kenneth David, *What Can Nanotechnology Learn From Biotechnology?* 2008.
Elke K. Arendt and Fabio Dal Bello, *Gluten-Free Cereal Products and Beverages*. 2008.
Debasis Bagchi, *Nutraceutical and Functional Food Regulations in the United States and Around the World*, 2008.
R. Paul Singh and Dennis R. Heldman, *Introduction to Food Engineering*, fourth edition. 2008.
Zeki Berk, *Food Process Engineering and Technology*. 2009.
Abby Thompson, Mike Boland and Harjinder Singh, *Milk Proteins: From Expression to Food*. 2009.
Wojciech J. Florkowski, Stanley E. Prussia, Robert L. Shewfelt and Bernhard Brueckner (eds) *Postharvest Handling*, second edition. 2009.